BIOETHICS

A Critical Issues in Bioethics Series Book from
The Center for Bioethics and Human Dignity

This volume launches the Center's second series of bioethics books. Whereas every book in the Center's well-established Horizons in Bioethics Series brings together an array of insightful writers to address important bioethical issues from a forward-looking Christian perspective, volumes in the Critical Issues in Bioethics Series have a different purpose. Each of these volumes features one or two authors bringing Christian perspectives into dialogue with other perspectives that are particularly influential today. This first volume addresses the field of bioethics broadly, while subsequent books will focus on particular topics such as end-of-life or genetic issues.

Both series are projects of The Center for Bioethics and Human Dignity, an international center located just north of Chicago, Illinois, in the United States of America. The Center endeavors to bring Christian perspectives to bear on today's many pressing bioethical challenges. It pursues this task by developing two book series, six audiotape series, six videotape series, numerous conferences in different parts of the world, and a variety of other printed and computer-based resources. Through its membership program, the Center networks and provides resources for people interested in bioethical matters all over the world. Members receive the Center's international journal, *Ethics and Medicine,* the Center's newsletter, *Dignity,* the Center's Update Letters, special World Wide Web access, an Internet News Service and Discussion Forum, and discounts on most bioethics resources in print.

For more information on membership in the Center or its various resources, including present or future books in the Critical Issues in Bioethics Series, contact the Center at:

The Center for Bioethics and Human Dignity
2065 Half Day Road
Bannockburn, IL 60015 USA
Phone: (847) 317-8180
Fax: (847) 317-8153
E-mail: cbhd@biccc.org

Information and ordering is also available through the Center's World Wide Web site on the Internet: http://www.bioethix.org

BIOETHICS

A Christian Approach
in a Pluralistic Age

SCOTT B. RAE

PAUL M. COX

WILLIAM B. EERDMANS PUBLISHING COMPANY
GRAND RAPIDS, MICHIGAN / CAMBRIDGE, U.K.

© 1999 Scott B. Rae and Paul M. Cox and
The Center for Bioethics and Human Dignity

First published 1999 by Wm. B. Eerdmans Publishing Co.
255 Jefferson Ave. S.E., Grand Rapids, Michigan 49503 /
P.O. Box 163, Cambridge CB3 9PU U.K.

Printed in the United States of America

04 03 02 01 00 99   7 6 5 4 3 2 1

Library of Congress Cataloging-in-Publication Data

Rae, Scott B.
Bioethics: a Christian approach in a pluralistic age / Scott Rae, Paul Cox.
p.   cm.   — (Critical issues in bioethics)
Includes bibliographical references.
ISBN 0-8028-4595-9 (pbk.: alk. paper)
1. Medical ethics.   2. Christian ethics.
3. Medicine — Religious aspects — Christianity.
I. Cox, Paul.   II. Title.   III. Series.
R725.56.R34 1999
241'.642 — dc21   99-15037
                                       CIP

Contents

Series Editors' Foreword

We live in an age when scientific knowledge has provided human beings with an unprecedented ability to manipulate life and death. In the West there has been a cultural shift from a so-called Judeo-Christian consensus to fragmented secular assumptions about the nature of human life, community, and "reproduction" as well as the practice of medicine and scientific research. There is little doubt that these changes in science and culture have fueled the controversies surrounding abortion, physician-assisted suicide, genetic engineering, the patient-doctor relationship, reproductive technologies, cloning, and the allocation of health care resources, to name just a few.

Bioethics is the interdisciplinary study of these and other issues of life and health. It involves an attempt to discover normative guidelines built on sound moral foundations.

The purpose of this series is to bring thoughtful and biblically informed Christian voices in bioethics into dialogue with other voices that are influential today. As Christians we believe that human persons are made in the image of God and for that reason their lives are sacred. We also believe that God's entire creation was made for a purpose, and we discover this purpose from the Holy Scripture as well as philosophical reflections on the nature of things. Because we live in a pluralist society, we believe that it is our responsibility to explain why all people should take Christian perspectives into account. Such is the case not least because these perspectives have shaped so much of Western culture, especially its assumptions about human dignity. Accordingly, the books in this series will be useful to those who do not share our theological commitments. They can be read side by side with books espousing secular or other perspectives and are ideal for bioethics courses in nontheological as well as theological settings.

Because bioethics is theoretical as well as practical, the authors in this series are committed to providing a principled case for their perspectives as well as suggestions and insights on how scientists and/or health care practitioners may employ these principles in a laboratory and/or clinical setting. In addition, we believe that pastors, students, professors, and others will profit from these books. C. S. Lewis warned of a future in which "Man's final conquest has proved to be the abolition of Man." The purpose of this series is to help forestall or even prevent such a future.

DENNIS HOLLINGER
Professor of Christian Ethics
Dean of College Ministries
Messiah College

FRANCIS J. BECKWITH
Associate Professor of Philosophy,
Culture & Law
Trinity Graduate School
Trinity International University

Acknowledgments

M any people contributed to making this volume what it is. We would be remiss if we did not give them the credit they are due. First and foremost, thanks to John Kilner and The Center for Bioethics and Human Dignity for giving us the opportunity to write this book. We are delighted to be included in this series and honored that we would write the first volume in it. Dr. Kilner has been a faithful friend and colleague in bioethics for some time, and we appreciate his encouragement and insightful commentary on earlier drafts. Similarly, the general editors of the series, Dennis Hollinger and Frank Beckwith, provided an enormous amount of helpful and perceptive critique that greatly strengthened our work. They will also enrich the succeeding volumes in this series.

Along the way, a number of medical professionals gave us their valuable time and invaluable comments on earlier drafts of the book. They saved us from going to press with some medical and technical aspects that were not adequately nuanced. We are grateful to them for their time and their friendship. Dr. Eugene Berman, with whom one of us (Scott Rae) has worked very enjoyably in bioethics at Providence St. Joseph Medical Center (Burbank, Calif.), was very helpful in chapters 6 and 8. These chapters are much improved as a result of his comments. His colleague Dr. Steve Hersch provided helpful material on chapter 7. Dr. Hersch and Scott's own experience in the ICU at St. Joseph's provided a good deal of the raw material for that chapter. Scott is appreciative to Dr. Hersch for the education he provided during that time. Scott is also very grateful to his longtime friend Dr. Andy MacFarlan for his invaluable insights on chapter 7. He made so many significant observations that are reflected in that chapter. Scott is especially grateful for his permission to use the narrative account of the dying process of his father-in-law, which closes chapter 7.

We both are grateful to our colleagues in the philosophy of religion and ethics program at Talbot School of Theology, Biola University, for their encouragement, support, and friendship. Dr. J. P. Moreland and Dr. Doug Geivett provide a great setting in which to go about our work. Our dean, Dr. Dennis Dirks, is very supportive of our writing, and Scott is very appreciative for the sabbatical leave in the fall of 1997 that enabled us to get a good start on the book.

Most of all we appreciate our families, who endure much so that we can pursue a ministry of writing. Scott thanks his wife, Sally, and three boys, Taylor, Cameron, and Austin, for their patience while we finished this project. Paul Cox thanks his wife, Linda, and daughters Rachal and Rebecca for similar patience. We gratefully dedicate this book to our families.

Introduction

It is widely held that the bioethics movement was born in a predominantly religious cradle.[1] Many of the early bioethicists were theologians driven by their religious views to become involved in the field. The early bioethical discussion was chiefly a theological one, since it dealt with issues at the beginning and ending edges of life. Clearly these were issues in which theologians were forced to new applications of their views, and as a result theologians had a great deal to offer in terms of the initial bioethical reflection. A seminal conference in 1968 to gather those engaged in ethical reflection on medicine is regarded by many as the birthplace of the discipline of bioethics.[2] As the beginning discussion broadened and matured, academic philosophers, lawyers, academic physicians, and medical practitioners all became seriously involved in the ongoing conversation. In that process, one can see the partial marginalization of religious voices in bioethics, though there remains today a strong Catholic presence in nonprofit health care with its vigorous advocacy for access to health care for the poor, protection for the unborn, and opposition to euthanasia. In addition, the pro-life movement, though not exclusively religiously based by any means, nevertheless includes a substantial contingent of religious voices, mainly Protestant evangelicals and Catholics. However, religious voices have been excluded by the "pluralism" and secularization of the academy in general, and thus as the bioethics discussion moves

1. David W. Smith, "Religion and the Roots of the Bioethics Revival," in *Religion and Medical Ethics: Looking Back, Looking Forward,* ed. Allen Verhey (Grand Rapids: Wm. B. Eerdmans Publishing Co., 1996), pp. 9-18.

2. Fruits of the conference are reported in Kenneth Vaux, ed., *Who Shall Live? Medicine, Technology, and Ethics* (Philadelphia: Fortress, 1970).

into the philosophical, medical, and legal academies, religious voices no longer carry much weight.[3] It is quite possible that the religious voices have contributed to their own marginalization, ironically, by their support for the development of a common language in which to express religious perspectives. One result of this development is that medicine has lost a valuable resource for self-correction, which is particularly needed in an era of managed care and marketplace medicine.

Our goal is that this book can provide an assessment of various approaches to bioethics that are particularly influential today, and then develop a framework for a Christian approach in comparison with these approaches. This book is not primarily issue oriented, though we will touch on numerous debated issues in bioethics. Rather we intend to provide an account of the primary theological notions that we consider critical to inform a Christian perspective on bioethics. These form a lasting framework which can assist people in addressing the many pressing issues in the field.

Part I (the first two chapters) takes into account that in the past twenty-five years many others have attempted to formulate coherent and compelling perspectives on bioethics. Many have recognized the need for theoretical foundations for bioethics as well as for reflection on the many pressing issues. Chapter 1 provides an outline and critique of some of the most significant religiously based frameworks for doing bioethics. We address Catholic, Protestant, and Jewish approaches to bioethics and take up representative figures in each of these religious traditions. From the Catholic perspective, we address the Ethical and Religious Directives for Health Care, which outline official Catholic Church teaching which guides health care delivery in Catholic facilities. Then we take up two major figures in Catholic bioethics. One dominant Catholic figure, Richard McCormick, interprets the Directives more broadly and approaches bioethics from more of a natural law position. We have also included by way of comparison a more conservative interpreter of the Directives, William E. May, whose views are consistent with a more literal understanding of the Directives.

Two Protestant theologians are also considered in this chapter, Paul Ramsey and James Gustafson. Both are well known in theological circles, and are widely read and very influential. They both reject the natural law approach — Ramsey favoring a covenantal approach and Gustafson, a theo-

---

3. This is the argument of Stephen Lammers, "The Marginalization of Religious Voices in Bioethics," in *Religion and Medical Ethics,* pp. 19-43. See also Daniel Callahan, "Religion and the Secularization of Bioethics," *Hastings Center Report* (special supplement: "Theology, Religious Traditions and Bioethics") 20, no. 4 (July-August 1990).

centric approach. Finally, representative Jewish interpreters are considered, and we note, interestingly, that the textual approach of the Jewish theologians has much in common methodologically with an evangelical ethic that gives primacy to the exegesis of the biblical text.[4]

By contrast, many schools of nonreligious bioethics have arisen and assumed dominance in the academic development of the field. We take up two representatives of very influential perspectives. The first is the principle-based approach of Tom Beauchamp and James Childress. Their use of the principles of autonomy, beneficence, non-maleficence, and justice has become a paradigm for a good deal of case consultation in bioethics in health care institutions around North America and Europe. We will argue that the principles have value for bioethics, but that they must ultimately be theologically grounded. We further critique this system for failing to give sufficient place to other moral considerations, such as moral virtues.

A second system is the postmodern system of H. Tristram Engelhardt, in which he attempts to formulate a moral system that is capable of handling the wide variety of views of morality in today's pluralistic culture. He contrasts the morality that one uses when among "moral friends" such as fellow members of a religious community, with that used when among "moral strangers," or those with whom one has little if anything in common when it comes to morality. He virtually despairs of being able to provide a content-full morality when among such a diverse population. We outline and critique his system and consider him a representative of those who struggle to make sense of bioethics in a postmodern world. We could have easily taken the entire book to address and critique the different systems of bioethics currently in use. However, those addressed here provide an adequate background against which to discuss various distinctive elements of a Christian approach.

Part II (chaps. 3–8) forms the main section of the book. Here we attempt to put forth the primary theological concepts that we believe should inform a Christian perspective on bioethics. Foundational to our approach are the notions of general revelation, the dominion mandate, and common grace (chap. 3). Through these lenses we assess medical technology and conclude that, generally speaking, it is a part of God's general revelation to the human race and its use is clearly part of the dominion mandate given to human beings as recorded in the Bible's opening chapters, Genesis 1–2. Health care, which is used to offset the effects of the entrance of sin into the world, is generally to be considered God's good gift to the human race. However, it

---

4. For the sake of length, we have not included various representatives of Islamic or other religious approaches to bioethics, though they warrant serious assessment.

does not follow from this that medical technology can be used apart from moral scrutiny. We apply such scrutiny to the more controversial technologies such as reproductive technologies, life-sustaining technologies, and human cloning. We attempt to address the issues from the perspective of theology, but bring broader considerations in as well to illustrate the common ground that a Christian approach has with other approaches at various points.

Undergirding the areas of patient dignity and rights are the theological views of a human person. Chapters 4 and 5 address the theological foundation for viewing human persons as intrinsically of inestimable worth. We take the notion of human beings as created in God's image as the grounding for attributing such significance to human beings. We further argue that the *imago Dei* and the incarnation strongly suggest that the Bible attributes personhood to the unborn from the earliest stages of pregnancy (chap. 4). We expand this argument in chapter 5 to make this controversial notion persuasive in philosophical terms more easily accessible to a pluralistic audience. There we argue for a substance view of a human person that holds a continuity of personal identity through change. In our view, this way of viewing a human person is most consistent with biblical teaching. Chapter 6 expands the discussion of personhood by carefully examining the notion of personal autonomy and its relationship to the common good. Throughout chapters 5 and 6, very specific illustrations demonstrate the concrete implications of the general analysis. Chapter 5 applies the substance view of a human person to infertility treatments, embryo and fetal research, the maternal-fetal relationship, and assistance in suicide. We then apply the broader discussion of chapter 6 to issues in everyday medical practice such as informed consent, confidentiality, cultural diversity, and the patient-physician relationship.

Chapter 7 takes up the issues around death and dying in greater depth. We view death in theological perspective as a conquered enemy. It is an unavoidable part of life under the curse of sin, and thus there can be limits on how aggressively we are to fight it. Moreover, death has been vanquished at the cross, and for believers it is the doorway into eternal life. Thus death, though evil, is not something to be resisted at every turn and at all costs. We apply this perspective to caring for the dying, which includes proper pain management (a moral imperative), clear and timely communication, and respect for a patient's wishes at the end of life. However, it does not include assistance in suicide. Physician-assisted suicide is not necessary for treating a patient's pain, and is already leading to harmful consequences in places where it is loosely legalized, such as the Netherlands.

Not only are these clinical issues important, but the broader context of health care delivery is also critical. As discussed in chapter 8, many ethical concerns are involved. What makes for a just health care system is still very much in debate, as the debate over health care reform in the 1990s made evident. The growth of managed care medicine in the United States and elsewhere has further raised questions about the justice of current systems. At the core of this discussion is the notion of distributive justice, and we attempt to bring a biblical perspective to a complex philosophical discussion. We then attempt to apply this perspective to the complex relationship between business and medicine, and managed care in particular.

Part III of the book (the final two chapters) explicitly engages the pluralistic culture in which health care is practiced today. Here our goal is to suggest some ways in which bioethics can be done in a postmodern, pluralistic setting. Chapter 9 is not a critique of postmodernism but an approach to bioethics in which we take distinctively Christian perspectives and argue for them in ways that are not entirely dependent on our theological view of the world. We take the controversial issue of surrogate motherhood as an example of how one might do this. Chapter 10 takes up a method for doing bioethical case consultation that we have used in specific health care settings such as hospital ethics committees. This model can be used irrespective of one's worldview and is well suited for use in culturally diverse environments.

Our hope is that the reader will find this book a stimulating and substantial contribution to developing Christian bioethics that can make a constructive contribution in a pluralistic world. May it further equip readers to articulate more effectively the elements of a Christian perspective on the many pressing bioethical issues in today's world.

PART I

INFLUENTIAL APPROACHES
TO BIOETHICS

CHAPTER 1

Religious Approaches to Bioethics

Introduction

For the past twenty years, moral philosophers and ethicists have been focusing much of their attention on the ethical questions raised by developments in the medical field. As would be expected, the discussions by these moral philosophers and ethicists have led to diverse opinions and methodologies concerning the resolution of questions and dilemmas raised in the realm of medicine. Religious or theological approaches have also been a part of these deliberations in bioethics. Indeed, religious perspectives were among the first responses to the ethical challenges of medicine. The response of religion to ethical issues raised by medicine should come as no surprise since "religious communities had long and worthy traditions of attention to the ordinary human events of giving birth and suffering and dying and support for the extraordinary tasks of caring for those giving birth, suffering, or dying."[1] The purpose of this chapter is to examine and evaluate how three Western religious perspectives approach the ethical questions raised by medicine. Though most religious systems have interacted with bioethics issues, there are three religious perspectives which are well developed and have been particularly influential in the development of bioethics as a field. They and their representatives have been selected here simply to illustrate significant reli-

---

1. Allen Verhey, ed., *Religion and Medical Ethics: Looking Back, Looking Forward* (Grand Rapids: Wm. B. Eerdmans Publishing Co., 1996), p. 2. Chapter 1 in this volume documents the birth of the bioethics movement in the cradle of Catholic, Protestant, and Jewish religious thought.

gious approaches today. No attempt has been made to provide an exhaustive survey of religious approaches or writers.

The three religious perspectives we will address in this chapter are Roman Catholic, Protestant, and Jewish. One particularly prominent approach within Roman Catholic moral theology is the natural law approach of Thomas Aquinas.[2] The claim of natural law is that there are objective moral truths that can be known by all human beings. Aquinas stated that these first principles of morality were discovered as reason reflected upon the basic inclinations of human nature itself. (For example, Pope Paul VI's *Humanae Vitae* (1968) condemns artificial contraception based upon a deductive approach from a Thomistic natural law first principle.) In recent years a movement has arisen within the ranks of Catholic moral theology to reformulate traditional natural law approaches.[3] One such reformulation has been done by Richard McCormick. Later in this chapter we will use McCormick as an example of a Catholic methodology to resolve issues related to bioethics. Although Catholic bioethics has been characterized by a natural law approach, Protestant thinkers generally have chosen a different method.

In general and for various reasons, Protestant moral thought has not embraced natural law approaches to doing ethics. Just as there are many strains of Protestant theology, so there are diverse methodologies to doing theological ethics. Protestant moral thought can be permeated by Reformation themes such as Luther's "the freedom of a Christian" or principles extracted from the Bible such as love (Christian love as exemplified in the life of Jesus).[4] Two prominent Protestant thinkers who have written extensively in the area of bioethics are Paul Ramsey and James Gustafson. Just as we will use Richard McCormick as an example of Catholic moral methodology, so we will use both Ramsey and Gustafson as illustrations of Protestant moral approaches to doing bioethics.

Although both Ramsey and Gustafson are Protestant in their Christian

2. Charles Curran, "Roman Catholicism," in *Encyclopedia of Bioethics*, ed. Warren T. Reich, vol. 4 (New York: Free Press, 1978), p. 1524.

3. For example, see John Finnis, *Natural Law and Natural Rights*, and Germain Grisez, *Christian Moral Principles*. These works both claim to constitute a new natural law theory that both recovers and avoids the supposed problems with Aquinas's natural law theory. For a critique of Finnis and Grisez, see Russell Hittinger, *A Critique of the New Natural Law Theory*. The text of *Humanae Vitae* may be found in Stephen E. Lammers and Allen Verhey, eds., *On Moral Medicine: Theological Perspectives in Medical Ethics*, 2nd ed. (Grand Rapids: Wm. B. Eerdmans Publishing Co., 1998), pp. 434-38.

4. For an overview of some of the various approaches taken by Protestant theological ethics, see James T. Johnson, "Protestantism: History of Protestant Medical Ethics," in *Encyclopedia of Bioethics*, ed. Warren T. Reich, vol. 3 (New York: Free Press, 1978), p. 1365.

orientation, only the former would affirm the classical doctrines of the ortho-dox faith as formulated in both the Nicene and Chalcedon creeds. However, even though Ramsey and Gustafson differ dramatically in their confessional and creedal stance as Protestants, they are two of the best representatives of mainline Protestant Christianity to have written in bioethics, though clearly other representatives could have been chosen.[5] The Christian perspectives se-lected here are by no means the only significant Christian voices. In fact, the present volume is part of a larger attempt to develop a more biblically based Christian voice in bioethics.[6]

While various movements within Judaism could easily receive separate treatment here, it will only be possible to examine the core elements that for the most part are held in common, plus the more detailed views of two illus-trative Jewish bioethicists. The foundation for doing Jewish bioethics is two-fold Torah: Scripture and tradition. Scripture is the written Torah and tradi-tion is the oral Torah.[7] Thus a Jewish approach to resolving ethical issues in the realm of health care is basically threefold: (1) locate the appropriate scrip-tural teaching; (2) ascertain the rabbinic commentaries on the text which are found in the Talmud; and (3) search out applications of scriptural principles to specific cases, whether legal or otherwise.

> Jewish ethics, particularly medical ethics, represents the accumulated wis-dom and intellectual labor of millennia, stretching from the Bible and the Talmud, through the codes of Jewish law, to the most recent and contempo-rary rabbinic essays and responsa. All are considered inspired by the Divine truths enshrined in the *Torah*, the eternal guide for Jewish conduct. While these laws claim our loyalty on the strength of their religious authority, they also express the moral truths of Judaism.[8]

Therefore disagreements in Jewish bioethics typically revolve around the in-terpretation and application of divine truth. Ethical discussions are theologi-cal deliberations.

Two prominent Jewish bioethicists are Immanuel Jakobovits and Fred Rosner. Their writings provide good illustrations of Jewish bioethics method-ology. Thus we will examine and evaluate their approaches to doing bioethics.

5. Among these are theologians Stanley Hauerwas and Gilbert Meilaender.
6. All the work of the Center for Bioethics and Human Dignity (Bannockburn, Ill.) is exemplary of this effort.
7. Reich, ed., "Judaism," in *Encyclopedia of Bioethics*, 3:1301.
8. Rabbi Dr. David M. Feldman and Fred Rosner, M.D., eds., *Compendium on Medi-cal Ethics*, 6th ed. (New York: Federation of Jewish Philanthropies of New York, 1984), p. 11.

Jakobovits is a rabbi and consequently emphasizes the rabbinic discussions and applications of texts to particular issues. For Jakobovits, these rabbinic deliberations of texts provide the context for their employment in the medical realm. Rosner, a medical doctor, carefully explains the relevant medical data and then employs generally accepted Jewish scriptural principles to the situation.

These three religious perspectives and their representative adherents exemplify a range of substantive and thoughtful approaches for consideration. There is also some degree of overlap in the various perspectives. Since these three religious positions are diverse, it seems best to choose some "reference point" from which to understand their respective procedures. One such reference point is the issue of autonomous refusal of lifesaving medical treatment. This is an oft-debated issue in bioethics, and McCormick, Ramsey, and Gustafson have written extensively on it.[9] Although Jakobovits and Rosner have not addressed this issue as extensively as their Catholic and Protestant counterparts, they have written material that is germane to the subject. Thus, by examining how each of these thinkers approaches the issue of refusal of lifesaving or life-prolonging medical treatment, we will gain insight into their respective methodologies.

Roman Catholic Bioethics

Catholic bioethics is officially governed by the church's Ethical and Religious Directives.[10] These serve as guidelines for health care practice in Catholic hospitals around the world. As one might expect, they are subject to a wide range of interpretations, from most strict, among more "conservative" Catholics, to a more flexible reading among more "liberal" Catholics. The Directives are grounded in the healing ministry of the church, which is seen in continuity with Jesus' healing ministry while on earth. The ministry of Catholic health care is rooted in the commitment to promote human dignity, care for the poor, and contributing to the common good. Health care from the Catholic perspective is to treat the whole person, not just disease, and thus there is a significant pastoral and spiritual component to it. The Directives uphold the importance of the patient-professional relationship, including informed consent, surrogate decision making, patient rights, and proper protection of hu-

---

9. It should be noted that McCormick and Ramsey have addressed this issue directly and extensively, while Gustafson has only approached it in an indirect manner.

10. The Directives were most recently revised in 1994 and published in *Origins* 24, no. 27 (15 December 1994): 449-61.

man subjects in medical research. The most controversial part of the Directives deals with issues at the beginning of life. Here they take a strong stand for the sanctity of human life from conception onward and prohibit nontherapeutic abortion and embryo research. The official Catholic view of marriage and procreation prohibits most reproductive interventions, birth control, and sterilization, unless clearly medically indicated. There is great debate in Catholic circles on these issues, and Richard McCormick represents a less rigid approach than many of his Catholic contemporaries.[11]

The Directives outline compassionate care for the dying, which includes things like proper pain management and a presumption in favor of life that prohibits assistance in suicide, but they also show respect for informed and competent refusal of life-sustaining treatment. Finally, the Directives suggest principles of cooperation in which Catholic hospitals can enter into joint ventures and partnerships with non-Catholic health care institutions without compromising the distinctives of Catholic health care. This section was added in the latest revision in response to the dramatic way in which the health care delivery system is changing. The Directives are grounded in a natural law approach that is consistent with the tradition of Catholic moral theology.

William E. May

Although this chapter will explore the views of Richard McCormick, it is important to mention that there are more conservative moral theologians within the Catholic Church. One such person is William E. May. In fact, May designates McCormick a "revisionist theologian,"[12] characterizing him and others as such because they want to adjust or revise certain Catholic moral stances as stated in the "Majority Report" of the Papal Commission for the Study of Population, the Family, and Natality. Furthermore, May believes the revisionist group employs a principle that ultimately undermines the case for moral absolutes: the "preference principle" or the "principle of proportionate good." This principle of proportionate good will be carefully examined when the discussion of McCormick ensues. May states:

> According to this principle it is morally right to intend a nonmoral evil, such as the death of an innocent person, if this evil is required by a "proportion-

11. The Catholic approach to reproductive technology will be addressed in more detail in chapter 3.

12. William E. May, *An Introduction to Moral Theology*, rev. ed. (Huntington, Ind.: Our Sunday Visitor, 1994), p. 111.

13

ately related greater good." Thus, as Richard A. McCormick says, "Where a higher good is at stake and the only means to protect it is to choose to do a nonmoral evil, then the will remains properly disposed to the values constitutive of human good. . . . This is to say that the intentionality is good even when the person, reluctantly and regretfully to be sure, intends the nonmoral evil if a truly proportionate reason [i.e., good] for such choice is present."[13]

In other words, according to May, McCormick and other revisionist theologians are denying the absolute ontic nature of moral acts. By placing acts within the context of the "proportionate principle," viewing the nature of human acts as a totality, and considering the historicity of human existence, certain acts are no longer immoral by their very nature. Thus May's position is in sharp contrast to that of McCormick.[14]

Richard A. McCormick

Richard McCormick is a leading figure among Catholic moral theologians. From 1965 until 1984 he wrote the influential "Notes on Theology" series in *Theological Studies*. Furthermore, he has consistently maintained the natural law approach of the Aristotelian-Thomistic Catholic moral tradition. In general he believes actions are to be judged on the basis of what values they advance and what values they denigrate within the context of an objective hierarchy of values. For McCormick, all moral choices must maintain a proper balance between values preserved and values lost. In this approach he believes he is emphasizing the contextual and consequence-recognizing side of Thomistic rationality. This is the side of Thomism that emphasizes the use of reason or intelligence to solve moral dilemmas instead of being subject to the "facts of life" or the "whims of nature." Thus a particular situation could arise whereby there would be a justifiable exception to a moral norm. For instance, according to McCormick's methodology, one could imagine a situation in which a decision would maintain a greater "proportion" of values and yet, in the same instance, not preserve all values. The exception would be based in maintaining a greater "proportion" of values. But what are these values that McCormick thinks should be kept at a certain proportionality, and how are they discovered?

13. May, *An Introduction to Moral Theology*, p. 114.
14. See the following articles by William E. May to see how a more conservative Catholic view looks at biomedical issues: "Feeding and Hydrating the Permanently Unconscious and Other Vulnerable Persons," *Issues in Law and Medicine* 3, no. 3 (winter 1987), and "Ethics and Human Identity: The Challenge of the New Biology," *Horizons* 3 (spring 1976).

McCormick discovers his values and explicates them in typical Thomistic fashion. The values are not located in reason but are discovered by reason when reason reflects upon the basic tendencies of human beings. According to McCormick, these basic inclinations are "the tendency to preserve life; the tendency to mate and raise children; the tendency to seek out other men and obtain their approval — friendship; the tendency to establish good relations with unknown higher powers; the tendency to use intelligence in guiding action; the tendency to develop skills and exercise them in play and in the fine arts."[15] He views these as the basic objective values and the first principles of moral reasoning. Moreover, he states that we not only discern "values" but also distinguish a hierarchy of goods. Therefore, according to McCormick, moral choice involves the advancement of some values over other values. Indeed, moral choice involves the realization of the highest good possible in a situation. All human beings have this ability to know these values because they are based in the basic tendencies or inclinations of human nature which all human beings share. Consequently, "Christian" ethics is human ethics.

In typical natural law fashion, McCormick states that the Christian faith offers no new content to these values discoverable by all human beings. Thus,

> there is a *material* identity between Christian moral demands and those perceivable by reason. Whatever is distinct about Christian morality is found essentially in the style of life, the manner of accomplishing the moral tasks common to all men, not in the tasks themselves. Christian morality is, in its concreteness and materiality, *human* morality. . . . The experience of Jesus is regarded as normative because he is believed to have experienced what it is to be *human* in the fullest way and at the deepest level. Christian ethics does not and cannot add to human ethical self-understanding as such any material content that is, in principle, strange or foreign to man as he exists and experiences himself.[16]

According to McCormick, Christianity only offers two things to the ethical task: (1) illumination of these basic human values; and (2) a complete worldview to encompass those values. However, Scripture is not a necessary component to doing ethics. (Scripture is important, however, as a revelation of those truths which are undiscoverable by human reason.)

When there is a conflict between the realization of all values in a situation,

---

15. Richard A. McCormick, "Theology and Biomedical Ethics," *Eglise et Theologie* 13 (1982): 313, reprinted in *Logos* 3 (1982): 25-45.

16. Richard A. McCormick, "The Judeo Christian Tradition and Bioethical Codes," in *How Brave a New World? Dilemmas in Bioethics* (Garden City, N.Y.: Doubleday, 1981), p. 9.

McCormick holds that we should always attempt to secure the highest value in the hierarchy of values. This is using what he calls "proportionate reason." When two or more basic values are in conflict, the only way in which one can maintain a proper proportion of values in this situation is to choose the course of action which does not entail a greater elimination of value. In other words, one must choose between the conflicting values based upon what is necessary to maintain basic goods.[17] Now the question becomes, How does McCormick handle a situation in which a person decides to deny a basic good such as life itself?

A much debated issue in bioethics is the relationship between a patient's autonomy and the exercise of beneficence by physicians or medical personnel.[18] Those involved in health care tend to believe that they know what is best for the patient. After all, in their mind, the patient contracted with them concerning health care. Furthermore, many physicians believe it is practically impossible to completely inform patients about their illnesses in such a way that they will know as much as the medical personnel involved in their care. Thus the patient should depend upon the physician and other health care professionals to make the medical decisions involving the health of the patient.

On the other hand, others argue that this way of thinking, known as paternalism, violates the self-determination of the patient. According to them, the freedom of self-determination is demanded by the principle of autonomy. By affirming autonomy one is showing respect for the dignity of that person. Autonomy is grounded in the notion that each individual has his or her own goals, belief system, and life plan. Thus that individual should be the one who makes the decisions concerning his or her life, not someone else. Nevertheless, some health care professionals still think their view of what is best for the patient is in the patient's best interests.

17. McCormick's proportionate reason sounds vaguely similar to the ethical theory of W. D. Ross. Thus it should be noted that McCormick sees a conceptual similarity between his views and the position of Ross. What makes this interesting is that Ross is a deontologist and McCormick works out of a teleological framework. Ross holds that moral conflicts are linked to relationships. Thus each situation implicitly contains *prima facie*, meaning conditional, duties. According to Ross, a person must hierarchically arrange these duties and make the decision that maintains the most important duty or duties. McCormick thinks what makes a duty more pressing is "that a more urgent good is at stake in some way." For McCormick's discussion of the relationship between himself and Ross, see Richard A. McCormick, "A Commentary on the Commentaries," in *Doing Evil to Achieve Good: Moral Choice in Conflict Situations*, ed. Richard A. McCormick and Paul Ramsey (Chicago: Loyola University Press, 1978), pp. 253f.

18. For a thorough discussion of the various forms that paternalism can take, see James F. Childress, *Who Should Decide? Paternalism in Health Care* (New York: Oxford University Press, 1982).

Therefore these health care professionals warrant paternalism on two grounds: (1) incompetency of the patient — that is, the patient is incapable of determining what is best for himself or herself;[19] and (2) that the patient's request is unduly harmful to his or her best interests. The first reason has been designated "weak" paternalism because it does not call into question the right of the patient to make his or her own decisions. Rather, it addresses the capability or competence of the patient. The second reason has been termed "strong" paternalism because it states that even though the patient is competent, the patient's decision should be voided and replaced with the judgment of the health care professional.[20]

McCormick's moral theory connects moral rights and duties to moral values that are to be realized. Thus the moral right of self-determination is linked to the moral value of human freedom. But, of course, central to his theory is the concept of a hierarchy of values. Because there is an ordering of values, the right of self-determination is potentially conditional upon the realization of other, more basic values. Consequently, McCormick's theory, in principle, could support a "strong" paternalism. In other words, the moral right of self-determination could be limited or suspended by the need to fulfill a more fundamental value.

McCormick addresses the issue of competent patients rejecting life-sustaining treatment in his article "The Moral Right to Privacy."[21] According to McCormick, Catholic moral theory has consistently coupled self-determination with the duty of preservation of life. However, Catholic moral thought places limits on this duty to preserve life. The Judeo-Christian position affirms that "life is indeed a basic and precious good, but a good to be preserved precisely at the condition of other values."[22] McCormick views the statement of Pope Pius XII that "[l]ife, death, all temporal activities are in fact subordinated to spiritual ends"[23] as portraying the conditional nature of the preservation of life. Spiritual ends for which "preservation of life" could be

19. See Ruth R. Faden and Tom Beauchamp, *A History and Theory of Informed Consent* (New York: Oxford University Press, 1986), for a discussion of informed consent and what it entails.

20. For an in-depth understanding of "weak" and "strong" paternalism, see Joel Feinberg, "Legal Paternalism," *Canadian Journal of Philosophy* 1 (1971): 105-24. See also Feinberg's *Social Philosophy* (Englewood Cliffs, N.J.: Prentice-Hall, 1973).

21. Richard A. McCormick, "The Moral Right to Privacy," reprinted in *How Brave a New World?*

22. Richard A. McCormick, "To Save or Let Die: The Dilemma of Modern Medicine," in *How Brave a New World?* p. 345.

23. Pius XII, *Acta Apostolicae Sedis* 49 (1957): 1031-32, cited in *How Brave a New World?* pp. 345f.

suspended include: (1) the sacrifice of one's own life for the "glory of God, salvation of souls, service of one's brethren, etc.";[24] and (2) the capacity to sustain human relationships. According to McCormick, we are told not only to love God but to love our neighbor as well. Thus, in his understanding, this means that a large portion of loving God is loving him through love to others. Therefore, if there no longer exists any possibility for human relationship, "life can be said to have achieved its potential."[25]

With the possibility of limiting the "preservation of life" as an absolute duty, we can return to the issue of competent patients rejecting life-sustaining treatment. McCormick affirms self-determination as a necessary means to the fulfillment of personal duty. In other words, generally speaking, patients are in the best position to discern which treatments have a "reasonable benefit" or which treatments would force an "unreasonable burden" upon them. Therefore self-determination becomes the only viable way for patients to achieve their personal duty to themselves. Consequently, however, self-determination is a "conditional" or "instrumental" good "precisely insofar as it is the instrument whereby the best interest of the patient are served by it."[26]

If underlying the value of self-determination is the basic good "the best interest of the patient," McCormick then thinks he can place some stipulations upon self-determination. He says the right of self-determination evaporates when its usage "is *de facto* and in the circumstances no longer to the overall good of the person involved." For instance, if a person should determine to commit suicide, that person is exercising his or her self-determination "in a way commonly regarded as destructive to self,"[27] and thus that person's right of self-determination is no longer sustained by its underlying good. Thus, if it should turn out that a patient wants to choose a course of action that would be against his or her best interests, intervention by an outside party would be morally acceptable.

In terms of a patient rejecting life-sustaining treatment, McCormick says,

> [T]he appropriate mix of values during dying, how one shall live while dying, belongs to the patient. And here patients may and do differ within the range of morally acceptable options.
>
> Of the three key values present (preservation of life, human freedom, lack of pain), some will choose to maximize freedom, others to minimize

24. McCormick, "Theology and Biomedical Ethics," p. 321.
25. McCormick, "To Save or Let Die," p. 349.
26. McCormick, *How Brave a New World?* p. 359.
27. McCormick, *How Brave a New World?* p. 359.

pain even with the diminution of freedom. Still others will manage their dying with a controlling view of the financial and/or psychological condition of their dear ones. . . . Treatment that conforms to such wishes and perspectives may be considered reasonable (morally appropriate), always allowing for legal appeal by physician or hospital if a patient is judged to be frivolously jeopardizing life.[28]

Hence McCormick indicates what is a proportionate reasoned decision and what is a nonproportionate reasoned decision. A proportionate reasoned decision would include such values as preservation of life, human freedom, and lack of pain. A nonproportionate reasoned decision would be a choice that was "frivolous." McCormick never defines "frivolous."[29] However, he does think rational people would be able to recognize a disproportionate choice and agrees to intervention by a third party in such cases. In fact, these potential outsiders would have no problem with paternalism because they would perceive it to be in the best interests of the patient. "Most people . . . would think that what is actually in a person's best interests ought to prevail over what the deluded or misguided person thinks is his best interests. In this sense . . . most people would be objective or normative in determining best interests, for best interests are best interests, not putative best interests."[30] Moral decision making is the result of common reflection and discourse within the community of God's people.[31] According to McCormick, this should not imply that the community is always correct, but rather that "a realistic individual will understand the dangers of trying to discover moral truth alone, of deciding what is right and wrong in isolation from a pool of wisdom and reflection far greater than the individual's."[32] Thus communities should familiarize and nurture the individual in moral development. Moreover, communities may at times have to correct the proportionate reason which individuals use. Consequently, individual self-determination is an instrumental good which can bring about the implementation of the basic good or goods. Nevertheless, this individual self-determination does not exist within a vac-

---

28. Richard A. McCormick, "The Quality of Life, the Sanctity of Life," in *How Brave a New World?* pp. 399f.

29. McCormick consistently equates the choices made by third parties for incompetent persons with the choices that competent persons should make for themselves.

30. Richard A. McCormick, "The Rights of the Voiceless," in *How Brave a New World?* pp. 107f.

31. Richard A. McCormick, "Notes on Moral Theology: 1977," in *Notes on Moral Theology, 1965-1980* (Lanham, Md.: University Press of America, 1984), p. 699.

32. Richard A. McCormick, "Notes on Moral Theology: 1978," in *Notes on Moral Theology, 1965-1980,* p. 768.

uum. The autonomy of the individual is complemented and augmented by the broader community, which provides further reflection and discernment so that the basic good or goods are brought about which truly are in the "best interests" of the individual.

In summary, a Catholic approach to bioethics typically is a natural law approach. It is a human ethic because any human being by reflection upon his or her basic inclinations should be able to promulgate the first principles of morality or, in McCormick's words, the basic goods or values of life. Moral decision making consists in making decisions that affirm and bring about these foundational values. If conflict should arise between the implementation of values such that it is not possible to realize all values in a situation, then one must make the decision that is proportionate.

Protestant Bioethics

Paul Ramsey

Before his death in 1988, Paul Ramsey was the Harrington Spear Paine Professor of Christian Ethics at Princeton University. Writing as a Christian ethicist, Ramsey produced a voluminous amount of material on the relationship between theology and bioethics. His first work, *Basic Christian Ethics* (1950), is a systematic treatment of theological ethics which Ramsey described as "an essay in the Christocentric ethics of the Reformation."[33] According to Ramsey, the central ethical principle of Christianity is "obedient love."[34] The foundation of this obedient love is twofold: (1) The meaning of love is explicated in the life and teachings of Jesus (this is the Christocentric portion of Ramsey's ethic). (2) The meaning of "obedient" as it relates to the concept of love is embedded in the faith relationship of the nation of Israel.

The principle to be derived from this love of Jesus and covenant relationship of Israel is the idea of righteousness. According to Ramsey, it is the biblical conception of righteousness which provides "the meaning and measure of full human obligation."[35] The appropriate response to God's covenant relationship is "grateful obedience or obedient gratitude." The righteousness of God, then, becomes the standard by which we should measure the right-

---

33. Paul Ramsey, *Basic Christian Ethics* (New York: Charles Scribner's Sons, 1950), p. xiv.

34. Ramsey, *Basic Christian Ethics*, p. xi.

35. Ramsey, *Basic Christian Ethics*, p. 3.

ness of all our human relationships. Therefore we should treat our fellow human beings "according to the measure of [their] real need" (which is the way God treats them).[36] Thus Ramsey's ethical position is not only centered in the biblical concept of covenant fidelity but is totally directed at meeting the real needs of our neighbor. It is not the "good" that one is trying to understand; rather, it is whose "good" one should be seeking. Accordingly, this is "the main, perhaps the only, concern of Christian ethics."[37]

Ramsey wants to make clear that he believes people naturally seek "the good" due to natural desire. However, love of one's neighbor may not be what we naturally seek, but covenant obedience requires that we seek the good of our neighbor. This is the "right" thing to do. Therefore Ramsey says "Christian ethics is a deontological (or principle-based) ethics, not an ethic of the 'the good.'" Only after the Christian's "right relation" of focusing in on his or her neighbor's needs does the Christian seek "as a secondary though quite essential concern . . . for his neighbor's sake to ascend whatever scale of values he might find reasonably creditable."[38] In contrast to McCormick, Ramsey does not believe that a moral theory can be teleological (outcome or result based), whereby one first determines the "good" or "goods" and then deduces how to attain and implement them. Ramsey makes this point extremely clear:

> *Agape* defines for the Christian what is right, righteous, obligatory to be done among men; it is not a Christian's definition of the good that better be done and much less is it a definition of the right way to the good. . . .
>
> Eschatology has at least this significance for Christian ethics in all ages: that reliance upon producing the *teloi* (the end, or result), or on doing good consequences, or on goal-seeking, has been decisively set aside. . . . The Christian understanding of righteousness is therefore radically non-teleological. It means ready obedience to the *present* reign of God, the alignment of the human will with the divine will that men should live together in covenant-love no matter what the morrow brings, even if it brings nothing.[39]

Ramsey thus rejects all forms of consequentialism in moral theory. The only good to be pursued is the neighbor's good, and any other good which might come about in seeking the neighbor's good is "as quite unintended consequence."[40]

36. Ramsey, *Basic Christian Ethics*, pp. 9, 14.

37. Ramsey, *Basic Christian Ethics*, p. 114.

38. Ramsey, *Basic Christian Ethics*, p. 116.

39. Paul Ramsey, *Deeds and Rules in Christian Ethics* (New York: Charles Scribner's Sons, 1967), pp. 108-9.

40. Ramsey, *Basic Christian Ethics*, p. 149.

In light of Ramsey's concept of covenant fidelity, which embodies pursuing the good of the other, we should not be surprised at the major focus of his discussions in bioethics. He continually focuses upon the demands of the physician to the patient or the researcher to the subject. Of course, it is possible to argue that a covenant also contains stipulations for both parties involved in the covenant relation. Nevertheless, Ramsey only emphasizes the responsibilities of the health care professional. Moreover, he uses the discussion of these responsibilities to make a larger argument for morality in general. Thus it appears that he is indirectly arguing against an overall decline in societal morality which is having an "overflow" effect upon the medical field.

For instance, in *The Patient as Person* Ramsey seeks to protect the idea of humanity's "sacredness" in the biological order from the threats of medical vitalism (the view that the body should be kept alive at all costs) and medical expediency.[41] In *Fabricated Man* he argues to preserve both the unitive and procreative aspects of marital sexuality and human parenthood that are increasingly under attack due to the development of reproductive technology.[42] In *Ethics at the Edges of Life* he attempts to straighten out our moral and legal reasoning as it pertains to active, involuntary euthanasia.[43] Ramsey's manner of argument is to express the positive obligations of covenant fidelity in negative or limiting terms. In other words, he often describes what we ought not to do instead of telling us what we ought to do.

The next area to address in Ramsey's ethic is the place of moral rules or moral principles. The principal and foundational norm of Ramsey's moral theory is *agape* understood as "obedient love." This love is a covenant-oriented love directed at the other or one's neighbor. At first it seems that Ramsey has no place for rules in his system, for he says that "Christians are bound by Jesus' attitude of sticking as close as possible to human need, no matter what the rules say, as the primary meaning of obligation. . . . Strictly speaking, this is a new 'principle' for morality only in the sense that here all morality governed by principles, rules, customs, and laws goes to pieces and is given another sovereign test."[44] However, Ramsey goes on to state that "Christian love in search of a social policy" may well need to utilize the prac-

41. Paul Ramsey, *The Patient as Person: Explorations in Medical Ethics* (New Haven: Yale University Press, 1970).

42. Paul Ramsey, *Fabricated Man: The Ethics of Genetic Control* (New Haven: Yale University Press, 1970).

43. Paul Ramsey, *Ethics at the Edges of Life: Medical and Legal Intersections* (New Haven: Yale University Press, 1978).

44. Ramsey, *Basic Christian Ethics*, p. 57. It is interesting to note that the title of the chapter from which this quote was extracted is "Christian Liberty: An Ethic without Rules."

tical wisdom of natural law traditions and other epistemic sources while at the same time insuring that, while *agape* "makes alliance or coalition with any available sources of insight of information about what should be done, it makes *concordat* with none of these."[45] Love continues to be the controlling partner in these linkups with other sources.

Furthermore, Ramsey develops a Protestant natural law that appears to develop independent moral norms that work alongside *agape*. In this development of natural law, Ramsey still rejects "traditional" Roman Catholic interpretations of natural law involving rational deduction of moral norms from a static and universal human nature. What bothers him about the Catholic natural law formulation is that "revelation has 'republished' the entire natural law and thereby made our knowledge of it certain and exact."[46] Ramsey develops his concept of Protestant natural law by saying that the principles of natural law are discovered "in the course of active reflection upon man in the context of moral, social, and legal decisions."[47] Thus he takes a phenomenological approach to the insights of his understanding of natural law, as opposed to the ontological necessity of Catholic moral theory. Consequently, the principles of Protestant natural law are acquired rather than being latently present, as understood by the Catholic natural law tradition.

Where does all of this leave Ramsey in relation to moral rules and principles? In *Deeds and Rules in Christian Ethics* he designates his position as "mixed agapism."[48] He calls it "mixed agapism" because *agape* can be related to principles of morality in two ways: (1) The concept of *agape* contains certain norms or practices which are guiding principles of morality. For example, certain "forms of steadfastness in responsibility one to another would seem to be the most likely inference from Christlike love. . . ." (2) Apart from *agape* there are "structures of life into which we are called; and practices into which every man is born who was ever born,"[49] and these structures have within them norms that provide people with moral rules and guiding principles of morality.[50] This is the mixture that makes up the idea of "mixed agapism." Ramsey says "that a proper understanding of the moral life will be one in which Christians determine what we ought to do in very great measure by determining which rules of action are most love-embodying, but that

---

45. Ramsey, *Basic Christian Ethics,* p. 344.

46. Paul Ramsey, *Nine Modern Moralists* (Englewood Cliffs, N.J.: Prentice-Hall, 1962), pp. 212f.

47. Ramsey, *Nine Modern Moralists,* p. 216.

48. Ramsey, *Deeds and Rules,* pp. 29, 117-20.

49. Ramsey, *Deeds and Rules,* p. 164.

50. Ramsey, *Deeds and Rules,* pp. 120, 122.

there are also always situations in which we are to tell what we should do by getting clear about the facts of that situation and then asking what is the loving or the most loving thing to do in it."[51] There is an "internal asymmetry" between these two sources of morality. This is what Ramsey seems to mean when he discusses "love transforming natural justice."[52]

When Ramsey involves himself in concrete ethical situations, he tends toward a rule-dominant approach. In fact, he believes this is consistent with the Christian faith and love which reveals the restrictive nature of moral rules:

> A position we might call "pure or general rule-agapism" would seem to be entailed in any conviction that in Jesus Christ the righteousness of God and the mystery of the ages, the meaning of the creation, of mature manhood, and the destination of man toward unfailing covenant with God and fellow man, have been made manifest. An unbinding love would seem the least likely conclusion one would reach if he seriously regarded the freedom of God's love in binding Himself to the world as the model for all covenants between men. Could anyone who perceives that God in total love and total freedom bound Himself to the world possibly view the implications of this love as unbinding to men?[53]

Thus, according to Ramsey, general rules are consistent with the freedom of *agape*, in that we should come to realize that some things are "as unconditionally wrong as love is unconditionally right."[54]

Therefore Ramsey's ethic of covenant fidelity or obedient love is in sharp contrast to McCormick's moral theory of value realization. For McCormick morality focuses around the realization of values, and for Ramsey covenant obedience is the central aspect of ethics. Furthermore, Ramsey grounds his natural law approach in the assessing of experience, whereas McCormick discursively perceives what is natively present. Ramsey wants to maintain the unconditional nature of love and the associated rules, while McCormick weighs the consequences to hierarchically fulfill the basic good or goods.

With an understanding of Ramsey's moral theory, we now need to examine his approach to the issue of competent patient refusal of life-sustaining treatment. In *The Patient as Person* Ramsey says that in the case where cure is no

---

51. Ramsey, *Deeds and Rules*, p. 5.
52. Ramsey, *Deeds and Rules*, p. 122.
53. Ramsey, *Deeds and Rules*, pp. 127f.
54. Ramsey, *Deeds and Rules*, p. 129.

longer possible, covenant fidelity requires "(only) caring for the dying."[55] Furthermore, when one weighs the benefits and the hardships involved in certain medical treatments, morality may demand the cessation of treatment:

> The "process of dying" is not the only condition for stopping the use of medical means, although when present it is a sufficient and morally obliging condition. Other conditions can make it morally right to stop the use of medical means, although the decision to do so may not be a strictly medical judgment. . . .
>
> . . . Even when he could succeed [medically], a doctor may and sometimes should allow his medical judgment to defer to a patient's estimate of the higher importance of the worth and the relations for which his life was lived.[56]

Ramsey does broaden the morally possible reasons for continuing or discontinuing treatment beyond the medical. In other words, the patient's choice may be based in factors other than medical success. Moreover, according to Ramsey, "Not every means for prolonging life, once it is successful and made available — even 'customary' medical practice — becomes thereby ordinary and mandatory upon both the patient and doctor. There are always broader human factors to be taken into account, and these always in Christian medical ethics kept the saving of life from being made an absolute and inflexible norm, a hardship inhumanly applied."[57] Thus, in Ramsey's mind, there could be a myriad of morally appropriate reasons for discontinuing treatment that have absolutely nothing to do with their medical potency.

In a later work, *Ethics at the Edges of Life*, Ramsey discusses five morally acceptable standards by which to decide upon the withholding or withdrawing of treatment: (1) ordinary/extraordinary treatment distinction; (2) standard medical care policy; (3) the right of the patient to refuse treatment; (4) medical indications policy; and (5) a quality-of-life-expected policy. However, according to Ramsey, "the significant moral meaning of these similar related standards can be reduced almost without remainder to a medical indications policy."[58] To make his position perfectly clear, Ramsey states:

> Why not say that the classification "ordinary/extraordinary" can simply be reduced to (1) a determination either of the treatment indicated or that there is not treatment indicated in the case of the dying, and (2) a patient's

---

55. Ramsey, *The Patient as Person*, p. 127.
56. Ramsey, *The Patient as Person*, pp. 136f.
57. Ramsey, *The Patient as Person*, p. 141.
58. Ramsey, *Ethics at the Edges*, p. 155.

right to refuse treatment? The answer to that question is that there are medically indicated treatments (these used to be called "ordinary") that a competent conscious patient has no right to refuse, just as no one has a moral right deliberately to ruin his health. Treatment refusal is a relative right, contrary to what is believed today by those who would reduce medical ethics to patient autonomy and a "right to die."

. . . A medical indications policy is applicable both to the non-dying and to the dying, to the conscious and the unconscious. Instead of a conscious non-dying patient's right to refuse treatment we need to emphasize his free and informed participation in medical decisions affecting him when there are alternative treatments.[59]

This appears to be a shift in Ramsey's thinking from his previous statements in *The Patient as Person*. This latter assertion by Ramsey seems to be placing the appropriate moral determinations totally within the confines of the medically possible. Or, as Ramsey puts it, the patient's self-determination does "not encompass the right . . . to assault the value of his own life with or without medical assistance."[60]

What appears to be a shift in Ramsey's earlier thought is in reality only an adjustment. For Ramsey there are only two possibilities in respect to death: "dying well enough" or choosing death as an end or means.[61] In Ramsey's mind this latter choice is plainly wrong since, according to "our religious faith[,] that life is a gift."[62] In addition, life is not only a gift, it is a trust. We do not own our life, we are stewards of our life. "What, then, does one choose in a medical-moral policy of allowing to die or refusing further treatment — if that is not dominion (or co-dominion) over human life instead of trusteeship or stewardship, if that is not based on a fundamental denial that life is a gift and a trust?"[63] Thus, all Ramsey has really done by invoking the metaphors of "gift" and "trust" is to unpack the covenant relationship that one has with God. It is important to Ramsey that patients understand that they have a duty to God since he was the one who gave them life. Nevertheless, Ramsey is not arguing that every refusal of treatment is morally objectionable — only those decisions to refuse treatment that encompass the idea that one is choosing death as an end or means. Therefore "a conscious, competent, 'incurable' patient would have a relative right to refuse treatment in

---

59. Ramsey, *Ethics at the Edges*, p. 156.
60. Ramsey, *Ethics at the Edges*, p. 158.
61. Ramsey, *Ethics at the Edges*, p. 149.
62. Ramsey, *Ethics at the Edges*, p. 146.
63. Ramsey, *Ethics at the Edges*, p. 147.

the course of shared decision-making concerning his or her case."[64] Ramsey is just placing checks and balances on the autonomy of the patient.

Ramsey appears to be trying to do three things in the decision-making process: (1) affirm the importance of the medical information; (2) affirm, in some sense, the autonomy of the patient; and lastly, (3) affirm the responsibilities of the patient in the "covenant" relationship with God. In the end, it does appear to be somewhat ambiguous as to what the patient is to do. However, Ramsey thinks he has provided the transcendent moral framework for each individual decision.

James M. Gustafson

A second Protestant Christian ethicist who has written widely on bioethics and is influential in his views is James M. Gustafson, Henry B. Luce Professor of Humanities and Comparative Studies at Emory University. He is concerned about "the importance of taking very seriously the kinds of precise and technical information required to make particular judgments and choices (while not losing sight of the difficulties in getting accurate information and ideologically unbiased interpretation), and the importance of making the moral arguments of Christians more rigorous both philosophically and theologically."[65] Gustafson has produced a systematic treatment of his approach in his two-volume work entitled *Ethics from a Theocentric Perspective*. In this work he wants to locate ethics within the divine will in such a manner that we "relate ourselves and all things in a manner appropriate to their relations to God."

Gustafson does not think those who do theology have consistently connected "ethics" and "theology." In other words, as they reflect upon the issues, say, in bioethics, there is little theological representation involved in their analysis. According to Gustafson,

> [M]uch theological or "religious" writing is directed to the justification of an enterprise in the eyes of persons who are not really interested enough to care whether the justification is adequate or not. (I worked for years on a book *Can Ethics Be Christian?* with the nagging sense that most persons who answer in an unambiguous affirmative would not be interested in my supporting argument, that a few fellow professional persons might be interested enough to look at it, and that for those who believe the answer is

64. Ramsey, *Ethics at the Edges*, p. 165.
65. James M. Gustafson, "A Theocentric Interpretation of Life," *Christian Century* 97 (1980): 754.

negative the question itself is not sufficiently important to bother about.) While theologians ought to continue to participate competently in the public debates about matters of technology and the life sciences, they would also do well to attend to the home folks who *might* care more about what they have to say. . . .

It is the "religious ethicists" who have most to be anxious about, in my judgment. They will have either to become moral philosophers with a special interest in "religious" texts and arguments, or become theologians: or "religious dimensions" theologians. Only indifference to what they are writing, or exceeding patience with inexcusable ambiguity, can account for the tolerance they have enjoyed.[66]

Gustafson's commentary on the state of religious ethics underscores his commitment to the need for religion to qualify morality.[67] According to Gustafson, one cannot reflect theologically without involving oneself in ethical reflection as well. Thus, how does Gustafson connect theology and ethics?

For Gustafson, theology is an activity of the practical reason which involves discerning that part of the human experience which is "religious." "Religious," to Gustafson, means "that dimension of experience (in which not all persons consciously share) that senses a relationship to an ultimate power that sustains and stands over against humans and the world."[68] Therefore this "ultimate power" that Gustafson refers to is never directly experienced by the self. Rather one engages it through an experience of something else.[69] The task of theology, then, is not only to ascertain what part of experience is religious, but also to infer from the religious dimension of experience the ultimate power's qualities and characteristics, purposes and intentions, and relations to the world.[70] According to Gustafson, "ethics like theology is also an activity of practical reason; it is a reflection on those dimensions of human experience denoted moral." Ethics seeks to "analyze the necessary conditions for moral activity" and to "indicate normatively what moral principles and values ought to govern human action." Religion qualifies moral experience when one decides to act in response to the ultimate power, and likewise, the *"theological* qualification of *ethics"* happens when one articulates the relation

---

66. James M. Gustafson, "Theology Confronts Technology and the Life Sciences," *Commonweal* 105 (16 June 1978): 386.

67. For a discussion by Gustafson on what qualification would look like, see James M. Gustafson, *Can Ethics Be Christian?* (Chicago: University of Chicago Press, 1975).

68. James M. Gustafson, *The Contributions of Theology to Medical Ethics,* pp. 5f.

69. Gustafson, *Contributions of Theology,* pp. 5f.

70. Gustafson, *Contributions of Theology,* p. 7.

of the ultimate power "both as a necessary condition for moral action, and as a necessary justification for moral values and principles that judge, prescribe, and govern action."[71] Hence Gustafson has defined the task and method of theology and its relationship to ethics.

Remembering that the ultimate power is discerned mediately through experience, Gustafson's theocentric ethics decides to change the foundation of "faith" from the cognitive realm to the realm of the affections. Gustafson thinks the focus of faith should be upon *piety,* the most central religious affection of all. By "piety" he means awe and respect. Furthermore, awe and respect mean that our religious affections may include both an attraction and a repulsion to the powers of God as we experience them. In other words, "both a love of God, the giver of the possibilities for value and meaning in life, and fear and anger in the face of conditions which frustrate human aspirations and threaten or deny human life"[72] are revealed in human experience.

Focusing on the "affective" part of human experience by which to come into contact with the ultimate, what sort of method, then, reveals this ultimate power? According to Gustafson, we begin to experience the ultimate when we ask certain kinds of questions about our experiences. Four questions need to be asked so that the religious significance of experience is revealed: (1) In whom or in what can we have confidence? (2) To whom or what do we owe loyalty? (3) For what can we, or ought we, to hope? and (4) What are the appropriate objects of human loves, desires, or aversions?[73] The areas of life in which these questions should be asked are nature, history, culture, society, and self.[74] These are the questions which will surface the ultimate in human experience. Nevertheless, Gustafson is quick to point out that some people ask and answer these questions in such a manner that they do not discover the ultimate's presence or power. Consequently, he concludes that there are "functional surrogates to religion as [he] understands it."[75]

Up to this point we have shown that Gustafson views theology beginning with human experience. The basis of faith is not located in the cognitive element of our being, but rather it is found in the affective part of us. These affective responses to human experience, when coupled with the appropriate questions, yield the presence and power of the ultimate. Our answers to these questions about affective responses to experience are couched in the symbols

71. Gustafson, *Contributions of Theology,* p. 13.

72. James M. Gustafson, *Ethics from a Theocentric Perspective,* vol. 1, *Theology and Ethics* (Chicago: University of Chicago Press, 1981), p. 204.

73. Gustafson, *Ethics from a Theocentric Perspective,* 1:224f.

74. Gustafson, *Ethics from a Theocentric Perspective,* 1:207-23.

75. Gustafson, *Ethics from a Theocentric Perspective,* 1:225.

and worldviews of the communities and traditions in which we have been exposed throughout our lives. To all of this Gustafson adds another element.

He says all of our religious symbols and ideas must be in concert with what the physical and social sciences have discovered. He contends: "The substantial content of theology, if it is not in perfect harmony with scientific knowledge, cannot be in sharp incongruity with it, and what we say about God must be congruent in some way with what we know about human experience and its objects through the sciences."[76] Thus the discoveries and claims of the physical sciences become the test for the tenets of theology. In other words, there must be congruency between the assertions of theology and the data of the sciences. In light of this need for congruency between theology and science, Gustafson thinks that certain traditional ways of speaking about God are still viable. Symbols like God as Creator, God as Sustainer and Governor of the "ordering" of creation, and God as Judge and Redeemer accurately portray God's relationship to humanity and the world.[77] Although Gustafson does accept the above-mentioned religious symbols, he rejects certain other traditional religious themes.

Since scientific conformity is the test for theological assertions, some traditional religious themes are considered implausible by Gustafson. For instance, the idea that humanity is the goal and the apex of creation does not fit with the current scientific evidence. Assuming that evolutionary theory is a correct interpretation of origins, Gustafson says "there was no particular merit in bringing [humankind] into being through such an inefficient and lengthy process."[78] Furthermore, science has shown that "as the beginning was without us, so will the end be without us." In addition, scientific evidence not only removes the centrality of humanity, but typical Christian eschatological symbols are unsupportable by science.[79] Likewise, science does not offer any evidence for the traditional language of "eternal life" or a "resurrection destiny."[80]

In explicating Gustafson's "theocentric ethics," the issue of Christology remains to be discussed. Some have suggested that his theology is not Christian due to his views on Christology.[81] He will admit that Christology is "the most critical doctrinal issue" if one claims to be doing Christian theology, but he states quite clearly that his project was not to defend traditional Christian-

76. Gustafson, *Ethics from a Theocentric Perspective,* 1:251f.
77. Gustafson, *Ethics from a Theocentric Perspective,* 1:236-51.
78. Gustafson, *Ethics from a Theocentric Perspective,* 1:267.
79. Gustafson, *Ethics from a Theocentric Perspective,* 1:268.
80. Gustafson, *Ethics from a Theocentric Perspective,* 1:183-84.
81. Gustafson, *Ethics from a Theocentric Perspective,* 1:273-74.

ity but rather to "find what can be most truly claimed about God."[82] Gustafson says his views about Christ are derived primarily from the synoptic Gospels. He negates the usage of the Epistles because their language, in describing Christ, is too "abstract," and abstract language does not invoke the affective response as well as a narrative does. In addition, he rejects "biblicistic views of revelation" and is "epistemologically suspicious" of christological concepts such as a "preexistent Christ."[83] For Gustafson, "Jesus incarnates theocentric piety and fidelity." The life and ministry of Jesus are insightful in that we "see and know something of the powers that bear down on us and sustain us, and of the piety and the manner of life that are appropriate to them." Jesus provides an "historical embodiment" of what God wants us to do.[84] Surely "the only good reason for claiming to be a Christian is that we continue to be empowered, sustained, renewed, informed, and judged by Jesus' incarnation of theocentric piety and fidelity."[85] Thus Jesus is only to be understood as a representation of someone who is allowing himself or herself to live under theocentric control. Jesus shows us how and what human experiences look like when they are theocentrically construed.

Therefore the practical moral question for a "theocentric" interpretation of the world is, What is God enabling and requiring us to be and to do? In addition, the requirements and enablement of God assume that we are participants in the processes and patterns of life.[86] We are to understand that we are not "spectators" to life and neither are we its "rulers." Gustafson says the traditional religious term that best expresses our relationship to life is "stewardship." "Stewardship" conveys the idea that we are "temporary, responsible custodians of, and contributors to, the realms in which we participate."[87] Since we are "stewards" or "participants" who are theocentrically organizing our lives and responding to the governance of God, we need to extract ourselves from a rule-centered mentality. This does not mean that Gustafson entirely removes moral rules or principles from his position. Rather he sees a fixation on moral rules that narrowly cover every situation as problematic for two reasons: (1) historical conditions change, and thus rules need to be general enough to flex with history; and (2) the divine governance of the world is not done through a fixed eternal order, but rather an ordering.

82. Gustafson, *Ethics from a Theocentric Perspective*, 1:275, 279.
83. Gustafson, *Ethics from a Theocentric Perspective*, 1:275 n. 65.
84. Gustafson, *Ethics from a Theocentric Perspective*, 1:276.
85. Gustafson, *Ethics from a Theocentric Perspective*, 1:276, 277.
86. James M. Gustafson, *Ethics from a Theocentric Perspective*, vol. 2, *Ethics and Theology* (Chicago: University of Chicago Press, 1984), p. 146.
87. Gustafson, *Ethics from a Theocentric Perspective*, 2:145.

Consequently, moral rules and principles "have to be open to revision and extension in the light of alterations in natural, social, historical, cultural, and individual conditions."[88]

Gustafson's theocentric ethics is not a rule-centered morality, nor does it provide the comfort of any type of moral theory, whether deontological or utilitarian:

> It does not relieve the anxiety of taking risks; it does not eliminate the need sometimes to act unjustly for the sake of a wider justice; it does not resolve the deep ambiguities of moral choices in certain particular conditions; and it does not eliminate the possibility of genuine tragedy as a feature of human moral experience. It does not provide a bland assurance that something good will issue from every circumstance of what is injurious to human welfare, that every "crucifixion" will issue in a glorious "resurrection," that all things work together for good for those who love God.[89]

To Gustafson, a moral theory takes one away from being a "participant" and makes one a spectator; one never really engages the situation. With moral theory in hand, a person takes on the posture of an ideal observer and thus begins to evaluate the situation from the position of God.[90] Instead, theocentric ethics is about "discernment."

Moral discernment to Gustafson is fundamentally a reflective, rational activity: "it is reflection on one's own motives and desires." We morally and reflectively evaluate the various means and consequences of our action. Nevertheless, in the end, Gustafson says our discernment results in "an informed intuition": "[I]t is not the conclusion of a formally logical argument, a strict deduction from a single moral principle, or an absolutely certain result from the exercises of human 'reason' alone. There is a final moment of perception that sees the parts in relation to a whole, expresses sensibilities as well as reasoning, and is made in the conditions of human finitude."[91] We assess the situation, we evaluate means and ends as well as consequences, and out of this reflective process we obtain a sense or an intuition of what we should do. But where is the divine governance in all of this?

Gustafson explains how one should discern the divine governance, and it will not be discovered in a timeless and changeless moral order. This does

---

88. Gustafson, *Ethics from a Theocentric Perspective*, 1:316.
89. Gustafson, *Ethics from a Theocentric Perspective*, 1:316f.
90. Gustafson, *Ethics from a Theocentric Perspective*, 2:146.
91. Gustafson, *Ethics from a Theocentric Perspective*, 1:338.

not imply relativism; rather, historical conditions change and thus moral rules and principles "need to be extended in their applications, may need to be revised, and in some instances may need to be radically altered." We should not look for the divine governance in the "moral details" of Scripture. The Bible contains the responses of people to the divine governance in their particular situation, and these responses should not be understood as exact ways to always react to the divine governance. According to Gustafson, the only thing that can be discerned about the divine governance is "the necessary conditions for life to be sustained and developed."[92] These necessary conditions form the bases for ethical reflection. Although theocentric discernment rejects the idea of static norms deduced from some immutable order of creation, it still places its moral determinations within "an objective 'reality' of which human life is a part."[93]

In summary, Gustafson's theocentric ethics wants to rescue ethics from anthropocentrism and return it to a theocentric approach. Theocentric ethics is concerned with discerning the divine will and participating in the divine ordering of creation. Central to the process of discernment is the concept of *piety*. Piety is the affective powers of our being discerning the divine ordering. Unlike natural law, theocentric ethics does not provide one with a set of "goods" or values which are hierarchically arranged. There are no specific rules or practices derived from *agape* or "covenant fidelity." Rather theocentric ethics requires that we understand that we are interactive participants in the divine ordering of the whole of creation. Thus we are to avail ourselves of the information obtained by the natural sciences. In the entire process of discernment, associated with theocentric ethics, we can never be objectively certain. Now, how does a "theocentric" approach try to resolve the issue of refusal of life-sustaining treatment by competent persons?

Unlike McCormick and Ramsey, Gustafson has written very little on the subject of life-sustaining treatment. In one sense this should not be surprising, since his "theocentric" ethic avoids giving absolute statements on many moral issues. The process of discernment includes too many factors related to particular circumstances for one to absolutize a certain decision. However, Gustafson does give us insight into how his position would approach this issue by his discussions of life and death and suicide.

When Gustafson discusses life-and-death, he tends to preface his comments with a quote from Karl Barth: "Life is no second God, and therefore the

---

92. Gustafson, *Ethics from a Theocentric Perspective*, 1:339.
93. Gustafson, *Ethics from a Theocentric Perspective*, 2:8.

respect due it cannot rival the reverence owed God."[94] Thus physical life is not an absolute value, and yet at the same time Gustafson is quick to say that life is the "indispensable condition for human values and valuing."[95] Therefore, on the one hand we should not worship life, but on the other hand we should not be quick to end life. According to Gustafson, there are four religious qualifications to consider about life-and-death: (1) Life should be accepted as a gift since we are dependent creatures. (2) Our life is of relative worth in comparison to the life of God. (3) We are stewards of our life and thus are responsible to God for how we treat life. (4) As participants in life, we must be "responsive to the developments and purposes which are being made possible for [us] under the power and gifts of life from God."[96] It is clear from these points that a theocentric ethic calls one to respect life because God created it and one should be open to those routes of life preservation that the divine governance reveals.

Nevertheless, medicine should be reminded that "death is as integral an aspect of human life as it is of all other biologic species." Therefore technologies whose sole goal is to prolong life "should be seriously questioned if the ultimate result is destined to be a grotesque, fragmented, or inordinately expensive existence." Gustafson never explicitly explains what a "grotesque, fragmented, or inordinately expensive" life would look like, but he is quite clear that death is not the enemy. In fact, he believes that a "sensitive, perceptive" physician will try and guide his or her patients to "a perspective in which the preservation of life is not their God."[97] Hence our gratitude for life as a divine gift does not imply that we should always, under all conditions and circumstances, try to maintain and sustain life. As we will soon see, Gustafson views some decisions for suicide as not only understandable and excusable but justifiable.

Suicide is one of four moral issues discussed extensively in volume 2 of *Ethics from a Theocentric Perspective*. For Gustafson there are certain "conditions of the human spirit" which make suicide seem engaging. He focuses on "the sense of tribulation, affliction, or despair; a sense of impossibility, or fatedness; a deep conflict of loyalties; a sense of aimlessness or purposelessness; isolation from necessary patterns of mutual interdependence; and an excessive sense of moral scrupulosity."[98]

---

94. Gustafson, *Contributions of Theology*, p. 60, and James M. Gustafson and Richard Landau, "Death Is Not the Enemy," *Journal of the American Medical Association* 252 (1984): 2458.

95. James M. Gustafson, "God's Transcendence and the Value of Human Life," in *Christian Ethics and the Community* (Philadelphia: Pilgrim Press, 1971), p. 140.

96. Gustafson, "God's Transcendence," pp. 142-43.

97. Gustafson and Landau, "Death Is Not the Enemy," p. 2458.

98. Gustafson, *Ethics from a Theocentric Perspective*, 2:201-6.

Theocentric discernment, then, would call us to remove those things which make suicide seem the most viable option. Not only does theocentric discernment call us to work at changing those conditions which lead to suicide, but we should also "restrain persons from the act [of suicide] if we have opportunity to do so." However, there are times when theocentric discernment seems to justify suicide:

> Alas, for all too many persons there are good and realistic grounds for the deepest despair: persons facing unrelievable pain and suffering of body and spirit, persons facing the bleakness of continuous poverty and unemployment, persons facing the loss of simple dignity. No ringing ideals, no cogent argument for an imperative of a duty to oneself, no charge of self-justification, and no counsel of possibilities will bring relief or hope. To deaths of such persons by suicide one must consent. The powers that bear down upon them are greater than the powers that sustain them. Neither moralists nor God ought to be their judge.[99]

Thus theocentric discernment may require that one sanction suicide as well as fight against it.

If there are situations in which suicide is justifiable and sanctioned, then there certainly could be conditions which would make the refusal of treatment acceptable. Are there any guidelines or signposts which would help someone to discern those suicides that should be stopped and those that should not be interfered with? Gustafson offers some examples from which one could extrapolate some guidance for proper discernment:

> Is suicide not only understandable and excusable but also justifiable when a person takes his or her life in the face of what is reasonably perceived to be unbearable and unrelievable suffering for oneself? . . . Kant argues that the taking of one's life to avoid misery to oneself is not justifiable. I argue to the contrary; physical life is not of ultimate value; many persons who suffer acutely are in no way accountable for their sufferings. Suffering is inflicted upon them, and it can be a morally proper choice to seek the relief of death for their own sake and for that of others.
>
> Again the conditions in which one would justify such a suicide are context-bound. The case of an adolescent boy whose aim in life is to be a great athlete and who is permanently disabled by an accident is quite different from that of a person who has undergone years of suffering, whose capacities to value life and contribute to others have been largely spent, and for

99. Gustafson, *Ethics from a Theocentric Perspective*, 2:201-6.

whom there are no courses of action available which can relieve the suffering. . . .

A special set of cases occurs where patients exercise their legal and moral right to refuse life-sustaining or even life-restoring medical procedures. Their passivity is a factor in their dying; they do, however, intend their deaths. . . . A moral evaluation is again context-bound; the case of an aged person who is ill and of a patient who can no longer tolerate the effects of a kidney dialysis regimen are different from that of a young adult whose injury precludes that one aspiration can be filled but does not rule out others. In the latter case, from my perspective, the patient's present and future possibilities for participation in life for his own sake and for the roles he can have in human communities would morally warrant an intrusion even against the patient's will. This, I know, raises legal issues and issues of medical morality as it is dominantly viewed in our time and culture. But like Thomas Aquinas, I believe that when a member of a human community who has prospects of functioning in significant ways in life is lost to the community this deprivation violates a common good and is a warrant for intervention.[100]

Notice several things from this passage. First, a deliberate choice for death, either for one's own sake or the sake of others, can be morally justifiable. Second, a person's potential and possible contributions to the human community are legitimate restrictions upon his or her autonomy. Third, life-prolonging interventions for the patient's own sake or for the common good may be justified.

Jewish Bioethics

Catholic moral theology typically believes it has a universal ethic in the natural law. Adherence to a natural law perspective gives one the ability to equate Christian ethics with human ethics, for Catholic moralists adhering to the Thomistic tradition believe it is possible for any human being to discern "right and wrong" by reason alone. Of course, that which reason discovers will never violate the information and precepts located in the special revelation of Scripture. Many Protestants, on the other hand, have questioned the ability of unaided reason to correctly apprehend morality. For these Protestant thinkers, the fallenness of human beings affects their reason in such a way that they cannot adequately discern the prescriptions of morality. Thus human beings must look to the revelation of God for direction in moral

100. Gustafson, *Ethics from a Theocentric Perspective*, 2:214-15.

matters. Obviously, this can be accomplished in a variety of ways. The two Protestant ethicists that this chapter has examined (Ramsey and Gustafson) develop an ethical position by extracting what they believe to be a central emphasis of Scripture — covenant fidelity and theocentric perspective, respectively — and apply these ideas to specific ethical decisions for adjudication. Jewish ethics in general and Jewish bioethics in particular choose a different path from both their Catholic and Protestant counterparts.

Jewish ethics is typically established by divine law in the revealed text of the Old Testament. The methodology utilized for ethical decision making is as follows:

> The basic scriptural norm is located, its rabbinic elaborations are traced through the Talmud and related literature, its authoritative structure is determined, relevant precedents (if there are any) are culled from the vast literature of legal responsa by individual rabbinic authorities, and finally the person accepted by a community of Jews as their legal authority frequently seeks the counsel of learned colleagues.[101]

Thus Jewish ethics in general and Jewish bioethics in particular are usually quite concerned with explicitly following the detailed divine mandates of God revealed in Scripture. These mandates are not discoverable prior to or apart from Scripture. Furthermore, Jewish ethics is generally not about the application of some general overriding perspective that one discovers in Scripture and then rationally applies to various dilemmas. Rather Jewish ethics typically searches for individual texts that might be applicable to a current ethical discussion and examines the commentaries and previous legal judgments of these texts to determine their meaning and applicability to the existing situation. This leads to the importance of Jewish law. Leaving out the emphasis on the rabbinical tradition, the Jewish emphasis on the text of the law may be closest to an evangelical Christian view which begins with the authority of Scripture.

Jewish law, known by the Hebrew term "Halakhah,"[102] is an all-inclusive system of normative law used to guide one's decision making within the Jewish religious context. It is a system of law grounded entirely in the Old Testament. In addition, it is dynamic in the sense that it can be expanded and

---

101. David Novak, "Judaism," in *Encyclopedia of Bioethics,* ed. Warren T. Reich, rev. ed., vol. 3 (New York: Macmillan, 1995), p. 1302.

102. The term "Halakhah" is derived from a Hebrew word which means "to go" or "to walk." For the best English definition, see "Halakhah" in the *Encyclopedia Judaico,* 7:1156-57, which states that Halakhah encompasses the legal dimension of Judaism and "embraces personal, social, national and international relationships, and all the other practices and observations of Judaism."

further developed by principles of interpretation and biblical interpretation. The idea of lawmaking through exegesis can be traced to Ezra's leadership at the beginning of the Second Commonwealth, about 458 B.C. Under Ezra the study of the Scriptures would become a prime obligation of every person and such study would be publicly institutionalized. For this idea to become functional, however, there needed to be a group of "teacher-scribes" who would copy the sacred text and teach and interpret it in a language that people could understand. This was a fundamental shift from what had previously transpired when the law had been confined primarily to the priestly class. Thus, when the public reading of Scripture occurred, the teacher-scribe was free to give interpretations and applications of the Scripture to the lives of the people. Ezra's concern for exposing the lives and decisions of the people to the Scripture was the beginning of the Halakhah which would guide and influence Jewish ethical decision making to the present.

The development and nature of Halakhah highlights the Jewish concern for doing the will of God as found in God's revelation. For embodied in the Halakhah are the careful deliberations and energetic argumentation concerning four things: (1) the substance of the law; (2) the basis for the law; (3) the source of authority of the law; and (4) the range and limits of the law's application. Underlying this quest of Halakhah is the idea that getting to specific answers concerning the dilemmas of life is not easy and will take strenuous intellectual exertion. Furthermore, human fallibility is acknowledged since Halakhah literature will record minority and dissenting opinions based upon careful biblical exegesis. Halakhah is a massive literary repository of the written records of exhaustive deliberations over ideas, propositions, social issues, legal rules, ethical norms, views about human policy and the nature of government. With this background in common Jewish ethical procedure and its emphasis upon the proper interpretation and exegesis of the Scriptures as found in the Halakhah literature, it is time to examine the approaches of two prominent Jewish ethicists.

Fred Rosner

Dr. Fred Rosner, noted hematologist and scholar, renowned bioethicist, editor of *Medicine and Jewish Law* and *Moses Maimonides: Physician, Scientist, and Philosopher* as well as author of *Modern Medicine and Jewish Ethics,* is a Jewish doctor applying Jewish ethical principles to medical situations. In *Modern Medicine and Jewish Ethics* his methodology is always the same, regardless of the issue under discussion. First, Rosner begins with a careful medical discussion of the subject. Second, he moves to the current ethical debate of the issue, showing argumentation from all sides of the topic. Third, he presents the ethical teachings of other religious traditions on the issue. Lastly, he examines the Jewish teaching on the particular question he is exploring. When Rosner is giving a Jewish perspective, he always begins with scriptural examples that would apply to the issue and follows those with talmudic sources of commentary and legal *responsa* on the Scripture.

Now that we understand the basis and methodology of Rosner's approach to bioethics, how does or how would he handle the issue of a competent person refusing life-sustaining treatment? Rosner includes in *Modern Medicine and Jewish Ethics*[103] a section entitled "The End of Life," nine chapters ranging in topics from euthanasia to embalming and cremation. Chapters 16, 17, and 18 are entitled "Euthanasia," "Heroic Measures to Prolong Life," and "Treatment of the Terminally Ill," respectively. From the contents of these three chapters we are able to deduce what Rosner would believe to be the Jewish ethical response to a competent patient refusing life-sustaining treatment.

In Rosner's chapter on euthanasia he discusses a Jewish ethical tension in relation to a *goses*, the Jewish term used to describe one who is in a dying condition. Such a person is, according to Talmud sources, to be treated as a living person in all respects. This means that

> One may not bind his jaws, nor stop up his openings, nor place a metallic vessel or any cooling object on his navel until such time that he dies, as it is written: *Before the silver cord is snapped asunder.*
>
> One may not move him, nor may one place him on sand or on salt until he dies.
>
> One may not close the eyes of the dying person. He who touches them or moves them is shedding blood because Rabbi Meir used to say: This can be compared to a flickering flame. As soon as a person touches it, it becomes extinguished. So too, whosoever closes the eyes of the dying is considered to have taken his soul.[104]

Thus, according to Jewish rabbinic authorities, one is never to hasten the dying process in any manner. However, one is also not to in any way slow down the departure of the soul from the body when a person is in the dying condition.

On delaying the departure of the soul from the body, Rosner quotes Rabbi Moses Isserles when he writes, "if there is anything which causes a hin-

---

103. Fred Rosner, *Modern Medicine and Jewish Ethics,* 2nd revised and augmented ed. (New York: Yeshiva University Press, 1991).
104. Rosner, p. 205.

drance to the departure of the soul, such as the presence near the patient's house of a knocking noise, such as wood chopping, or if there is salt on the patient's tongue, and these hinder the soul's departure, it is permissible to remove them from there because there is no act involved in this at all but only the removal of the impediment."[105] Thus we have the tension between "not hastening death" and at the same time "not hindering the departure of the soul." To help clarify this tension, Rosner is quick to point out that the Jewish understanding of a *goses* is someone who has three days or less to live. This definition is certainly more narrow than the typical understanding of a person who is terminally ill; the standard definition of terminally ill is that a person has six months or less to live.

Thus the Jewish approach in treating the incurably ill person, whose death is imminent, is utilizing medical courses of action in which "one is certain that in doing so one is shortening the act of dying and not interrupting life."[106] Consequently, on the one hand medical personnel are to do everything to keep from hastening the death of the dying patient, while on the other hand they are not obligated or required "to initiate artificial support and/or other resuscitative efforts if it is obvious that the patient is terminally and incurably and irreversibly ill with no chance of recovery."[107] Rosner concludes his discussion by summarizing the traditional Jewish attitude toward euthanasia with a quote from Rabbi J. David Bleich, who states:

> The practice of euthanasia — whether active or passive — is contrary to the teachings of Judaism. Any positive act designed to hasten the death of the patient is equated with murder in Jewish law, even if the death is hastened only by a matter of moments. No matter how laudable the intentions of the person performing an act of mercy-killing may be, his deed constitutes an act of homicide. . . .
>
> In discharging his responsibility with regard to prolongation of life, the physician must make use of any medical resources which are available. However, he is not obligated to employ procedures which are themselves hazardous in nature and may potentially foreshorten the life of the patient. Nor is either the physician or the patient obligated to employ a therapy which is experimental in nature.
>
> . . . The attempt to sustain life, by whatever means, is naught but the expression of the highest regard for the precious nature of the gift of life and of the dignity in which it is held.

105. Rosner, p. 207.
106. Rosner, p. 208.
107. Rosner, p. 209.

... Only the Creator, who bestows the gift of life, may relieve man of that
life, even when it has become a burden rather than a blessing.[108]

Rosner's Jewish approach to understanding the nuances concerning the topic
of euthanasia illustrates three things: (1) All decisions, including medical,
about human life must be made within and in concert with a religious
Judaistic worldview. (2) The major interpretive key to knowing what actions are thus appropriate is found within rabbinic discussions and commentaries of applicable scriptural texts. (3) The sanctity of human life is of pivotal
weight to Jewish bioethical decision making.

Building upon the information on euthanasia, Rosner directly addresses the treatment of the terminally ill in chapter 18, which, in keeping
with his Jewish approach to bioethics, is appropriately entitled "Rabbi Moshe
Feinstein on the Treatment of the Terminally Ill." In other words, Rosner
would never consider examining any bioethical issue apart from reference to
a rabbinic judgment. Pertinent to our discussion, Rabbi Feinstein addresses
the issue of a terminally ill patient who refuses treatment.

Rabbi Feinstein follows typical Jewish ethical methodology in examining a patient who refuses life-sustaining treatment: scrutinize all possible scenarios. The first possibility as to why someone would refuse treatment could
be linked to a lack of confidence in his or her physician. In this case "one
should seek out another physician in whom the patient does have trust."
However, it could be that the patient has "given up." If this is the situation,
Feinstein says the patient should be persuaded to go on with treatment. Nevertheless, according to the rabbi, a physician should not pressure a patient to
continue treatment if the coercion itself could hasten his or her death or if
treatment will be of no benefit to the patient. Feinstein does believe there are
two kinds of instances where a patient should be coerced to receive lifesaving
surgery or treatment. If the result of the surgery would only leave the patient
with a handicap, the patient must be convinced to undergo the surgery. If the
patient cannot be persuaded of the need of the surgical procedure, then the
patient should be forced to undergo the surgery because "every patient is obligated to seek healing even if such healing includes major surgery."[109] The
second kind of scenario in which a patient should be coerced to receive treatment involves the probability of the success of the treatment. Feinstein states,
"if the patient refuses the dangerous therapy, one need not force him to accept it unless there is a better than 50 percent chance that the treatment may

---

108. Rosner, pp. 211, 212.
109. Rosner, p. 238.

arrest or reverse the disease process."[110] Thus Feinstein believes major surgery or treatment should be forced upon patients, terminally ill or otherwise, only when there is a chance for cure. Therefore, according to Rabbi Feinstein, one should only utilize those medical treatments which have strong possibilities of cure. If the treatments under consideration will only prolong suffering, one is not obligated to undergo them.

Such a view emphasizes the importance of the sanctity of human life in Jewish teaching. For Rosner, "The physician is given Divine license to heal but not to hasten death." Furthermore, according to Rosner,

> When a physician has nothing further to offer a patient medically or surgically, the physician's license to heal ends and he becomes no different than a lay person. Every human being is morally expected to help another human in distress. A dying patient is no exception. The physician, family, friends, nurses, social workers, and other individuals close to the dying patient are obligated to provide supportive, including psychosocial and emotional, care until the very end. Fluids and nutrition are part and parcel of that supportive care, no different than washing, turning, talking, singing, reading, or just listening to the dying patient. There are times when specific medical and/or surgical therapies are no longer indicated, appropriate, or desirable for a terminal, irreversibly ill dying patient. There is no time, however, when general supportive measures can be abandoned, thereby hastening the patient's demise.[111]

Clearly, if Rosner thinks this is the approach of the Jewish physician, it would also apply to the patient. Thus the patient is required to do all he or she medically can do up to the point that any further medical intervention would be of no avail. Proceeding in this manner maintains the sanctity of human life. It does not hasten death; at the same time it does not hinder the soul's release from the body.

Immanuel Jakobovits

Rabbi Immanuel Jakobovits, in his work *Jewish Medical Ethics*, confirms the analysis and approach of Rosner. However, unlike Rosner, Rabbi Jakobovits provides a rich religious texture to his discussions. According to Jakobovits,

110. Rosner, p. 239.
111. Rosner, p. 242.
112. Immanuel Jakobovits, *Jewish Medical Ethics* (New York: Bloch Publishing, 1975), p. xxxi.

"Religion and medicine have been in alliance with each other in every land, among all peoples. . . ."[112] Nevertheless, for Jakobovits medicine has not entirely and thus fully appreciated the factor that religion brings to the relationship. This is especially true of the Jewish religion.

At the heart of traditional Jewish faith is the relationship between the divine directions and physical health. In other words, the sanctions of revelation are not only given to spiritually sanctify the person, but these divine mandates are also given as a protection of physical health. According to Rabbi Jakobovits, medicine has emphasized the therapeutic whereas the Jewish faith focuses upon the prevention of illness by following the ethical dictates of the Creator. Therefore one important element of Jewish ethical thinking is to link disease or sickness with certain behaviors or practices which lead to poor health. However, just because there is a connection between certain behaviors and illness does not mean that Jewish ethical thinking believes that all disease or illness is tied to irresponsible or immoral behavior, or that every illness or disease can be avoided. Nevertheless, one important element of Jewish bioethics is the idea that some sickness is directly related to misconduct.

Rabbi Jakobovits also views illness as a "misfortune" which must be struggled against.[113] In other words, whether one is sick and suffering due to one's own conduct or ill through no fault of one's own, the appropriate response is to fight the illness. As Jakobovits writes, "Whether pain be looked upon as an instrument of divine punishment or not, it is clearly a curse."[114] Consequently, people who are sick are supposed to do everything within their power to regain their health. This, of course, would include availing themselves of all suitable medical treatment and technology.

Even though Jews, according to Jakobovits, regard disease, illness, or sickness as a curse, they also view it as having the potential to bring one closer to God. Jakobovits states that the Jewish religious perspective "subscribes to the belief in the atoning power of physical suffering and in its moral motivation."[115] In other words, there can be a providential side to being physically afflicted. Illness can be part of God's providential care for the person who is sick. Regardless of how one got his or her particular malady, one can rest assured that God is providentially using the illness to further reveal his divine presence and to morally develop the character of the person who is ill or suffering. Of course, this "providential" attitude to sickness and suffering raises a most difficult dilemma: What is the role of medicine if God is somehow using a per-

113. Jakobovits, p. 1.
114. Jakobovits, p. 103.
115. Jakobovits, p. 1.

son's illness in an overarching divine purpose for that person's life? Or, as Jakobovits puts it,

> Every religious system has recognized this inner conflict between the essentially divine (and therefore providential) character of disease and the human efforts, through medical treatment, to mitigate or, if possible, to frustrate its effect. For the monotheistic faiths this problem was particularly acute. The solutions offered, which varied widely and significantly, materially affected the entire course of medical history, often in its most decisive aspects.[116]

Jakobovits clearly recognizes the problem for a religious perspective such as his that believes God is directly involved in and using the illness of a patient for divine purposes. If God is somehow using sickness and suffering, what role then do medical personnel play?

Jakobovits states that there have been three answers given to this dilemma: (1) fatalism; (2) dominion; and (3) divine sanction. Fatalism asserts that the one who is ill should accept that illness from God and do nothing about it. Since the sickness is directly from God, to fight against it would be to fight against God. According to Jakobovits, this view "appealed to the ascetic tendencies of certain small Jewish sects." Thus mainline Judaism never held to this sort of fatalistic conclusion regarding medical intervention. A dominion perspective holds that it is the "prerogative and duty of man to harness his intelligence and the resources of nature in his conquest of disease as in his striving for prosperity."[117] This solution was preferred by some Jewish thinkers, including the great Maimonides. The third outlook on the dilemma, divine sanction, believes that "God expressly granted man the right to cure disease in the Bible, and it was on the strength of such scriptural sanction that the physician was permitted to practice his art."[118] Jakobovits views this as the Jewish foundation for medical practice. The God who is involved in the sickness and suffering of a patient is also the one who commands that people do everything within their power to heal themselves of their affliction. Furthermore, ". . . the physician's right to heal is a religious duty and . . . he who shirks this responsibility is regarded as shedding blood."[119]

Therefore, according to Jakobovits, a person who is sick, regardless of the illness, is to do everything possible to regain his or her health. Furthermore, physicians and health care workers have a divine mandate to use their educa-

116. Jakobovits, p. 2.
117. Jakobovits, p. 2.
118. Jakobovits, p. 3.
119. Jakobovits, p. 7.

tion, training, skills, and experience to care for and hopefully cure the person who is afflicted with a malady. Keeping these thoughts in mind, what would Rabbi Jakobovits say about a patient who refuses life-sustaining treatment? How would he describe a Jewish ethical position on this type of scenario?

Judaism as a religion puts an emphasis on life in this world. Therefore it is extremely important which actions one performs in this life and that one has the maximum amount of time to act. Consequently, "Judaism urges every caution to ensure that his [the patient's] last preparations for death shall not aggravate his condition or compromise his will or ability to live."[120] Thus patients who refuse life-sustaining treatment would be "compromising their ability to live." In fact, those caring for a terminally ill patient are not to discuss death in his or her presence, for this might cause the person to lose the determination to live. Jakobovits states:

> The rabbis insisted on maintaining the patient's hopefulness not merely by withholding information of his imminent death, but by positive means to encourage his confidence in recovery. The Midrash remonstrates with the prophet Isaiah for telling King Hezekiah, when he was "sick unto death": "Set thy house in order; for thou shalt die and not live" (2 Kings xx.I). On the contrary, "even when the physician realizes that his patient approaches death, he should still order him to eat this and not to eat that, to drink this and not to drink that; but he should not tell him that the end is near."[121]

According to this understanding, Judaism could not imagine or condone a patient refusing life-sustaining treatment just to hasten his or her death. A decision to hasten one's death would not be utilizing one's decision making in a correct manner, nor would it be a maximizing of life. However, there is more to be said here.

In Jakobovits's discussion of euthanasia, he states that Judaism is against any form of active euthanasia. Moreover, active euthanasia is designated as an act of murder.[122] However, "Jewish law sanctions, and perhaps even demands, the withdrawal of any factor — whether extraneous to the patient himself or not — which may artificially delay his demise in the final phase."[123] Thus the only time in which patients can refuse treatment for their condition is when their death is imminent. Patients who are terminally ill, but whose death is not imminent, do not fall into this category. Judaism, accord-

120. Jakobovits, p. 7.
121. Jakobovits, pp. 120-21.
122. Jakobovits, p. 123.
123. Jakobovits, p. 124.

ing to Jakobovits, is not without sympathy for those who were both incurably ill and in a state of severe suffering. In fact, death is seen as a release from this situation. Nevertheless, it must be a death that is accomplished by the disease or by God, and not by the actions of human agents.

Consequently, Rabbi Jakobovits does his ethical analysis within a worldview which attests to a special revelation which provides ethical guidelines for human actions. If there is not a direct statement of Scripture that explicitly covers an action, then one looks to rabbinic *responsa* for guidance. For within the *responsa* are examples of scriptural principles applied to particular cases. From these casuistic examples one gleans direction and guidance for one's choices. In this view Jewish ethical thinking and methodology revolve around the fact that God has revealed how he wants each human being to live. Moreover, since this life is a preparation for the next one, the choices one makes have eternal consequences. Consequently, it is extremely important to Jewish thinking that each ethical choice be a reflective one with its basis in God's revelation and the covenant that God made with Israel.

Review and Evaluation

Clearly there is a diversity of approaches toward doing bioethics by the above-examined religious ethicists. McCormick emphasizes the Thomistic natural law tradition and buttresses his methodology with Scripture and insights from the social sciences and human experience. Ramsey begins with Scripture and then develops a Protestant version of natural law by showing that human experience needs the concept of "covenant fidelity." Gustafson stresses the divine ordering in human experience which can be exemplified by scriptural symbols that match our human experience and the findings of the sciences. Rosner and Jakobovits place the source of bioethics in the revelation of God in the Law of Moses and its application to particular situations reflected in the *responsa* of the rabbinic community.

Not only is there a diversity as to the source of each of these religious ethical approaches, but the bases of moral decision making vary as well. McCormick's natural law theory wants to maintain that there are objective values which can be perceived by all persons. Indeed, not only are objective values able to be known, but one also possesses the ability to recognize an objective order of values. Thus one should choose to realize and/or avoid the decimation of the highest good or the most basic value. In contrast, Ramsey states that one must make choices that are in concert with the principle of covenant fidelity. Gustafson presents decision making as a reflection of values, rules, and character formation. Rosner and Jakobovits view moral choice as grounded in the direct application of the appropriate scriptural command to the situation facing the person.

Furthermore, each of these thinkers is trying to avoid what he perceives as a problem for ethics. McCormick wants to remove the possibility of ethics becoming a total reflection of a person's values or preferences disguised in moral language. Thus he emphasizes an objective realm of values beyond the individual which guides and directs subjects in their decision making. As concerned as McCormick is with subjectivizing morality, Ramsey is concerned with "exceptions" to moral decisions. In other words, he believes that if ethics becomes tied up with the consequences of an act, then there will always be exceptions to rules and principles. A rule or principle is open to violation because it would prohibit the maximization of some good. Gustafson is concerned to avoid the rampant "anthropocentrism" in ethics. According to him, persons are to enlarge their "wholes" so that they are able to accommodate the divine ordering of creation. For Gustafson, we are to relate all things to the divine purposes in the world. Rosner and Jakobovits want to avoid ambiguity in moral decision making. By adhering to the direct commands of Scripture and their application to specific situations, one is removed from "flexible" decision making. Rosner and Jakobovits's approach is a more direct usage of Scripture as opposed to applying the meaning of symbols and ideals to particular decisions.

All of these religious approaches to doing bioethics have strengths and weaknesses. McCormick's natural law approach offers a human ethic which needs little adherence to any religious position for usage or implementation. Its underlying assumption is that human beings have the capacity to arrive at what is good via a reflection upon their basic inclinations. However, there are two problems inherent in McCormick's position. First, we may all agree on the general basic human inclinations that McCormick elucidates. The problem, however, is when one attempts to develop specific actions which would fulfill these general inclinations. For example, Thomas Aquinas and McCormick would say that one of the three general inclinations of humankind is a natural inclination to propagate the species. Reason reflects on this and promulgates the precept that the species is to be propagated and children educated. We doubt there would be any disagreement up to this point. However, the next step both Thomas and McCormick would doubtless take would be to say that this is best accomplished inside a monogamous, heterosexual relationship. In our particular culture there are pockets of people who would take issue with this way of fulfilling the general precept of propagating the species. For instance, lesbian couples would argue that they have the right to have children, and by utilizing reproductive technologies they are able to make this a reality. Based upon a natural law precept, how would or could McCormick marshal a response based upon natural law? In other words, the strength of natural law is in its identification of agreed-upon general principles. The weakness of natural law is when it attempts to become more definite and specific. It is then that natural law falls prey to the proverb "There's more than one way to skin a cat." This leads to a second problem associated with natural law approaches.

All natural law methodologies seem to fall prey, ultimately not generally, to the very thing they are trying to avoid, subjectivism. At the general level of identifying universal principles, natural law works quite well. Nevertheless, general principles are, at the end of the day, general principles, and thus never give the kind of specificity most people need in terms of an exacting moral decision. Since general principles themselves, then, do not elicit specific content, the content must be provided by the subject making the decision. This subjective, particular content is usually reflective of the historical-cultural location of the subject. This idea was recognized by Reinhold Niebuhr in his critique of natural law. Niebuhr writes, "The fact remains, nevertheless, that reason is not capable of defining any standard of justice that is universally valid or acceptable. . . . In short, it is not possible to state a universally valid concept of justice from any particular sociological locus in history. Nor is it possible to avoid either making the effort or making pretenses of universality which human finiteness does not justify."[124] Thus the very thing natural law wants to accomplish, a universally binding approach, is difficult to achieve. Since each individual person operates out of and is part of a "particular sociological locus," it will be that locus that fills in the specific details of the application of the general precepts of the natural law.

Of course, as was stated earlier, Paul Ramsey hopes to avoid "exceptions" to moral rules by his concept of "covenant fidelity." Ramsey insists that *agape* as expressed through covenant fidelity should be the central moral principle guiding behavior. It is the example of God's covenant fidelity to us that provides the example or model for our attitude and behavior toward others.

On the issue of *agape* being expressed through the vehicle of covenant fidelity, it appears that the demands of morality for everyone, whether Christian or not, have risen to benevolence as opposed to non-maleficence. Ramsey needs to temper his demands of morality to include the ever present egoism of the agents involved. At best we should hope for and expect justice

---

124. Reinhold Niebuhr, "Christian Faith and Natural Law," in *Love and Justice,* ed. D. B. Robertson (Gloucester, Mass.: Peter Smith, 1976), pp. 48, 49.

from unregenerate men and women, not love. Justice discriminates according to what one deserves, whereas love is nondiscriminating and offers the other what he or she does not deserve or more than he or she deserves. Love can and should remain an ideal which drives justice to be more than it should be, but to expect the responses characteristic of love by people who are not a part of the community of God's people is to be overly idealistic. For the world justice, not love, is the appropriate standard. For God's people love is the standard set by Jesus.

A second critique of Ramsey has to do with his approach to Scripture. He rightly draws the concept of covenant fidelity out of the teaching of Jesus and the Old Testament as the central concept in Christian ethics. But he seems hesitant to bring other resources of specific texts of Scripture to bear on bioethical issues in the way that Jewish ethics typically does. Though giving more weight to Scripture than Gustafson, Ramsey reflects a less than orthodox view of the inspiration and authority of Scripture. While his view of covenant fidelity is clearly rooted in biblical teaching, Ramsey seems to reject a more textual approach to bioethics that would be consistent with a higher view of Scripture. He rightly attempts to avoid simplistic proof texting and to emphasize central theological concepts. However, he appears hesitant to draw upon more specific ethical guidance in the Bible.

Gustafson's "theocentric" approach has two major problems: (1) At the end of the day it becomes overly intuitive and thus highly subjective and impractical. (2) It can become just another form of utilitarianism. Remember that the responsibility inherent in theocentric ethics is discerning, participating in, and relating all things in accordance with God's purposive ordering of creation. This is more than a simple assignment; it may be virtually impossible. Even Gustafson himself alludes to the almost impossible nature of his ethic when he frequently quotes a line from Milton's *Paradise Lost* which says, "So little knows/Any, but God alone, to value right/The good before him. . . ."[125] The question is not whether God may know right from wrong or good from bad; the question is, how do we know? If all things are ultimately to be theocentrically related, then somehow or another we need to have some way of doing this. Gustafson is right to say that we need to recognize that all of creation is to relate itself appropriate to its relation to God. This is the material principle in his ethic. But how does one work this principle out in practical situations? Where does the content come from to fill in the gaping blanks of what to do? This is what leads to an overdependence upon intuition and thus subjectivism.

125. Gustafson, *Ethics from a Theocentric Perspective*, 2:279-319.

Gustafson's theocentric ethics provides an air of responsibility and seriousness to moral decision making. He is extremely clear that the problem with current religious theories of ethics is that they are all too anthropocentric. We must expand our horizons and "pick up" on the divine ordering in creation and "get in step" with God. This sort of approach heightens the moral awareness, but it does not provide any specific moral guidance. The rules, systems, and principles Gustafson rejects offer far more concrete guidance in ambiguous situations. He wants to speak in broad terms about God's divine ordering, but he has nothing specific to say about typical moral decisions. He offers no real possibility of constructing a systematic ethic. Therefore each person is left to "sense" how he or she perceives God ordering any particular situation that he or she is faced with. Thus theocentric ethics can easily dissolve into anthropocentric ethics — the very thing Gustafson wants to avoid.

Another problem for Gustafson's theocentric ethics is its similarity to utilitarianism. His concern for the relations between "parts" and "wholes" leaves his theory, at times, sounding a lot like a reworked utilitarianism. This point becomes extremely clear in the following quote:

> In wartime presumably the enemy is an "unjust aggressor" against one's own nation; by weak analogy a preventable disease is an aggressor against the health of the community. It is arguable, at least, that where the risk of death is not as high as it is during combat, or where the maximum harm falls short of the risk of death, there are grounds for putting some (nonconsenting) persons at risk for the sake of prospective benefits to others.[126]

Thus, according to Gustafson, the well-being of the "wholes" may be more important than the rights of the "parts." It should be noted, however, that Gustafson would define the "common good" as a collective value held by the community. This common good, at least in his view, should not be understood as an aggregate of individual goods. Of course, what he hopes to avoid by defining "common good" in this way is the possibility of linking his theory to that of utilitarianism which, in some forms, would see decision making linked to the act which brings about the greatest amount of good for the greatest number of people. Nevertheless, how is one to understand putting at risk people who have not agreed to being put at risk for a larger number of people, that is, "the community," except within the framework of utilitarianism? In fact, act-utilitarianism basically states that the moral thing to do is to perform the act that maximizes the good for the greatest number of people

126. Gustafson, *Ethics from a Theocentric Perspective,* 2:309.

considered. This is exactly what Gustafson appears to be suggesting in the quote cited above. Due to the utter ambiguity of theocentric ethics, it can become any theory it wants. And in this particular instance it resembles utilitarianism. Of course, give Gustafson another specific scenario that needs moral guidance, and theocentric ethics could look like deontology or even virtue theory.

In contrast to the previous three theories under discussion, Jewish bioethics typically offers specificity to the decision-making process. As was stated earlier, Jewish ethics is traditionally grounded in a covenant with God. This covenantal concept has many ramifications, but the one that is most important for our evaluation is:

> Because God gave the Law, it can speak to every area of life, including many that fall outside of the jurisdiction of other legal systems. Jewish law sets an order not only for society but also for private lives of an individual and a family, and it assumes competence to regulate even the speech patterns and thoughts of Jews. So, for example, it includes rules which determine even the shoe that you are to tie first when getting dressed and the position in which you are to sleep, and it specifies with remarkable particularity the duties incumbent upon spouses to each other, including even the number of times that a man must offer to have sex with his wife. . . . These are all areas which legal systems dare not to touch, let alone regulate, but Jewish law exercises jurisdiction on these subjects because its author is God (however that authorship is understood), and God has the power, the right, and perhaps even the obligation to address these crucial areas of life.
>
> . . . The Covenant model nicely describes both the wide range of concerns treated by Jewish law and the specificity of its rules: a covenant has specific clauses, and when God is the author, they can cover the whole gamut of human experience.[127]

Some believe that this kind of covenantal understanding leads to a casuistic approach that both removes individual self-determination from ethical decisions and is "too limited to address problems found in such areas as biomedical ethics."[128] These critics think the case analysis and precedent approach of Jewish ethics should be replaced by the development of principles which reflect the rich theological heritage of Judaism and be applied to often complex issues surrounding bioethics.

127. Elliot N. Dorff and Louis E. Newman, eds., *Contemporary Jewish Ethics and Morality* (New York: Oxford University Press, 1995), p. 65.
128. Dorff and Newman, p. 177.

At first glance this seems to be a reasonable criticism of Jewish ethics in general. However, this sort of criticism may misunderstand typical Jewish methodology. Jewish ethics does develop principles, but they are grounded in specific doctrines and narratives of Scripture buttressed by precedents of applications. For example, Judaism traditionally holds to the doctrine of the "infinite value of human life." This doctrine was the basis of both Rosner's and Jakobovits's deliberations concerning the issue of "refusal of life-sustaining treatment." A principle that develops out of this doctrine is "integrity of life," which means that human life, however tenuous, is sacred and invaluable. Therefore the obligation incumbent upon everyone is to protect, preserve, and save any life, even when that life is marginal and has only a brief span of time to continue. Consequently, no life can be taken or compromised by another human being.

Thus, utilizing Rosner's and Jakobovits's discussions as a backdrop, one could construct a Jewish methodology of ethics in the following manner: (1) Start with the appropriate doctrine of Scripture. (2) Utilize principles which legitimately flow from that doctrine. (3) Do a careful examination of the ethical situation. (4) Make application of the principle or principles. (5) Carefully examine and study prior applications of the principle or principles under consideration. This approach avoids playing "fast and loose" with an isolated principle. By examining previous cases, it gains guidance and has installed a "check" on the implementation of its principle or principles. Two things are gained by contemplation of previous cases: analogies and proper means of application.

Conclusion

There is great variety and richness in the religious approaches to bioethics. Religious reflection on bioethical issues provides a rich reservoir of resources not only for religious believers but also for the culture at large, providing centuries of thought on these issues that is just as relevant today as when these resources were originally written. It is unfortunate that in a good deal of the public policy discussion of bioethics, the contribution of religious voices is not sought or heard. To be sure, religious reflection on complex issues has at times not been helpful, but public policy is formulated today in a way that appears to be biased against the contribution of religious perspectives and fails to appreciate the productive contribution these various perspectives can make.

We will draw upon some of these perspectives throughout the book as we attempt to develop a viable Christian approach. For instance, we find the Jewish methodology just discussed helpful in several respects. Further we will develop some overriding theological concepts that inform many bioethics issues, as Ramsey and Gustafson try to do. We will also employ a natural law approach in our desire to communicate Christian bioethics to an increasingly secular society. Our approach will essentially be a blend of key theological concepts such as the place of general revelation, the image of God, the common good, and eternal life, plus some textual analysis of key passages of Scripture, which will inform our key theological notions. We will not attempt to reduce Christian ethics to one key principle, such as covenant fidelity. Rather, we will bring a number of key theological concepts to bear on the critical bioethics issues of the day.

Before developing this approach, we should note that bioethics has developed significantly as a discipline in the past twenty years and has grown apart from its original religious roots. Though religious voices are still as present as ever, public bioethics has become more secularized in its approaches. The discipline of bioethics has reflected on most of the key ethical issues facing health care independent of religious perspectives. Public policy is increasingly informed by these nonreligious perspectives, and they have overtaken religious views in terms of influence in the bioethics community. Accordingly, in the next chapter we must consider some of the dominant perspectives in the secular bioethics community.

CHAPTER 2

Secular Approaches to Bioethics

Introduction

Currently the prevailing influence on or predominant approach to bioethics is secular in nature. In one sense this is a rather recent phenomenon. Originally moral theology occupied the center of moral discussions concerning medicine. Allen Verhey observes that "there are long and worthy traditions of theological reflection" about the issues and dilemmas in the realm of medicine, and thus it should not be surprising that "religious thinkers played an important role in the 'renaissance of medical ethics' in 1965 to 1970."[1] Nevertheless, Verhey notes that this "renaissance" was followed by the "enlightenment" of biomedical ethics. The "enlightenment" project was concerned with developing a purified "public" sphere of discourse over against the particular, and was done

> sometimes to justify but always to identify and apply moral principles that all people can and must hold independently of their particular communities and histories, quite apart from their specific loyalties and identities, unbiased by any particular narrative which they remember or by any partial vision of human flourishing for which they hope. There was, for a time [in biomedical ethics], an enlightenment suspicion of particular traditions, an enlightenment confidence in the progress of human science and unqualified human reason, and an enlightenment celebration of individual auton-

1. Allen Verhey, "Talking of God — but with Whom?" *Hastings Center Report* (special supplement: "Theology, Religious Traditions and Bioethics") 20, no. 4 (July-August 1990): 21.

54

omy over against the "authority" of priest and politician and that new figure of arbitrary dominance, the physician.[2]

This "enlightenment" project in bioethics has thus marginalized theological
and religious discussions pertaining to the questions raised by the medical
field. In fact, this marginalization of theological and religious perspectives
had been accomplished by 1989, when the primary question at a Hastings
Center symposium on "Religion and Bioethics" was, "What significance, if
any, does [religion] hold for the ways we now do bioethics?"[3]

The result of this "enlightenment" project is a completely secular view
of bioethics. This "secular" approach is characterized by several factors. First,
for the most part it perceives ethical theories as primarily reduced to deontological and utilitarian theories of ethics. Second, it develops principles
and rules from the application of these two theories to the various scenarios
faced by the medical community. Third, it usually, then, identifies four major
biomedical principles: (1) autonomy; (2) non-maleficence; (3) beneficence;
and (4) justice. Lastly, the kinds of cases that are examined are ones that ro-
tate around three major areas of consideration. Leon Kass classifies these
cases in the following manner:

> Biomedical technologies can be usefully organized into three groups ac-
> cording to their major purpose: (1) control of death and life; (2) control of
> human potentialities; and (3) control of human achievement. The corre-
> sponding technologies are: medicine, or those parts of medicine engaged in
> prolonging life and controlling reproduction; genetic engineering; and
> neurological and psychological manipulation.[4]

The perspective of this secular approach is to explicate universal rules and apply
them to particular cases. It is what Edmund Pincoffs calls "Quandary Ethics":

> That the business of ethics is with "problems," i.e. situations in which it is
> difficult to know what one should do; that the ultimate beneficiary of ethi-
> cal analysis is the person who, in one of these situations, seeks rational
> ground for the decision he must make; that ethics is therefore primarily
> concerned to find such grounds, often conceived of as moral rules *and the*

2. Verhey, p. 21.
3. Daniel Callahan and Courtney S. Campbell, preface to special supplement, "Theology, Religious Traditions and Bioethics," of *Hastings Center Report* 20, no. 4 (July-August
1990): 1.
4. Leon R. Kass, *Toward a More Natural Science: Biology and Human Affairs* (New
York: Free Press, 1985), p. 19.

principles from which they can be derived; and that metaethics consists in the analysis of the terms, claims, and arguments which come into play in moral disputation, deliberation, and justification in problematic contexts.[5]

This is the typical way contemporary ethical theory views ethics. As a caveat, initially the approach of those doing biomedical ethics from the secular viewpoint was characterized by "description" of dilemmas as opposed to providing "prescriptions" of what one ought to do. The Hastings Center would be a good example of discussing and describing dilemmas without directly offering prescriptions or "oughts." The two most prominent examples of the secular approach which applies universal principles to dilemmas in medical ethics are Tom L. Beauchamp and James F. Childress's *Principles of Biomedical Ethics*[6] and H. Tristram Engelhardt's *The Foundations of Bioethics*.[7] This chapter will explicate, examine, and evaluate the approach of Beauchamp/Childress and Engelhardt. Beauchamp and Childress take a conventional liberal approach to doing ethics, while Engelhardt expresses a more minimalist standpoint. Furthermore, Beauchamp and Childress assume a modern "enlightenment" approach to their perspective, while Engelhardt works out his position within the context of a postmodern mentality.

The Approach of Beauchamp and Childress

Beauchamp and Childress perceive the role of bioethics as the application of principles or rules to the issues created by the practice of medicine. They state, "we are mainly concerned with interpreting principles and developing general moral action-guides for use in the biomedical fields. . . ." Normally this would be perceived as the methodology of applied ethics. However, for reasons later to be discussed, Beauchamp and Childress want to distance their approach from that of applied ethics by naming their endeavor "practical ethics." According to Beauchamp and Childress, their method has been "misleadingly called *applied ethics*." Rather,

> The term *practical* refers to the use of ethical theory and methods of analysis to examine moral problems, practices, and policies in several areas, in-

5. Edmund Pincoffs, "Quandary Ethics," *Mind* 80 (October 1971): 552.
6. Tom L. Beauchamp and James F. Childress, *Principles of Biomedical Ethics*, 4th ed. (New York: Oxford University Press, 1994).
7. H. Tristram Engelhardt, Jr., *The Foundations of Bioethics*, 2nd ed. (New York: Oxford University Press, 1996).

cluding the professions and public policy. Often no straightforward movement from theory or principles to particular judgments is possible in these
contexts, although general reasons, principles, and even ideals can play
some role in evaluating conduct and establishing policies. Theory and
principles are typically invoked only to help develop action-guides, which
are also further shaped by paradigm cases of appropriate behavior, empirical data, and the like, together with reflection on how to put these influential sources into the most coherent whole.[8]

Thus the structure of their process of "practical ethics" is to analyze the theoretical bases of morality in general and then to construct the world of medicine correspondingly. The reason, also, that Beauchamp and Childress believe
that we can apply general ethical principles to medicine is because their
model assumes that medicine is value-neutral, that is, that there are no inherent moral relationships within medicine as such.

In the latest edition of *Principles of Biomedical Ethics*, Beauchamp and
Childress have made what *appear* to be major adjustments in the mechanics
of their ethical approach. Previously their approach was best understood
when viewing their moral justification process. They arranged their system
around four tiers which were hierarchically arranged. According to Beauchamp and Childress, justification begins with "Particular Judgments and
Actions" which are based in "Rules" which are applications of "Principles"
which are ultimately grounded in and flow from "Ethical Theories."[9]
Beauchamp and Childress defined their terms in the following manner:
"*Judgments* express a decision, a verdict, or conclusion about a particular action. . . . *Rules* are more specific to contexts and more restricted in scope. . . .
Principles are more general and fundamental than moral rules and serve to
justify the rules. . . . *Theories* are integrated bodies of principles and rules and
may include mediating rules that govern choices in cases of conflicts."[10] Previously, then, ethical theories themselves were self-justifying. Biomedical ethics was simply the application of theories to the medical realm, which produced a set of principles. In the fourth edition of their work this has changed
somewhat.

The adjustment the two authors made in their most recent work relates
to moral justification. Their previous approach had depended upon a form of

8. Beauchamp and Childress, 4th ed., p. 4.
9. Tom L. Beauchamp and James F. Childress, *Principles of Biomedical Ethics*, 3rd ed.
(New York: Oxford University Press, 1989), pp. 6ff. In fact, Beauchamp and Childress illustrate this process with a diagram that portrays the upward flow of justification.
10. Beauchamp and Childress, 3rd ed., p. 7.

deductivism which "holds that justified moral judgments are deduced from a preexisting theoretical structure of normative precepts that cover the judgment."[11] Now, however, Beauchamp and Childress find that moral justification needs to be more eclectic. They describe three methods of moral justification in which they "defend a version of the third that incorporates important parts of the other two." Important as this may be for understanding how they "justify" their particular approach of "practical ethics," it has not changed their overall position. For, as Beauchamp and Childress say, "The upshot of our analysis of coherence and specification is the following: One goal of a moral theory, and central to its account of justification, is to move from general levels of theory to particular rules, judgments, and policies that are in close proximity to everyday decisions in the moral life."[12] In other words, Beauchamp and Childress are still starting with theories and applying these theories to the questions, issues, and dilemmas surfaced by the medical realm. Just as before, the application of these ethical theories, and their new justification, yields the same four principles: (1) autonomy; (2) non-maleficence; (3) beneficence; and (4) justice. Thus their approach is substantially the same, regardless of the change in moral justification. For, "Although rules, rights, and virtues are of the highest importance for health care ethics, principles provide the most abstract and comprehensive norms in the framework."[13]

In addition, Beauchamp and Childress want it understood that the four principles of biomedical ethics are subject to what they call *specification* and *balancing*. By the term "specification" they mean that when one utilizes a principle, one "must also be able to specify the content in a way that surpasses ethereal abstractness, while also indicating the cases that properly fall under the principles. If a principle lacks adequate specificity, it is empty and ineffectual."[14] The kinds of factors that help a principle develop specificity are "efficiency, institutional rules, law, and clientele acceptance." Moreover, things like "the demands of political procedures, legal constraints, uncertainty about risk, and the like"[15] are necessary for specifying both what is an example of an appropriate usage of the principle as well as what considerations need to be accounted for when applying the principle. Beauchamp and Childress illustrate what specification looks like in the following manner:

---

11. Beauchamp and Childress, 4th ed., p. 14.
12. Beauchamp and Childress, 4th ed., p. 31.
13. Beauchamp and Childress, 4th ed., p. 37.
14. Beauchamp and Childress, 4th ed., p. 28.
15. Beauchamp and Childress, 4th ed., pp. 28f.

As a simple example of specification, consider again the rule "Doctors should put their patients' interests first." A fact of life in modern medicine in the United States is that patients sometimes can afford the best treatment strategy only if their physicians falsify information on insurance forms, or at least only thinly spread the truth. It follows from a proper understanding of the rule of patient-priority that a physician should act illegally by lying or distorting the description of a patient's problem on an insurance form. Our rules against deception and for patient-priority are not categorical demands, and they stand in need of specification to give fuller, more concrete moral advice to physicians who wonder whether they should deceive payers, and, if so, under which conditions.[16]

Thus, according to Beauchamp and Childress, specification means that the content of an application of a principle must cohere with other relevant norms. This method makes it possible to adjust the outcome of a principle's usage, but it also means that "all moral norms are, in principle, subject to such revision, specification, and justification."[17]

Moreover, just as principles need "specification," principles also need "balancing." Specification addresses the "substantive development of the meaning and scope of norms," whereas "balancing consists of deliberation and judgment about the relative weights of norms."[18] Indeed, according to Beauchamp and Childress, principles are thus *prima facie* binding. In other words,

Prima Facie obligation indicates an obligation that must be fulfilled unless it conflicts on a particular occasion with an equal or stronger obligation. A prima facie obligation is binding unless overridden or outweighed by competing moral obligations. Acts often have several morally relevant properties or consequences. For example, an act of lying may also promote someone's welfare, and an act of killing may involve the relief of pain and suffering as well as respect for a patient's request. Such acts are at once prima facie wrong and prima facie right, because two or more norms conflict in the circumstances. The agent must then determine what he or she ought to do by finding an actual or overriding (in contrast to prima facie) obligation. . . . An agent's actual obligation in the situation is determined by the balance of the respective weights of the competing prima facie obligations (the relative weights of all competing prima facie norms such as beneficence, fidelity, and justice).[19]

16. Beauchamp and Childress, 4th ed., p. 29.
17. Beauchamp and Childress, 4th ed., p. 30.
18. Beauchamp and Childress, 4th ed., p. 32.
19. Beauchamp and Childress, 4th ed., p. 33.

Therefore principles, rules, or duties are not absolute in the sense that they can never have exceptions. However, there are some rules, due to either the nature of the act they prohibit or the definition of the terms involved in the prohibition, that do not need balancing or cannot be balanced away by any other norm. For example, "gratuitous infliction of pain and suffering" is virtually absolute due to the nature of the act being prohibited. Murder also receives an absolute status due to the fact that murder means "unjustified killing."[20]

Knowing that they need to situate their approach of "*prima facie* principles" within an ethical theory, Beauchamp and Childress identify their theory as "Principle-Based, Common Morality Theory."[21] When the discussion of theory arises in their work, they are careful to insure that they are not misunderstood as to how their approach fits into "theory language":

> Occasionally we refer to our system and to arguments in this book as a *theory*. A word of caution is in order about this use of the word *theory*. This term is commonly used in ethics to refer to each of the following: (1) abstract reflection and argument, (2) systematic reflection and argument, and (3) an integrated body of principles that are coherent and well developed. . . . We have attempted in this book to construct a coherent account adequate for the particular subject of biomedical ethics, but we do not claim to have developed or to presuppose any particular comprehensive ethical theory in ways suggested by (3). We engage *in theory* . . . , and so in abstract reflection and argument (1). We also present an organized system of principles, and so engage in systematic reflection and argument (2). But, at best, we present only some elements of a comprehensive *general* theory (3).[22]

Typical of their eclectic approach to doing ethics, Beauchamp and Childress want to avoid being pigeonholed into any comprehensive ethical theory. For, in their mind, this would keep them from making the necessary adjustments that any complex moral situation requires. They seem to want to remain "consistently inconsistent." An overarching, comprehensive ethical theory would require consistent application of the central motif of the theory across all situations, and this is exactly what Beauchamp and Childress want to avoid. Nonetheless, as they have stated, their approach does fit best within a "Principle-Based, Common Morality Theory." So, what is a "Principle-Based, Common Morality Theory," and how does it operate?

20. Beauchamp and Childress, 4th ed., p. 32.
21. Beauchamp and Childress, 4th ed., p. 100.
22. Beauchamp and Childress, 4th ed., p. 45.

We have already seen that the approach of Beauchamp and Childress for doing biomedical ethics involves the usage of four main principles: autonomy, non-maleficence, beneficence, and justice. These are the four principles that need to be applied, specified, and balanced in relation to any issues, questions, or dilemmas surrounding the medical field. According to Beauchamp and Childress, their four principles are ultimately grounded in and flow from a "common morality." This idea of "a common-morality takes its basic premises directly from the morality shared in common by the members of a society — that is, unphilosophical common sense and tradition." It could be that some of the elements shared by a common morality are also shared by philosophically oriented ethical theories. Nevertheless, "common-morality ethics relies heavily on ordinary shared moral beliefs for its content, rather than relying on pure reason, natural law, a special moral sense, and the like."[23] Although this common morality elicits principles, these principles are to be understood as pluralistic. This means that the principles developed within the framework of a common morality do not need to fit within some overall, transcendent perspective which would arrange and adjudicate the respective principles. For example, all principles of obligation flowing from utilitarianism need to meet the criteria of "utility." "Utility" is the overall perspective and point of reference.

It appears that there are certain assumptions within the Beauchamp and Childress project that should be explicated. First, moral reasoning involves analyzing the logical and linguistic structures of moral language. This methodology elicits the meaning of "moral" and basic moral intuitions. Second, phrases such as "common morality" can refer to and mean the same as "intuition." The idea of common sense or intuition can be used to describe unprovable moral assumptions. Third, morality is ultimately a rational exercise, and moral language and moral reasoning are the same for all rational beings. Herein the term "rational" means that there are rational rules and principles which are universalizable to all rational beings. Fourth, ethics is a science that studies objective moral principles and organizes them into a coherent whole.

The Approach of Engelhardt

Beauchamp and Childress still retain many of the elements of the "enlightenment" project in their approach to biomedical ethics, but the same cannot be

23. Beauchamp and Childress, 4th ed., p. 100.

said of Engelhardt. Engelhardt is attempting to construct a basis for bioethics in the midst of a postmodern culture and world. The problem he sees for bioethics in a postmodern setting can be seen in the following statements:

> This is not a book in applied ethics. More accurately, this is not a book that applies a particular, canonical, concrete, content-full moral understanding to health care. Instead, there is a swarm of alternative ethics ready to give rise to a babble of conflicting bioethics. This circumstance constitutes the foundational moral challenge of all health care policy. It brings the very field of bioethics into question.
>
> Rather than sharing one morality, we confront strikingly different concrete moral visions and accounts of moral obligations, rights, and values. Each account asserts its own priority. . . . When asked how to justify these diverse moral understandings, some appeal to considerations of consequences; others appeal to principles of right and wrong that are independent of outcomes. It is because of this cacophonous plurality of bioethics that contemporary health care policy is framed. The diversity of moral visions and justifications challenges the coherence of maintaining that there is a secular bioethics.
>
> This book recognizes the impossibility of discovering the secular, canonical, concrete ethics. The *Foundations of Bioethics* attempts instead to secure a content-less secular ethics. Given the limits of secular moral reasoning, all that is available is a means (within certain constraints) of giving moral authority to common undertakings without establishing the moral worth or moral desirability of any particular choices. The project of securing as much universality as possible for the claims of bioethics has roots in the Enlightenment project of establishing a universal content-full ethics and a moral community of all persons outside of any particular religious and cultural assumptions. . . . This book focuses on the failure of this project to discover a canonical, content-full ethics for bioethics to apply.[24]

Therefore Engelhardt is looking for a foundation, so to speak, where there can be no foundation for bioethics. This problem of "foundation" is linked to the failure of the modern enlightenment project.

According to Engelhardt, "The West entered modernity with robust expectations from reason."[25] Once Western society separated itself from a religious perspective, it looked to a universal rationality to fill in the gap left by the extraction of a common religious vision. However, the hopes of modernity have been slaughtered at the altar of confusion and diversity. Instead of

24. Engelhardt, pp. viif.
25. Engelhardt, p. 4.

reason providing one moral vision, it provided many outlooks. Engelhardt observes:

> Rather than philosophy being able to fill the void left by the collapse of the hegemony of Christian thought in the West, philosophy has shown itself to be many competing philosophies and philosophical ethics. The attempt to sustain a secular equivalent of Western Christian monotheism through the disclosure of a unique moral and metaphysical account of reality has fragmented into a polytheism of perspectives with its chaos of moral diversity and its cacophony of numerous competing moral narratives. This circumstance as a sociological condition, reflecting our epistemological limitations, defines postmodernity. Secular rationality appears triumphant. But it has become many rationalities. It is not clear whether it can give moral or metaphysical orientation.[26]

In this kind of postmodern environment, how can one do ethics, much less biomedical ethics? This leads Engelhardt to further define the landscape of a postmodern culture before offering a solution.

Engelhardt's analysis leads him to make three important distinctions. The first is between a content-full morality and a purely procedural morality. On the one hand, a content-full morality means that one possesses a morality that offers "guidance regarding what is right or wrong, good or bad, beyond the very sparse requirement that one may not use persons without their authorization." On the other hand, a procedural morality means that persons turn over the moral authority to others with their consent. The second distinction is between "moral friends" and "moral strangers." Moral friends are such because they share a common morality with all of its built-in assumptions and thus are able to resolve moral controversies and disagreements based upon a common foundation. In contrast, moral strangers do not share a common morality and thus must resolve moral conflict by a common agreement. A third distinction made by Engelhardt weaves these distinctions into a complete tapestry. He contrasts community with society. A "*community* is used to identify a body of men and women bound together by common moral traditions and/or practices around a shared vision of the good life, which allows them to collaborate as moral friends." A society, however, is "an association that encompasses individuals who find themselves in diverse moral communities."[27] Engelhardt concludes that we must recognize that we live in a *society,* not a community.

26. Engelhardt, p. 5.
27. Engelhardt, p. 7.

This *society* will contain both moral friends and moral strangers. Therefore Engelhardt wants to offer a "secular means for coming to terms with the chaos and diversity of postmodernity."[28]

Since we are left at the brink of nihilism, controversies can only be resolved by one of the following options: "(1) force, (2) conversion of one party to the other's viewpoint, (3) sound rational argument, and (4) agreement." Engelhardt does not believe argument and conversion are workable options since they both fail to speak with rational authority across the great diversity of moral viewpoints. The only options remaining are force and agreement. Engelhardt does not necessarily rule out force as a viable option, but finds that the use of force is not prudent or enlightened, for moral confrontations are linked to moral differences and thus must be resolved in a way that involves analytical reflection. Thus "[a] goal of ethics is to determine when force can be justified."[29] Consequently, Engelhardt believes that we are left with only one real option in the midst of this ethical and philosophical malaise: agreement. By "agreement" he means:

> If one cannot establish by sound rational argument a particular concrete moral viewpoint as canonically decisive (and one cannot, because the establishment of such a viewpoint itself presupposes a moral viewpoint, and that is exactly what is at stake), then the only source of general secular authority for moral content and moral direction is agreement. To rephrase the point, because there are no decisive secular arguments to establish that one concrete view of the moral life is better morally than its rivals, and since all have not converted to a single moral viewpoint, secular moral authority is the authority of consent. Authority is not that of coercive power, or of God's will, or of reason, but simply the authority of the agreement of those who decide to collaborate. This basis for morality is available in the notion of ethics as a means of securing moral authority through consent in the face of intractable content-full moral controversies. If one is interested in collaborating with moral authority in the face of moral disagreements without fundamental recourse to force, then one must accept agreement among members of the controversy or peaceable negotiation as the means for resolving concrete moral controversies.[30]

Agreement, then, provides a way to resolve moral controversies rather than the use of force. Therefore "secular moral authority is the authority of per-

---

28. Engelhardt, p. 10.
29. Engelhardt, p. 67.
30. Engelhardt, p. 68.

mission."[31] In the model being proposed by Engelhardt, ethics becomes "consent" to "agreement" which leads to negotiating moral disputes. This methodology provides a means for moral strangers to live together in a postmodern world without ever trying to resolve their ultimate moral commitments.

However, Engelhardt's description of the current moral situation and the solution to this postmodern dilemma causes both an epistemological and a sociological splitting of the self. Consequently, for Engelhardt, "The moral life is lived within two dimensions: (1) that of a secular ethics, which strives to be content-less and which thus has the ability to span numerous divergent moral communities, and (2) the particular moral communities within which one can achieve a content-full understanding of the good life and of content-full moral obligations." The first tier, secular ethics, could be designated the public sphere. Accordingly, the second tier would be identified as the private sphere. This schemata recognizes that people are to understand that they live in two realms: public and private. For Engelhardt, this understanding not only removes the apparent clash between these two realms, but it also makes possible a procedural answer to the confrontation of the public and the private. The public realm is content-less and thus allows those of diverse moral communities the freedom to *personally* exercise their own particular moral commitments. In addition, it does not allow any particular moral community to set the moral agenda for the rest of society. For example, the public realm "can establish secular rights of patients to refuse even lifesaving treatment." Nevertheless, the private realm "will indicate when one ought to exercise that right."[32]

According to Engelhardt, rational beings are able to extract themselves from their a-rational moral commitments, particular to their community, and enter a neutral location (the public arena) for the sole purpose of resolving moral controversy. The impetus and reason, why these rational beings leave their individual moral communities, is because they want to avoid the possibility that any one particular moral community will utilize force and impose its respective moral outlook upon all communities. Since conversion and rational argument are not workable solutions and the use of force is unpalatable, the answer that the members of the respective moral communities seek will be found through the vehicle of consensus. In general, the concept of consensus will be supported because of its apparent reasonableness as the only answer to the dilemma of extreme pluralism. The moral authority exe-

31. Engelhardt, p. 69.
32. Engelhardt, p. 78.

cuted by consensus will flow from its link to being the most reasonable solution. Consensus undergirded by reason and moral authority will create a set of procedures which will be agreed upon by all participants in the "peaceable community." Engelhardt describes this peaceable community and its ties to morality in the following way:

> In short, the notion of the peaceable community as fashioned by the principle of permission is a cardinal element in the lives of persons. One embraces it as soon as one attempts to talk about morality across moral communities. Not to adopt it is to lose the basis for coherent moral discourse in a secular, pluralist society. The principle of permission grounds the morality of mutual respect in the sense that it requires that others be used only with their consent.[33]

The "peaceable community" is shaped and held together by the fact that all particular moral communities "consent" to give their "permission" to each and every other particular moral community to be moral in the way they so choose. This does not mean, however, that "anything goes." Rather, what makes the larger society "peaceable" is that all have agreed upon the procedures by which the extreme plurality of the society will be adjudicated. Of course, these procedures, agreements, or contracts must be rational in the sense that all members and potential members are willing to consent to them by virtue of their rationality. Therefore the foundation of these procedures is in the structures of rationality and not in the particular tastes or preferences of individual moral communities.

The basis, according to Engelhardt, which makes morality possible is the cardinal moral principle of mutual respect, and "mutual respect becomes understood as using others only with their permission." Mutual respect with its derivative of permission will be the source of the moral life because it is connected "to the very enterprise of being a person." Engelhardt believes that the more closely one links the foundation of one's ethic to being a person, "the more firmly it can be generally justified."[34] Moreover, the procedures that are mutually agreed to by the members of the peaceable community can be articulated into the form of universal principles. These principles function as tools to casuistically resolve moral dilemmas. The bioethical principles that Engelhardt perceives coming out of these mutually agreed-upon procedures are the same principles identified by Beauchamp and Childress. However, Engelhardt structures the relationship between the principles much differently.

33. Engelhardt, p. 108.
34. Engelhardt, p. 104.

The four biomedical principles developed by Beauchamp and Childress were *prima facie* principles. For example, they do not perceive autonomy as somehow having an *a priori* priority over the other three principles. They maintain that "respect for autonomy, then, has only prima facie standing and can be overridden by competing moral considerations."[35] In other words, there are actions which affirm autonomy and yet could violate the principles of beneficence or non-maleficence. In Engelhardt's framework, the moral life is governed by the formal principle of autonomy and is to be differentiated and yet somewhat connected to beneficence. As Engelhardt puts it,

> Reflections on autonomy lead to the justification of a morality of mutual respect, whose sanctions are the loss of the grounds for respect and for protest against defensive and punitive actions by others. Reflections on the morality of beneficence, however, focus on the morality of common welfare. To affirm the morality of beneficence is to affirm the enterprise of the common good, of the fabric of mutual sympathies, which fashions the morality of welfare. To reject beneficence outright is to lose all claim to the sympathies of others. . . . In summary, violations of the principle of permission justify circumscription of the autonomy of the offender. Violations of the principle of beneficence eliminate claims by the offender to the kind of beneficence rejected for others.[36]

The peaceable community is grounded in autonomy, for "the cardinal moral principle will be that of mutual respect in the common negotiation and creation of a concrete moral world."[37] Thus the principle of autonomy is the only morally necessary principle required for the coherence of the moral world. All conduct is to be evaluated in light of the principle of autonomy, and autonomy can override all other factors. Nevertheless, an autonomous individual can relinquish his or her autonomy in two ways: (1) willingly, that is, by expressing consent; or (2) by performing an action that violates another person's autonomy. Those who choose to use force against another person, thus violating that person's autonomy, are placing themselves outside the confines of the moral community. This, then, puts those who violate the autonomy of others in the position of having force used against them.

As to beneficence, Engelhardt views it in a typical manner: promoting the good of others. Although the principle of beneficence is important be-

35. Beauchamp and Childress, 4th ed., p. 126.
36. Engelhardt, p. 104. It is important to note that Engelhardt will use "mutual respect" and "autonomy" interchangeably.
37. Engelhardt, p. 104.

cause it gives meaning and content to morality, the principle itself cannot be justified within pluralist secular society. Unlike autonomy, "the principle of beneficence needs to be specified within a *particular* moral community in order to be of any practical use."[38] In other words, if one is to promote the "good" of someone, that good will have to be defined by that someone and the community he or she has chosen to belong to. This is the reason why Engelhardt believes autonomy or permission has ultimate priority over beneficence. For example, a Jehovah's Witness may require a blood transfusion to save his or her life. Notwithstanding, due to that person's religious perception of the "good," he or she refuses the transfusion. The hospital staff, however, does not hold the views of the Jehovah's Witness and believes they should transfuse this person. Notice how the principle of beneficence is being interpreted differently by the hospital team and the Jehovah's Witness. The physicians and nurses want to act benevolently toward the patient, but their view of the "good" is strikingly opposed to the position of the patient. Thus, if the team chooses not to transfuse the patient, Engelhardt would say they may have acted in a nonbeneficent manner "without being in conflict with the minimal notion of morality."[39] In other words, the physicians and nurses may not have shown beneficence, that is, promoting their concept of the good, toward the patient, but they did maintain the principle of autonomy.

Consequently, in contrast to Beauchamp and Childress, who believe an autonomous act could be immoral, Engelhardt maintains that all actions with respect to autonomy are legitimate. For Engelhardt, immoral acts are acts that violate the principle of autonomy "because the core of secular moral legitimacy is authorization." When a moral agent breaches the principle of beneficence, however, he or she has only committed an act that is morally improper.[40] The principle of autonomy guarantees individuals the right to do what is wrong. It is important to note, however, what Engelhardt means by "wrong" or "immoral."

> One should note here the moral sanctions for misconduct. Secular morality lacks the sanctions of the law and of religion. It cannot of itself execute, imprison, fine, or damn to hell. Secular morality can demonstrate that certain ways of acting justify blameworthiness or impede the realization of the goals of the actors. Secular morality can also show when defensive or punitive force is justifiable. But in itself it has no physical force. The sanctions of

38. Engelhardt, p. 109.
39. Engelhardt, p. 105.
40. Engelhardt, p. 110.

morality are tied to its justification. To use unconsented-to force against the innocent is incompatible with holding that others are wrong in using such force against oneself, or meaning anything more by terming another wrong or blameworthy than that one dislikes the other's conduct and wishes that he and others would refrain from it. In short, the notion of the peaceable community as fashioned by the principle of permission is a cardinal element in the lives of persons. One embraces it as soon as one attempts to talk about morality across moral communities. Not to adopt it is to lose the basis for coherent moral discourse in a secular, pluralist society. The principle of permission grounds the morality of mutual respect in the sense that it requires that others be used only with their consent.[41]

With these reflections in hand, one can now reappraise the sanctions for immorality. First, as has been noted, philosophical arguments will not deliver the sanctions available through certain religious arguments. Philosophers will not be able to demonstrate that particular forms of immorality will lead to eternal pain. Nor does philosophy have the sanctions of the law. It cannot provide fines, imprisonment, or the lash. The arguments examined earlier show that acting against the very notion of the peaceable community makes one blameworthy in the eyes of rational beings anywhere in the cosmos. As a result, one loses any ground for protesting against their defensive, punitive, or retaliative force. As soon as one is interested in ethics as an alternative to the resolution of moral disputes through force, one has committed oneself to mutual respect. And, if one rejects the principle of mutual respect, one cannot rationally protest when others respond with force. Since the questions regarding the sanctions for immorality are intellectual, the sanctions are intellectual. . . . Reflections on autonomy lead to the justification of a morality of mutual respect, whose sanctions are the loss of the grounds for respect and for protest against defensive and punitive actions by others. . . . In summary, violations of the principle of permission justify circumscription of the autonomy of the offender. Violations of the principle of beneficence eliminate claims by the offender to the kind of beneficence rejected by others.[42]

The concept of "wrong" or "immoral" is connected to being a member of a peaceable community. Assuming, again, that conversion and rational argumentation cannot be the basis of a peaceable community, then agreement is the only possible way to avoid the use of force. Thus autonomous individuals will limit their autonomy based upon their relationship to the overall com-

41. Engelhardt, p. 108.
42. Engelhardt, p. 111.

munity. However, this is not to say that certain autonomous acts are immoral or wrong in and of themselves. The sort of position that views certain acts as inherently immoral, according to Engelhardt, would fit within the confines of religion, law, or the morality of particular communities residing within the larger society.

As was stated earlier, Engelhardt basically adheres to the same four principles of biomedical ethics as Beauchamp and Childress. However, he subsumes non-maleficence and justice under the principle of beneficence; non-maleficence, he says, is "a special application of the principle of benefi-cence." He links non-maleficence to the principle of beneficence by viewing the former as denying others what they believe to be a "good" they want but that will ultimately harm them. "Harm," of course, would be defined within the particular individual's view of the good. For example,

> Consider a college sophomore who at the end of a passionate love affair reads Goethe's *Die Leiden des jungen Werther* and comes to the house of a friend to borrow a sixteen-gauge shotgun with which to commit suicide. Although the principle of permission would not forbid the provision of the shotgun on request, the principle of nonmaleficence would. Medical exam-ples may include requests for unjustified surgical procedures, drugs, or other treatments. It will be obligatory or supererogatory to do others their good, as long as the provision of that good in terms of one's own moral sense is not seen on balance to be a harm.[43]

Thus a person has the right to ask for help to perform an autonomous act. However, this act demands that the potential helper not only factor in the principle of beneficence (helping to promote the good the person desires) but must also consider the principle of non-maleficence (what the helper believes to be a harm). Consequently, non-maleficence is intimately joined to benefi-cence and cannot be understood or utilized apart from it.

When it comes to understanding the principle of justice, again as with non-maleficence, Engelhardt joins justice with the principle of beneficence. For Engelhardt, "justice can be understood as being at root a concern with beneficence."[44] To Engelhardt distributive justice is, after all, deciding how to do the good. When one discusses "doing good," one is talking about acting ac-cording to the principle of beneficence. Thus justice fits neatly under benefi-cence. What this means is that the properties according to which distribution takes place have become relative to each particular community's view of the

43. Engelhardt, p. 114.
44. Engelhardt, p. 121.

good. Moreover, if justice is a subset of beneficence, then are we obligated to act beneficently and thus justly?

Engelhardt concludes his chapter entitled "The Principles of Bioethics" by saying that we have two major moral principles: permission (autonomy) and beneficence.[45] Nonetheless, he introduces another principle later in his work, the principle of ownership, which seems to play a more significant role than even beneficence in terms of moral discrimination. As we will soon see, this principle of ownership "is a special expression of the principle of permission."[46] The idea of ownership flows from the fact that "labor transforms an object from a mere object to an entity fashioned by the ideas and will of a person," and furthermore, "by rendering the object a product, it is brought into the sphere of persons and their claims."[47] According to Engelhardt, there are at least three entities where someone can claim ownership: (1) ourselves (there is nothing we can imagine as having a stronger ownership of); (2) other persons (since others own themselves, they can transfer their personal ownership to another person); and (3) what one produces (which could include such entities as children and animals). Engelhardt finds that he is indebted to both Locke and Hegel for his understanding of ownership.

The principle of ownership, which is a special application of autonomy, forces Engelhardt to explain his views on personhood. He forthrightly states that "not all humans are equal." Indeed, he goes on to say that "persons, not humans, are special."[48] The basis of this conception of persons is secular morality. Moreover, he draws a further distinction between two kinds of persons: "persons in the strict sense" and "persons in the social sense." The former are characterized as self-conscious, rational, free, and moral. As Engelhardt explains,

> It is persons who are the constituents of the secular moral community. Only persons are concerned about moral arguments and can be convinced by them. Only persons can make agreements and convey authority to common projects through their concurrence. To choose, to make an agreement, is to be conscious of what one is doing. It requires the self-reflexivity of self-consciousness. Otherwise, there is a happening, not a doing. The choice to agree or disagree, to convey authority or to withhold authority, requires an appreciation of this basic difference involved in choosing. In this sparse sense, the self-consciousness of a moral agent must be rational.

45. Engelhardt, pp. 121f.
46. Engelhardt, p. 164.
47. Engelhardt, p. 155.
48. Engelhardt, p. 135.

It must include seeing the *ratio,* the relationship between choices and their consequences or significance. Further, for an agent to be an authority giver or withholder, rather than merely an effect of forces, it must be regarded as imputable, not simply as caused. It must be free. Finally, the agent must be a *moral* agent, possessing moral rationality in the sense of being able to appreciate that actions can be tied to a sense of blameworthiness or praiseworthiness. . . . This concept of person (as well as of moral competence) is thus defined wholly within the practice of moral strangers resolving moral controversies by agreement, by giving and withholding morally authoritative permission.[49]

Engelhardt's concept of a "person in the strict sense" is ultimately linked to his idea of "moral strangers." For it is only moral strangers who are able to form a society around agreement and the principle of autonomy. In other words, only a person in the strict sense can become part of a mutual agreement and exercise autonomous decision making. To be able to exercise autonomy and enter into mutual agreement, persons will need to have Engelhardt's four characteristics of a person in the strict sense.

"Persons in the social sense" comprise the rest of humanity. Engelhardt describes these "persons" in the following manner: "(1) humans who in the past were persons in the strict sense (e.g., individuals now suffering from severe Alzheimer's disease); (2) humans who are likely to become persons and have been brought within a social role giving them social standing (e.g., infants); and (3) those humans who have not, and never will, become persons in the strict sense (e.g., the profoundly mentally retarded)."[50] These persons in the social sense are not entities that have intrinsic moral standing. Rather, their personhood is conferred upon them for "social considerations." They will need to have their personhood justified by whether there is a usefulness to the community to do so. Persons in the social sense have no autonomy to protect or offend. The only forms of protection available to these "persons" are: (1) the beneficence of some particular moral community; (2) the moral status ascribed to them by persons who own them; and (3) the utilitarian benefit accorded by the secular moral community.

The distinction between persons in the strict sense and persons in the social sense plays out in the following way within an Engelhardtian society. If a member of a particular moral community believes fetuses are persons, then the society makes it possible for that person to choose not to practice abortion. In other words, that person is able to maintain his or her values and be-

49. Engelhardt, p. 136.
50. Engelhardt, p. 148.

liefs concerning personhood. In sharp contrast, however, if one is a member of a particular moral community that does not believe fetuses have moral status, then the society will allow that person to practice abortion. The only human entities to be protected by society are those that fit into the category of persons in the strict sense. Of course, it is possible a society might decide to confer status on those that are human but are not persons. According to Engelhardt, the basis of this conferral would be the "utilitarian benefit" to the entire society.

This discussion of persons in the strict sense and persons in the social sense relates to Engelhardt's principle of ownership because the latter derive their rights from the autonomy of their owners. Thus someone would violate the autonomy of the owner if that person acted contrary to the owner's views concerning a person in the social sense. An immoral act would be committed if it violated the autonomy of the owner. Nonetheless, if there is no owner, there can be no immorality as it relates to the person in the social sense.

> Because the only source of moral authority for moral strangers is permission, it follows that one may not use persons without their permission. . . . This is to say that the foundational element of the principle of ownership (and indeed of the principle of political authority) is the principle of permission. The principle of ownership (as well as the principle of political authority) is a special expression of the principle of permission. In particular, the principle of ownership focuses on the circumstance that persons are not only their bodies, but in that which they produce.[51]

At the core of morality is permission or autonomy. Persons in the social sense are human entities who have either been produced by persons in the strict sense or have in one way or another turned "authority over themselves to others and in doing so convey authority over their own bodies."[52]

Consequently, Engelhardt's "foundation of bioethics" revolves around the principle of permission or autonomy. The principle of permission makes morality possible between moral strangers. Moreover, it is autonomous persons that constitute the moral sphere and its conditions. Indeed, all other principles of bioethics are ultimately grounded in the principle of permission, and in fact are justified and qualified by the principle of permission.

51. Engelhardt, pp. 163f.
52. Engelhardt, pp. 163f.

Evaluation: Beauchamp and Childress

Beauchamp and Childress have provided an extremely well oiled approach to doing biomedical ethics. They have carefully and meticulously elucidated four principles (autonomy, non-maleficence, beneficence, and justice) to guide decisions and resolve dilemmas faced by the medical community. Furthermore, they have illustrated the importance of "balancing" these principles when two or more principles come into play in a situation. The weakness of their position is not related as much to the principles per se as to their justification for the principles.

Beauchamp and Childress are most explicit when they state that "any theory that eventuates in moral judgments that cannot be brought into reflective equilibrium with pretheoretical commonsense judgments will be considered seriously flawed." They clarify what they mean by a "common morality" theory when they state that it "is not merely a systematization of commonsense judgments or that all *customary moralities* qualify as part of the *common morality*."[53] It appears, then, that by common morality theory they mean a theory that derives principles from other principle-based ethical theories justified by a coherence theory of truth. This latter element makes their theory "pretheoretical" in that it is not just one theory with a transcendent criterion that must be met in all decision making. In addition, the idea behind a common morality relates to the theory's ability to be universalized, that is, the theory's ability to extend to the public and not be limited by any particular community. This makes the theory "commonly" accepted. What do Beauchamp and Childress mean when they state that their theory is justified by a coherence view of truth?

Simply put, a coherence theory of truth means that one accepts certain propositions or statements as correct if they cohere with one or more accepted presuppositions which are known to be true or accepted as true. Thus, if Beauchamp and Childress are justifying their common morality theory within a coherence model, what must moral judgments and statements cohere with? For them the concept which all moral principles must cohere with is "reflective equilibrium." This is suggested by their explanation "that convergence toward truth, not simply justification, is achieved by coherence (using an ideal such as reflective equilibrium)."[54] What do they mean by "reflective equilibrium"?

---

53. Beauchamp and Childress, 4th ed., p. 100.
54. Beauchamp and Childress, 4th ed., p. 27.

According to Beauchamp and Childress, their idea of the concept is grounded in the views of John Rawls, who describes it thus:

> I now turn to the notion of reflective equilibrium. The need for this idea arises as follows. According to the provisional aim of moral philosophy, one might say that justice as fairness is the hypothesis that the principles which would be chosen in the original position are identical with those that match our considered judgments and so these principles describe our sense of justice. But this interpretation is clearly oversimplified. In describing our sense of justice an allowance must be made for the likelihood that considered judgments are no doubt subject to certain irregularities and distortions despite the fact that they are rendered under favorable circumstances. When a person is presented with an intuitively appealing account of his sense of justice (one, say, which embodies various reasonable and natural presumptions), he may well revise his judgments to conform to its principles even though the theory does not fit his existing judgments exactly. He is especially likely to do this if he can find an explanation for the deviations which undermines his confidence in his original judgments and if the conception yields a judgment which he finds he can now accept. From the standpoint of moral philosophy, the best account of a person's sense of justice is not the one which fits his judgments prior to his examining any conception of justice, but rather the one which matches his judgments in reflective equilibrium. As we have seen, this state is one reached after a person has weighed various proposed conceptions and he has either revised his judgments to accord with one of them or held fast to his initial convictions (and the corresponding conception).[55]

Thus the process involved in attaining reflective equilibrium means that one begins with some conception of what one thinks is true. One then compares and examines one's conception in light of other positions. After carefully examining other viewpoints, one may revise one's position or maintain one's original conception. For Beauchamp and Childress, then, the process of justification must meet this test and cohere with the idea or process of reflective equilibrium. Although Rawls designates this approach as reflective equilibrium, it seems it could just as easily be termed "intuitive equilibrium." In other words, it is the examiner himself or herself who must feel comfortable with the final decision. For Rawls, in the above quote, says, "When a person is presented with an intuitively appealing account of his sense of justice . . . he

---

55. John Rawls, *A Theory of Justice* (Cambridge: Harvard University Press, 1971), p. 48.

may well revise his judgments to conform to its principles even though the theory does not fit his existing judgments exactly." In Rawls's entire explanation of the process of reflective equilibrium, neither he nor Beauchamp and Childress ever describe what the "reflective" part of reflective equilibrium involves other than that it is a "state" reached after comparing various conceptions. If this is correct, this means that the ultimate arbiter of the position held by Beauchamp and Childress is "intuition." If this is the case, then there is ultimately no rational way to justify any set of principles as superior to any other set of principles. In the end, cohering to reflective equilibrium only means cohering to one's own subjective, intuitive grasp of what one thinks is correct. Moreover, how would Beauchamp and Childress, much less Rawls, justify the concept of reflective equilibrium as an ultimate criterion by which all principles and moral conceptions must cohere?

Consequently, it would seem that Beauchamp and Childress have constructed a system of ethics that is ultimately grounded in a combination of intuition and self-evidence. By intuition a person directly apprehends something as being true or morally correct. Of course, developing the capacity to be immediately aware of something being true or morally correct may require certain innate capacities to be developed. Nevertheless, after a person gains such knowledge, it is just a matter of intuiting, that is, being immediately conscious of or directly aware of something being right or morally legitimate. Thus Beauchamp and Childress would say, if we are correct in our analysis of their position, that we are simply aware that a principle such as autonomy is correct. No other consideration could possibly bring about a state of reflective equilibrium. As to self-evidence, Beauchamp and Childress would ultimately have to argue that there is a necessary connection between, say, non-maleficence and rightness that makes non-maleficence self-evidently morally sound. Therefore reflective equilibrium can be understood as "seeing" the necessary connection between a certain moral principle and it being either morally right or morally wrong. The problem for Beauchamp and Childress is that their scheme of principles is not subject to rational or empirical justification because their principles are like the axioms of formal logic, which are intuitive or self-evident.

If a position or theory cannot rationally or empirically justify its starting points, then the system has no real way of being universally accepted. If there are competing ethical theories and they are to be resolved by reflective equilibrium, it would seem that acceptance would be based in an arbitrary acceptance of one theory or position over another. Alasdair MacIntyre illustrates this point of the inability to resolve moral discussions rationally when he discusses the moral debate that surrounds three very volatile issues:

(1) just-war theory; (2) abortion; and (3) the control of schools and medical care by either the public or the private sector.

> The first is what I shall call, adapting an expression from the philosophy of science, the conceptual incommensurability of the rival arguments in each of the three debates. Every one of the arguments is logically valid or can be easily expanded so as to be made so; the conclusions do indeed follow from the premises. But the rival premises are such that we possess no rational way of weighing the claims of one as against another. For each premise employs some quite different normative or evaluative concept from the others, so that the claims made upon us are of quite different kinds. In the first argument, for example, premises which invoke justice and innocence are at odds with premises which invoke success and survival; in the second, premises which invoke rights are at odds with those that invoke universalizability; in the third it is the claim of equality that is matched against that of liberty. It is precisely because there is in our society no established way of deciding between claims that moral argument appears to be necessarily indeterminable. From our rival conclusions we can argue back to our rival premises; but when we do arrive at our premises argument ceases and the invocation of one premise against another becomes a matter of pure assertion and counter-assertion. Hence perhaps the slightly shrill tone of so much moral debate.[56]

MacIntyre's point applies to Beauchamp and Childress's project in the following manner: When two very different and even contradictory conceptions of moral principles are both justified by reflective equilibrium, how does one decide between the two theories based upon reflective equilibrium? For example, to Beauchamp and Childress the principle of autonomy certainly coheres with the ideal of reflective equilibrium. And yet, the principle of autonomy might not cohere with the reflective equilibrium of a person in Chinese society. In other words, what creates reflective equilibrium for Beauchamp and Childress may be linked to the fact that they are a part of a society which places a high value on personal freedom. Using the concept of reflective equilibrium as the ideal with which all developed moral positions and principles must cohere places their "principles of biomedical ethics" in an unjustifiable position and, ultimately, makes their viewpoint strictly an option for those who may already hold to their existing presuppositions.

A second area of concern regarding the position of Beauchamp and

56. Alasdair MacIntyre, *After Virtue,* 2nd ed. (Notre Dame, Ind.: University of Notre Dame Press, 1984), p. 8.

Childress involves their approach to the field of medicine. Their assumption is that the participants in health care are able to turn their questions, issues, and dilemmas over to the ethicist who, with his or her ethical tools in hand, will promptly offer a set of principles which will elicit solutions to the problems raised by the medical field. Arthur Caplan designates this approach the "engineering model." He depicts this model as one which "discourages close attention to the realities of illness and anxiety for patients and their families. By locating moral competence in the applied ethicist, the engineering model discounts the realities — of the sick role, of the inability to cope with fear, of the experience of pain, and so on — that are so important in understanding moral issues in medicine. Moral expertise has wandered from moral reality."[57] Although the point of Caplan's article was only to show the limitations of the engineering paradigm when applied to medicine, he does indicate that something is transpiring in the realm of medicine that cannot be captured by any general ethical theory or broad set of principles. What may be more important than giving health care workers a set of principles is teaching them to be the kind of persons they must be to properly function in the health care arena. Moreover, health care workers need to remember the goal or end of medicine more than they need principles by which to solve supposed ethical dilemmas. Most of the questions, issues, and dilemmas raised in the medical arena can be resolved by reminding health care workers of the aim of their work as well as helping them develop the appropriate character traits that undergird and facilitate that end. While Beauchamp and Childress indicate an awareness that character is important, their focus on principles prevents them from according it adequate weight. For Beauchamp and Childress, the relationship between, say, the physician and the patient is primarily contractual. The duties of this contractual relationship flow from the "principles of biomedical ethics" rather than from the nature of the activity of care and healing. The nature and the end of the practice of medicine cannot be reduced to a set of principles, which is what Beauchamp and Childress have attempted to do.

Evaluation: Engelhardt

As was explained earlier in this chapter, Engelhardt pictures medicine as participating in the rampant pluralism of the society in which it is im-

---

57. Arthur Caplan, "Can Applied Ethics Be Effective in Health Care and Should It Strive to Be?" *Ethics* 93 (January 1983): 318.

planted. According to him, "contemporary bioethics is thus set against a background of considerable skepticism, lost belief, persisting convictions, a plurality of moral visions, and mounting public policy challenges."[58] Furthermore, medicine becomes a "peaceable community" where bioethics articulates the philosophy of secular pluralism. Moreover, those involved in the medical realm, like their counterparts in a secular, pluralistic society, come to the medical realm with their particular agendas and views of the "good." Like society at large, the medical field is strewn with autonomous people who are seeking to advance their agendas as moral strangers. Thus the relationships become characterized by negotiation, since for the most part there is no shared moral vision. Consequently, "fair procedures of negotiation will form the basis for resolving tensions among competing views of proper actions."[59]

The two principal players in the health care arena are the physician and the patient. Furthermore, according to Engelhardt, these players usually meet as moral strangers. This postmodern medical world sets off a whole series of elaborate scenarios concerning physician and patient.

> Circumstances are, however, complex, for there is not one unambiguous sense of the health care professions or of the medical profession. Postmodernity and the fragmentation of moral narratives touches to the core of the professions. Although there will be the possibility for a general abstract understanding of what it means to be a physician or nurse, a concrete understanding will be available only within a particular community of physicians, nurses, or other health care professionals and their view of the morally proper life and of the good practice of their profession. Thus, as patients negotiate with health care professionals about their treatment and care, they will need to determine the professional commitments of those with whom they are about to enter into the agreement for care and treatment. A woman of liberal moral persuasions will need to know, for example, whether the gynecologist with whom she is considering developing a patient-physician relationship holds views against sterilization and abortion. So, too, it will be prudent for someone diagnosed with disseminated cancer to know the physician's views regarding the use of narcotics and other drugs in the control of pain. For example, will the physician be willing to give sufficient pain medication in order to avoid the patient's feeling pain instead of relying on minimal amounts of medication so that the patient must request pain medication and experience pain between doses.

58. Engelhardt, p. 6.
59. Engelhardt, p. 289.

Similarly, an individual diagnosed with amyelotrophic lateral sclerosis or Lou Gehrig's disease (a fatal degenerative neurological disease) who does not wish to be preserved to the very end will need to establish a relationship with a neurologist who will support the patient's desires for minimal or no treatment toward the end of the disease's course. In order effectively to fashion a health care contract, the patient will need to know the moral and professional ideals of the physician. So, too, the physician will need to understand the patient's expectation from care.[60]

As moral strangers, the physician and patient must be extremely careful in their relationship with each other. There is no longer any room for assumptions as patient meets physician and as physician meets patient.

At this juncture it is important to point out that Engelhardt's entire project, and its ramifications, is built upon the fact that we must accept a postmodernistic view of reality. His concept of "moral strangers" and "moral friends" is predicated upon the idea that we, as a culture, no longer share the same moral vision and thus are either moral friends or moral strangers. According to Engelhardt, given the postmodern scenario, everything reduces to negotiation or force, including the medical realm. In a very interesting and safe way, he has described this postmodern world in somewhat romantic terms; that is, this is not a world to be frightened of, rather it is a world to be understood and then approached in an appropriate manner. In other words, in one sense one can be optimistic because now one knows how things are and thus how one should operate and navigate. Engelhardt's *Foundations of Bioethics* has tamed this postmodern world for us so that we now know how to correctly live and survive in a medical world thoroughly inundated with postmodernistic thinking. Nevertheless, his solutions do not mesh with his analysis.

Postmodern thought drinks deeply from the well of Nietzsche, who concluded in the nineteenth century what is technically called nihilism. Nietzsche would have agreed with the analysis of Engelhardt that once Western civilization eliminated its organizing principle — God or in particular Christianity — it was left with no basis for values. Thus the appropriate conclusion is that there is nothing but individual subjects who promote their subjective values or ideas of the good. Though Engelhardt, in light of his own personal religious commitments, would never identify himself as a "nihilist," his analysis of Western society is nevertheless identical with a "nihilistic" conclusion. Furthermore, Engelhardt acts as if this analysis will

---

60. Engelhardt, p. 294.

cause people to see that they must negotiate between conflicting subjective values or ideas of the good. However, this is not the conclusion of Nietzsche or other thinkers who have arrived at the postmodern conclusion. David Harvey describes the problem of the postmodern situation a little differently than Engelhardt does:

> We find writers like Foucault and Lyotard explicitly attacking any notion that there might be a meta-language, meta-narrative, to meta-theory through which all things can be connected or represented. Universal truths, if they exist at all, cannot be specified. Condemning meta-narratives . . . as "totalizing," they insist upon the plurality of "power discourse" formulations (Foucault) or of "language games" (Lyotard).[61]

In other words, postmodernity does not lead to negotiation, it inevitably leads to deception through language and imposed values through the use of power. The fundamental flaw in Engelhardt's conclusion is that in the face of conceptual and methodological relativism — which is what postmodernity is — people will not adjust their "good" via negotiation. Rather the situation will be, as Nietzsche and others have said, that each person will attempt to posit his or her values upon everyone else. Given the nature of postmodernity, why would anyone choose to negotiate when they can have their good realized by deception (using language to their advantage) or by imposing their good on others (using power)?

If Engelhardt is correct, moral strangers are really living in a Hobbesian world where everyone is in one way or another trying to get his or her way with everyone else. Again, why would someone accept Engelhardt's solution to the situation? Why would someone adopt his "good," the good of negotiation? For example, let's imagine a gynecologist who believes it is not "good" that certain infants with certain human faults live. Let's further imagine that one of that doctor's patients is carrying an infant who has one of those characteristics that the gynecologist thinks make an unborn child a candidate to be aborted. In discussions with the patient, it has come to the gynecologist's attention that she is a devoutly religious person who does not believe abortion is a legitimate medical procedure unless the life of the mother is at risk. Since clearly the doctor and patient in this scenario are moral strangers, what

61. David Harvey, *The Condition of Postmodernity* (Oxford: Basil Blackwell, 1989), pp. 44-45. For more on the implications of Nietzsche's thought for bioethics, see Stephen N. Williams, "Bioethics in the Shadow of Nietzsche," in *Bioethics and the Future of Medicine: A Christian Appraisal*, ed. John F. Kilner et al. (Grand Rapids: Wm. B. Eerdmans Publishing Co., 1995), pp. 112-23.

obligates the doctor to disclose his or her position to the patient concerning her unborn child? Engelhardt would say it is the principle of permission or autonomy. Why, however, given a postmodern setting, is it not just as viable for the gynecologist to hide his or her views and manipulate the patient with medical language such that she would accept an abortion? What would keep the gynecologist from giving the information to her in such a manner that she believes carrying this child to term will endanger her life? Telling a patient what one's position is assumes one believes in "truthfulness." Since the doctor and patient hold different perspectives on reality, truth itself is conditioned by one party's idea of the "good." This scenario reduces living to a nightmare. Nonetheless, that is the kind of life one will need to make preparation for if Engelhardt is correct.

Furthermore, Engelhardt believes that mutual respect will make it possible for negotiation to work. Mutual respect is the idea that each party in the negotiation process will simply agree to the nonuse of others without their consent and each person involved in negotiation will acknowledge that each person may agree or refuse to negotiate. Again, this is not only a rather romantic outlook on the postmodern setting, it is a romantic outlook on human nature as well. One could easily classify Engelhardt's position as "romantic pessimism." He is pessimistic about the possibility of obtaining content for morality in a postmodern setting while at the same time being extremely optimistic about a procedural process that will serve as a basis for adjudication between moral strangers. To put this point into a popular expression, "What is wrong with this picture?" Faith L. Lagay picks up on what the real possibilities are in this negotiation process:

> I worry, however, that the presence of only a constraining principle (nonuse of others without their consent) in the absence of any welfare consideration of beneficence fails to safeguard morality adequately. Seeking only to resolve moral dilemmas without force, value-stripped negotiators might agree on a course of action that none, individually views as moral. Such a result is all the more possible if negotiators are able, as in Engelhardt's ideal scenario, to leave their individual moral communities behind them when entering into negotiation.
>
> . . . The procedural bioethic thus serves as a political expedient for keeping the peace rather than serving a common morality.[62]

---

62. Faith L. Lagay, "Secular? Yes; Humanism? No: A Close Look at Engelhardt's Secular Humanism Bioethic," in *Reading Engelhardt: Essays on the Thought of H. Tristram Engelhardt, Jr.,* ed. Brendan P. Minogue, Gabriel Palmer-Fernandez, and James E. Reagan (Dordrecht, Netherlands: Kluwer Academic Publishers, 1997), p. 242.

Lagay is correct in her analysis that what will probably come out of negotiation may have absolutely nothing to do with morality. It is odd that Engelhardt thinks he can begin with an extremely pessimistic outlook and end up with a most romantic ending.

Moreover, Engelhardt's ultimate principle of permission or autonomy does not naturally follow from a postmodern viewpoint. Instead autonomy is linked to modernity, where reality could be known and understood by reason. In particular, the concept of autonomy is linked to the moral musings of Immanuel Kant, an Enlightenment philosopher. Kant argued that what gives every person dignity is neither social status nor special talents nor accomplishments but the innate power of reason — the capacity of each individual to think and choose, not only to shape his or her own life but also to protect and promote reciprocal respect by enacting laws that form the legal structure of life for everyone. In Kant's liberal political theory, the power of autonomy is what gives every person moral authority and status against the power of the state. The institutions of society must be regulated by laws based on reason; only these kinds of laws will consistently protect freedom and ensure justice. This is a far cry from Engelhardt's postmodern world, but it is the basis of autonomy or permission. For ultimately, autonomy or permission is based on a consistent, universal view of rationality.

Not only are there problems between Engelhardt's analysis and his solution, there are also difficulties with his view of personhood. As was explained earlier in the chapter, Engelhardt places persons into two classes: persons in the strict sense and persons in the social sense. Persons in the strict sense are true persons while persons in the social sense need to have their personhood bestowed upon them. According to Engelhardt, a true person is someone who can exercise autonomy, and only autonomous persons are capable of mutual respect. Since the composition of a moral community requires personal beings, the required characteristics for the status of a person are "self-conscious, rational, free to choose, and in possession of a sense of moral concern."[63] Those entities which do not possess these characteristics are not persons in the strict sense. Engelhardt states that "fetuses, infants, the profoundly retarded, and the hopelessly comatose provide examples of human nonpersons. They are members of the human species but do not in and of themselves have standing in the secular moral community." He states what he means even more strongly when he writes:

> It is nonsensical in general secular terms to speak of respecting the autonomy of fetuses, infants, or profoundly retarded adults, who have never been

63. Engelhardt, p. 136.

rational. There is no autonomy to affront. Treating such entities without regard for that which they do not possess, and never have possessed, deposits them of nothing that can have general secular moral standing. They fall outside of the inner sanctum of secular morality.[64]

In the above quote, Engelhardt could not be more clear on his views of personhood. Although his defense of personhood is tied to autonomy, it is also derived from his assessment of the fetus and other such human entities in terms of potentiality and probability.

Engelhardt presents potentiality in a rather straightforward manner. He says that "if fetuses are only potential persons, they do not have the rights of a person." By way of analogy he argues that "if X is a potential president, it follows from that fact alone that X does not have the rights and prerogatives of an actual president."[65] At this juncture there seem to be two problems associated with Engelhardt's explanation of potentiality. First, a potential person can be easily confused with a possible person. A possible person is an entity that could, under certain causally possible conditions, become an actual person (or at least part of one — for example, a human sperm or egg), but a potential person is a being that will become an actual person in the normal course of events or development. Using Engelhardt's example, most Americans are possible presidents, but we do not salute one another because of that. However, a potential president is one who has won the election and is preparing to be inaugurated. Potential presidents do get saluted, and some of this additional respect is a recognition not just of their current abilities but of the high office and sacred trust they are in the process of attaining. Likewise, although an embryo or especially a not-yet-implanted zygote might be spontaneously aborted, the chances are very good that it will achieve personhood and thus should be treated as such.

The Aristotelian argument of the essential connection between potentiality and actuality[66] strengthens the conceptual basis to argue for an equiva-

64. Engelhardt, p. 139.
65. Engelhardt, p. 142.
66. Aristotle's rather technical analysis of the potential in relation to the actual in the *Metaphysics* and his reflections on biological development in *On the Soul* and *On the Generation of Animals* provide a basis to explain the relationship of a developing biological entity to the mature member of the kind or sort it has the potential to become. For Aristotle the potential and the actual are the same being. Potential being and actual being of a biological organism can be considered different modes or ways of understanding the same thing or substance. This follows from Aristotle's notion of sensible substance as an integral union, or a composite of matter and form. For Aristotle a sensible thing or substance is and exists in three senses: (1) as matter it is potentially, but not actually, a "this"; (2) as

lence of moral value and status between embryos and fetuses as potential rational beings and human adults as actual rational beings. In this view the full value of the adult is implicit in the unborn because they are just different modes or senses of the same fundamental kind or sort of being. This ontological identity is presupposed by the fact that the fullness of human life is implicit in its living genetic mechanism as an integral and necessary part of its biography and complete meaning. Consequently, in contrast to Engelhardt, it follows that the human individual is properly described and valued as a rational being from its conception to its death irrespective of its growth and development of the physical characteristics, or the formation of the personality or self, which is ultimately required for rational awareness. In other words, Aristotle's analysis leads one to confess the following state of affairs: to kill the fetus is to kill the baby, to kill the child, to kill the young adult, to kill the adult, and thus to kill the older person. For the full value of the person is in every stage of development. Moreover, Aristotle could say, "Killing the potentiality kills the actuality."

---

form it is actually a "this"; and (3) as a composite of the two it exists as a kind of unity of which alone there can be generation and destruction. As a form, a sensible thing already contains its own principle of actuality within itself, even though as matter it is on the way to becoming a composite substance. Thus form is the essence of each thing and Aristotle designates it formal substance. Form is not, itself, generated or made in each individual, but the sensible thing, as a composite substance, is generated from the form which provides its identity or name. Hence a sensible thing already is an actuality in a significant sense as soon as there is sufficient reason to judge that the form from which it generates and takes its identity and name has become an integral part of its being. Aristotle's analysis provides a reasonable ontological foundation for the claim that the living genetic mechanism of members of the human species constitutes a biogenetic nature or essence. It follows from Aristotle's argument that the formal principle or nature from which and by which rational beings come into being, take their identity, grow and develop is present at the inception of each human individual.

The application of Aristotle's unifying formula that potential rational beings and actual rational beings are the same in regard to their fundamental kind of being adds further clarity and theoretical justification to the contention that the very meaning of the potentiality of a living thing is that it already is a certain kind of being which will develop in accordance with its proper kind. Moreover, the fundamental kind or sort a living "this" is, is determined at its inception by the initial actualization of its potential to be a living thing of that kind or sort. On the other hand, it also follows that potential human persons are different, in regard to the degree of actualization of their potential for growth and development, including neurological development. However, they are on the way to becoming substances in Aristotle's third sense of being as composite. Nonetheless, since this growth and development presupposes and proceeds from the primary actualization of the composite as a being of that kind, this being on the way does not, itself, imply deficiency of identity.

Moreover, the fetus's potential for personal function does not make him or her a person. Rather, it is because he or she is a person that he or she has this inherent capacity to function as a person. Engelhardt casts his objection to the fetus being a person in the following manner: first there is a potential person, which then becomes an actual person as that potential is actualized. The error of Engelhardt's position is that potentiality can only be applied to functioning, not to being. There is no such thing as a potential person. As to being or essence, either one is a person or one is not; one either has or does not have that nature or essence. Indeed, the only reason someone can function as a person is because he or she is a person. Thus one is first a person, from the actual moment of conception, and because of that fact one has the "basic inherent capacity" to act and function as a person.[67] The primary and most basic reality, then, is being a person. Robert Joyce puts it this way:

> A person is not an individual with a *developed* capacity for reasoning, willing, desiring, and relating to others. A person is an individual with a *natural* capacity for these activities and relationships, whether this natural capacity is ever developed or not — i.e., whether he or she ever attains the functional capacity or not. Individuals of a rational, volitional, self-conscious nature may never attain or may lose the functional capacity for fulfilling this nature to any appreciable extent. But this inability to fulfill their nature does not negate or destroy the nature itself.[68]

Therefore the moral status of the person or his or her personhood is unaffected by the extent to which that particular person is functioning or not functioning as a person. A person's moral standing and personhood is rooted in that person's nature, not in his or her achievements or physical progress. Herein lies the alternative to Engelhardt's mistake of distinguishing between "persons in the strict sense" and "persons in the social sense."

Conclusion

The principles of biomedical ethics developed by Beauchamp and Childress can be very helpful when applied to medical dilemmas, problems, and ques-

---

67. For a fuller discussion of this argument, see Stephen Schwartz, *The Moral Question of Abortion* (Chicago: Loyola University Press, 1990).

68. Robert E. Joyce, "When Does a Person Begin?" in *New Perspectives on Human Abortion*, ed. Thomas W. Hilgers, Dennis J. Horan, and David Mall (Frederick, Md.: University Publications of America, 1981), p. 347.

tions. Nevertheless, their approach suffers from two problems: (1) the grounding of their entire project; and (2) the inherent idea that medicine is somehow value-neutral. Utilizing a coherence theory of truth for justification, they have chosen what they designate as "reflective equilibrium" to be the arbiter by which all else must cohere. As discussed earlier, reflective equilibrium ultimately becomes the intuition of the particular person performing the justificatory process. Thus justification is reduced to subjectivity. Of course, the issue of grounding one's position is a difficulty for all secular approaches. As to medicine being value-neutral, Beauchamp and Childress seem to overlook the fact that there is an asymmetry of power between the caregiver and the patient. The fact that the health care professional wields an extreme amount of power over the patient points to the fact that medicine is inherently moral. Thus the state of medicine uncovers the importance of two factors which must be addressed by anyone discussing ethics in the biomedical realm: the character of the professionals and the balance of power needed by the patient. In other words, if the character of the caregiver is not addressed and the patient has no way of gaining a balance of power, then the medical realm will always be, in one way or another, an extremely frightening place to be sick.

To Engelhardt's credit, he forthrightly develops his approach within a postmodern setting. His exposition of postmodern thought and ensuing analysis are very insightful. Unfortunately he tries to sanitize a situation that cannot be disinfected. If Engelhardt is correct, then life in the world, especially in the medical world, will be our worst nightmare. Whereas Engelhardt believes that one can produce an ethic in a postmodern environment — the principle of permission or autonomy — earlier thinkers such as Nietzsche find that belief overly optimistic if not ridiculous. At least Beauchamp and Childress give themselves some hope by assuming the modernist emphasis on the power of reason. In sharp contrast, Engelhardt assumes the postmodernist death of rationality and then tries to be rational. One cannot build something upon nothing. In the end, perhaps the saddest observation is that of Engelhardt himself: "The contrast between general secular morality and content-full moral commitments is stark and disappointing."[69] The challenge facing bioethics today is indeed immense.

---

69. Engelhardt, p. 257.

PART II

PILLARS OF A CHRISTIAN APPROACH

CHAPTER 3

Medical Technology in
Theological Perspective

Introduction

Medical technology has been developed and applied at a truly astounding rate in the past thirty years. Its widespread application has increased longevity and has virtually conquered numerous diseases that routinely caused death or severe disability in the past. To be sure, this increase in longevity has at times been accompanied by a deteriorating quality of life; that is, medicine is more skilled than ever at keeping people alive with increasingly poor quality of life. But most people would consider the advances in medical technology to be highly beneficial, making life better for society as a whole. Virtually no one wants to go back to the early part of this century before the development of antibiotics, vaccines for childhood diseases, and life-sustaining technologies such as ventilators and dialysis.

But some of the advances in medical technology have put into the hands of human beings decisions that were once considered left to God. For example, the availability of life-sustaining technology has forced decisions on physicians, patients, and their families about withdrawing these technologies that heretofore were believed to be in God's hands because medicine had little ability to delay death. Similarly, with many of the new reproductive technologies, decisions about procreation which were once considered left to God are now being made by couples. Infertility is no longer considered an irreversible condition, or even a curse, and can be treated by a variety of reproductive technologies. The use of many of these technologies has raised the emotion-

91

ally charged question of whether their practitioners and patients are "playing God." That is, are they taking over areas that should be God's domain?

Take, for example, the spectrum of reproductive technologies now available to infertile couples. From intrauterine insemination (IUI) (especially using donor sperm) to in vitro fertilization (IVF) to the newest technologies involving sperm injection, critics charge that these new technologies have taken the awe and mystery out of procreation and reduced it to a cold technological process that, for people who utilize them, has separated the intimate act of sexual relations from procreating a child.[1] Technologies that involve fertilization outside the body, such as in vitro fertilization, are said to be examples of "playing God" with sperm and eggs and should not be done. Other critics cite the new and growing practice of sperm injection as an example of "playing God," since that technology replaces the normal process of natural selection for the sperm, in which defective sperm are unable to reach or penetrate the egg. Critics further point out the rare cases in which women who have lost their husbands extract their sperm posthumously and use artificial insemination to conceive children. In addition, critics insist that the development of artificial wombs, which will likely be a reality in the next thirty years, further renders the natural and God-ordained connection between sexual relations and procreation obsolete, and precludes what the normal gestational environment has to offer the developing child.

Or consider the genetic revolution. In the past few years there has been an explosion of both genetic technologies and genetic information. Prenatal genetic testing has enabled couples to see the genetic makeup of their unborn children, and in many cases they make decisions to end their pregnancies on the basis of such information rather than leaving the development of these children up to God. The Human Genome Project has opened up a new world of diagnostic information for patients at risk from hundreds of different genetic links and predispositions. Genetic engineering has raised the prospect of curing genetic disease and enhancing the genetic code of one's children.

---

1. See, for example, the official Catholic documents *Humanae Vitae* (1968) and *Instruction on Respect for Human Life in Its Origin and on the Dignity of Procreation (Donum Vitae)* (1987), where this critique is made. These have been reprinted in a wide variety of anthologies in bioethics. *Humanae Vitae* can be found in Stephen E. Lammers and Allen Verhey, eds., *On Moral Medicine: Theological Perspectives in Medical Ethics*, 2nd ed. (Grand Rapids: Wm. B. Eerdmans Publishing Co., 1998), pp. 434-38. The Vatican *Instruction* of 1987 can be found in Richard T. Hull, ed., *Ethical Issues in the New Reproductive Technologies* (Belmont, Calif.: Wadsworth Publishing, 1990), pp. 21-39, and Kenneth D. Alpern, ed., *The Ethics of Reproductive Technology* (New York: Oxford University Press, 1992), pp. 83-97.

Use of each of these technologies has raised questions of the moral appropriateness of manipulating the human genetic code, particularly in those cases in which the newly acquired trait would be passed on to succeeding generations.[2] Critics have charged that genetic engineers are "playing God" with the building blocks of life. This is especially the case with genetic technologies that do more than correct defective genes. The technologies that enhance already existing traits are said to be cases of tinkering with God's design for each individual person, or trying to improve on God's blueprint for people.

Perhaps the clearest example of these charges of "playing God" is the recent and controversial area of human cloning.[3] In 1993, when infertility researchers first cloned human embryos, the 8 November issue of *Time* magazine captured the visceral reaction of many people to this news. Cloning was the cover story that week, and on the cover of the magazine was a modified reproduction of Michelangelo's painting of the creation, in which the finger of God touches Adam's finger and through that touch God extends the breath of life into him and he becomes alive. *Time* artists altered the painting and, instead of God touching one person, he is touching five identical clones of Adam at the same time. The point clearly was that there was something wrong with human beings copying in the lab what God had already created in the body. The researchers who first cloned the embryos were widely criticized on various talk shows and in the national media for "playing God" in the lab. When Scottish scientists cloned an adult sheep successfully in 1996, raising the prospect of adult human cloning, similar concerns were raised and criticisms leveled at the scientific community. Critics insist that the combination of available reproductive technologies with human cloning is on the horizon, and that procreation can occur without sex, men, or women. With reproductive technologies, sex is not necessary for procreation. With cloning, men are not necessary for procreation, and with artificial wombs, when available, women would not be necessary. When that occurs, the reproductive revolution will be complete, and the critics' charge that technology will have completely usurped God's place in procreation.

Similar concerns about "playing God," though somewhat muted in recent years, are raised about the withdrawal of life-sustaining technology, particularly with newborns and the elderly. Some pro-life advocates charge that

2. This is known as "germ line therapy" as opposed to somatic cell therapy, in which the trait is not passed on to succeeding generations.

3. This and other religious objections to cloning are documented in National Bioethics Advisory Commission (NBAC), *Cloning Human Beings: Report and Recommendations of the National Bioethics Advisory Commission* (Rockville, Md.: NBAC, June 1997), pp. 39-61.

withdrawing life support, particularly medically provided nutrition and hydration, is tantamount to making life-and-death decisions that ultimately belong only to God. A best-selling exposé of abuses of technology in neonatal intensive care units around the country was titled *Playing God in the Nursery*.[4] The author charged that physicians were prematurely withdrawing life-sustaining technology from seriously ill newborns.

The degree to which these charges of "playing God" are true varies with the technology under consideration. It also varies with one's theological view of technology in God's economy. The place of technology theologically begins with the dominion mandate in Genesis 1–2 and the doctrines of general revelation and common grace. Questions about these technologies per se depend on the place of technology in general in God's order. Even if our theology affirms technology in general as a blessing of God, questions still remain about the use of any particular technology. Thus we may find that the Scripture affirms technology as God's good gift to the human race. But we may also find that theological principles give cause for caution in the application of any given technology, particularly those that touch life and death so closely.

Theological Setting for Medical Technology

The backdrop for the biblical teaching on technology begins in the creation account in Genesis 1–2. As man and woman stand at the pinnacle of God's creation, God charges them to exercise dominion over his creation (1:27-28). Their mandate was to subdue the earth and be its master, unlocking its resources for their benefit and the benefit of their successors, and in a sense continuing the spirit of creation by being co-creators with God in unlocking the secrets of the creation for the benefit of the human race. The responsibility God gave to Adam and Eve to work the garden (2:15) involved utilizing nature to meet their needs, and a part of that process was uncovering the hidden aspects of creation to provide for them. The command to exercise dominion was a positive commandment to master the creation. Dominion over creation clearly was to be an effort of the entire human race together, since the commands to multiply and populate the earth and to exercise dominion over the earth (1:28) are closely related. Though the account in Genesis 1–2 does not specifically spell this out, it is clear that God would provide for them all the tools they need to exercise proper dominion over creation. It would be

4. Jeff Lyon, *Playing God in the Nursery* (New York: Norton, 1985).

out of character for God to issue a command to them to have dominion over creation and fail to give them the necessary equipment to fulfill such a mandate.

The command to subdue the earth takes on added complexity after the entrance of sin into the world in Genesis 3. As part of the curse of sin, God makes it clear that Adam's role in subduing the creation to provide for his material needs will be much more arduous and difficult (vv. 17-19). Similarly, one of Eve's roles in subduing the creation, giving birth to children, will also be more difficult and painful (v. 16). Thus, exercising dominion over creation after the fall involved dealing with the effects of the entrance of sin into the world. Dominion now involved working toward restoring the creation to its original glory, even though that goal would never be fully accomplished until the Lord's return. Dominion now involved working toward improving the creation, or reversing the effects of the entrance of sin.[5] The most important of these effects was the new reality of death (vv. 2-3), which was universal in its scope (Rom. 5:12). That is, after the fall death, decay, and deterioration faced every person, and a significant part of dominion over the creation involved dealing with death and disease, which was the cause of death in most cases, so that humankind could alleviate the harshness of life after the fall.

Dominion over creation was not the only part of the creation mandate in Genesis 1–2. Human beings' God-given right to subdue the creation for their benefit did not give them the privilege of abusing the creation and treating it without regard to the consequences they would bring. Human beings did not have the privilege of "rape and pillage" over the creation. They were to exercise responsible dominion over it. God gave the human race dominion over creation as stewards over it. Dominion did not bring ownership of creation, since God owns the land (Lev. 25:23). Rather it brought responsibility for creation as a trustee. At creation, human beings were charged with both dominion and stewardship. Creation was theirs to use for their benefit, but it ultimately belonged to God and they were responsible to him for its proper use.

God provided human beings with the resources necessary for accomplishing the task of exercising dominion over creation. These resources came

---

5. It is probably going too far to say that the original command to exercise dominion was a command to improve on the creation, or be continual co-creators with God. Given the original perfection of creation prior to the fall, it is hard to see how it could be improved. But after the fall, dominion involved the work of restoration, and it could be said that from that point on humankind's responsibility for dominion involved efforts to improve on the fallen state of creation, even though humankind could not reverse its general fallenness.

from creation itself in the form of natural resources, and from humankind it-self in the ingenuity and initiative necessary to take advantage of all that the creation had to offer. That ingenuity and wisdom come from God as his gifts in his revelation to the human race. The Scripture is clear that God revealed himself and his wisdom both in Scripture and outside of Scripture. God's rev-elation of his wisdom outside of Scripture is commonly known as "general revelation." That is, it is available generally to all people and is not revealed exclusively to the community of God's people. The Scripture itself teaches the concept that God reveals himself and his wisdom outside of the pages of his Word. For example, in the Old Testament the concept of God's wisdom is closely related to the notion of general revelation. In the wisdom literature (Job through Ecclesiastes), there are two sources of God's wisdom: (1) natu-ral, or outside of Scripture, and (2) revealed, in Scripture. Both are legitimate and authoritative.

Scripture affirms that there is a fixed order that governs the physical world, the world of nature (Jer. 31:35-36; 33:20-21, 25-26). This order is also known as the laws of nature and has been discovered by the hard sci-ences, such as physics, astronomy, chemistry, and biology. This is reflected in creation psalms like Psalm 19 which praise God for the way he has re-vealed himself in creation. This is God's ordering wisdom that is embedded in creation. In Proverbs 8:22-31 it is clear that God's wisdom was intimately bound up with creation (3:19-20). God's wisdom was "engraved" or em-bedded into the creation from the very beginning. God's ordering wisdom is expanded in Proverbs 8:32-36 to include interpersonal and especially moral knowledge.[6] It is embedded in nature and can be discovered by rea-son. The writer draws conclusions about one's character and morality based on adherence to God's wisdom that is embedded in creation, suggesting that God's wisdom in creation includes moral knowledge. We could sum-marize it in a diagram:

6. One can make a good case out of the same texts in the wisdom literature for the concept of natural law, or God's general revelation in the area of moral values. Central to bioethics are the principles of autonomy, beneficence, non-maleficence, and justice devel-oped by Beauchamp and Childress (see their *Principles of Biomedical Ethics,* 4th ed. [New York: Oxford University Press, 1996]) and laid out in chapter 2 above. The fact that these are such widely held values is not an accident, but comes from natural law. For further reading on the concept of natural law in Christian ethics, see Scott B. Rae, *Moral Choices: An Introduction to Ethics* (Grand Rapids: Zondervan, 1995), and Michael Cromartie, *A Preserving Grace: Protestants, Catholics, and Natural Law* (Grand Rapids: Wm. B. Eerdmans Publishing Co., 1997).

God's Cosmic Wisdom/General Revelation

laws of nature over physical world   laws of nature over human behavior
technology/physical sciences   human/social sciences

Thus Scripture and God's natural wisdom, or general revelation, are two sides to God's wisdom. Even though the wise sage who was responsible for discovering and collecting the Wisdom Books of the Old Testament, particularly Proverbs, is under inspiration, this does not negate the fact that the sage gained these insights from his own observations. Two specific proverbs make the link between the sage's observations and moral conclusions drawn from them. In Proverbs 6:6-11 the sage observes the diligence and forethought of the ant, and draws a conclusion about diligence and laziness. Likewise, Proverbs 24:30-34 draws the identical conclusion, repeated verbatim, from observation of a lazy person and the consequences of that action. Thus observations of both the physical and interpersonal worlds are some of the sources for gleaning God's natural wisdom and drawing appropriate moral conclusions. Thus the goal of the sage was to discover and transmit those values embedded in creation through God's cosmic wisdom. There are, then, two aspects to God's wisdom in the Scripture: general revelation, outside of Scripture, and special revelation in the Scripture.

This idea of general revelation is closely related to the notion of what is called "common grace," or God's grace that is bestowed commonly, or on all humankind, irrespective of one's membership in the community of God's people. For example, the apostle Paul reminds his audience of philosophers on Mars Hill that God causes the rain to fall on the just as well as the unjust (Acts 14:17). He points out that the things that are necessary for people to survive, such as sunlight, crops, and water, are the result of God's general blessings, or his common grace.

The knowledge and skill that are necessary to develop the kinds of technologies that enable humankind to subdue the creation are part of God's general revelation and common grace. Humanity did not acquire the ingenuity and skill to develop sophisticated technology on their own apart from God. It is not an accident that these technologies came to be so useful in humankind's exercise of dominion over the creation. They are the gifts of God. Though it is true that humankind provided the initiative and perseverance to develop these technologies, the ability and the knowledge come from God. Thus technologies that generally improve the lot of the human race and specifically help reverse the effects of the entrance of sin into the world are part of his general revelation and common grace. The skill and expertise needed to bring about these creation-subduing technologies come ultimately from God and are his good gifts to bring creation under humankind's control.

This is particularly the case when it comes to medical technology. Since death is one of the primary consequences of the entrance of sin into the world, and disease is the primary cause of death and physical deterioration, medical technologies that bring cures to diseases and other afflictions are among God's most gracious gifts to the human race. Since death and disease are so closely connected, medical technology that alleviates disease is a very significant part of humankind's exercise of dominion over the creation. The healing ministry of medicine and the proper use of medical technology have contributed greatly, particularly in this century, to humanity's effective subduing of the earth. Through medical developments, many diseases have been once and for all conquered. Many childhood diseases which took the lives of children prematurely can now be prevented by simple vaccinations. Other diseases for which there had been no cure are now cured by administering antibiotics. Heart disease is now treatable through the development of a variety of surgical instruments and techniques. To be sure, there are still diseases that have no cure, such as many types of cancer and AIDS. Ultimately medical technology cannot conquer death, and it is an illusion to pursue technology to that end. There will always be diseases that will cause death. If the medical community finds cures to some, there will always be others that will cause death. Thus, in an ultimate sense, the development of medical technologies brings only partial and temporary victory over death. That is, medical technologies only partially and temporarily reverse the principal effect of the entrance of sin into the world, which is death. They have thus contributed to humankind's effective dominion over the creation, but they also reflect the limits imposed on humankind's dominion due to the entrance of sin in the world.

A further effect of sin in the world is that humankind is not only capable but also quite skilled at misusing technology. It can be used for destructive ends or for self-interest at the expense of the common good. Things like weapons of mass destruction and industrial processes that irreparably damage the environment are examples of the mixed blessing of many technologies. Even medical technology can be misused. Simple surgical techniques to treat a woman who has suffered a miscarriage can be used to perform abortions. Drugs that can relieve pain and alleviate suffering in cancer patients can also be used on the streets by addicts. Life-sustaining technology can be employed past the time it is beneficial to the patient, resulting in worse suffering, a deteriorating quality of life, and a painful delay of an inevitable death.

We must distinguish between the use of any particular medical technology per se and its intended or actual use in practice. That is, it is possible to see virtually any medical technology as a part of God's common grace to humankind. But that does not exempt it from moral assessment of its uses. It may be that some technologies have so few morally justifiable uses that it would be better for the medical community not to have developed that technology at all. Or some technologies may be so dangerous in their normal, intended use that their use in general is problematic. For example, one can argue that certain types of cloning are so potentially harmful to the fetus that cloning should not be attempted at all. A further caution in the use of these sophisticated medical technologies, especially for elective purposes such as assisted reproduction, has to do with the potential for technology to control and the prospect of the erosion of moral values as society seeks enhanced techniques to achieve inadequately examined ends. This emphasis on technology can lead to what Jacques Ellul calls "technical autonomy," in which the technology functions in a moral vacuum, with its practitioners accepting few if any limits on its use or development from moral and spiritual values.[7]

With these cautions in mind, we can see medical technology as part of God's common grace to assist humankind in fulfilling its role in properly exercising dominion over the creation. There are many medical technologies, such as antibiotics, which have such clearly beneficial uses that no moral questions about their normal use can be raised. But with the more controversial technologies, such as those used in reproductive and genetic engineering, society must make a moral evaluation about their intended uses. Society should avoid being taken captive to the technological imperative, which suggests that nothing should stand in the way of science and the application of technology. Just because a technology is available does not suggest that it should necessarily be used or not have significant limits placed on its use. We should note that even good uses of technology are still infected by the entrance of sin into the world. Even good uses of medical technology can have negative effects, and the presence of sin in the world does make for more ambiguity and complexity in evaluating the uses of any particular technology.

Medical technology can be seen as an aspect of God's general revelation or common grace to the human race to equip it to more effectively exercise dominion over the creation by reversing the effects of the entrance of sin into the world, namely, disease. The Ethical and Religious Directives for Health

---

7. For further discussion of this provocative point, see Jacques Ellul, *The Technological Society*, trans. John Wilkinson (New York: Vintage Books, 1964), and *The Technological Bluff*, trans. Geoffrey W. Bromiley (Grand Rapids: Wm. B. Eerdmans Publishing Co., 1990).

Care of the Catholic Church summarize the place of medical technology within God's economy. The preamble states, "This sharing (in dominion over creation) involves a stewardship over all material creation (Gen. 1:26) that should neither abuse nor squander nature's resources. Through science the human race comes to understand God's wonderful work; and through technology it must conserve, protect and perfect nature in harmony with God's purposes."[8] The Catholic Church's official teaching correctly sanctions the general use of medicine as part of God's provision to human beings, though, as will become clear in the remainder of this chapter, not without moral limits.

Application to Reproductive, Genetic, and Life-Sustaining Technologies

Within the general acceptance of medical technology as the good gift of God revealed through general revelation, there are some new reproductive, genetic, and life-sustaining technologies that raise difficult questions for both medical professionals and the public at large. We begin with the presumption that medical technology that helps alleviate the effects of the entrance of sin into the world is a good thing and comes from God. But that does not mean that all potential uses of any technology are exempt from moral examination, nor are all uses of a particular technology morally appropriate. Each technology and each potential use of it are the legitimate focus of moral scrutiny.

Reproductive Technologies

In the last twenty years reproductive medicine has made stunning progress in treating infertility. A variety of new, expensive, and sophisticated techniques now enable couples to procreate when previously their only options would be adoption or remaining childless. Infertility physicians have given the "gift of life" to couples who had essentially given up hope for having a child of their own. These techniques range from relatively simple ones such as artificial insemination, both with the husband's and donor sperm, to more complicated ones such as the in vitro fertilization family of technolo-

8. United States Catholic Bishops, "Ethical and Religious Directives for Catholic Health Care Services," *Origins* 24, no. 27 (15 December 1994): 449-64, at 452.

gies,[9] to very complex technologies involving sperm injection. Reproductive arrangements such as surrogate motherhood are neither new nor particularly complex technologies, though there are arrangements that involve IVF.[10] What is new about surrogacy is the presence of lawyers and contracts in the area of procreation.

The strongest critique of reproductive technology has come from Roman Catholic theologians, who come to the issue out of a natural law framework.[11] Two official Catholic documents summarize the church's opposition to most reproductive interventions, *Humanae Vitae: On the Regulation of Birth,* issued in 1968, and *Instruction on Respect for Human Life in Its Origin and on the Dignity of Procreation.*[12] This latter is often referred to as *Donum Vitae* and was issued in 1987.

The crux of the Catholic argument is the doctrine of the essential unity of sexual relations in marriage. Every individual "marriage act," that is, sexual encounter in marriage, must be open to the possibility of creating new life. This is because when God designed sexual relations, he invested sex with two inseparable aspects, the unitive and the procreative. These are both parts of the essential structure of the sex act, neither of which can be separated from the other. *Humanae Vitae* states:

> That teaching [that every sexual act must be open to procreation], is founded upon the inseparable connection, willed by God and unable to be broken by man on his own initiative, between the two meanings of the conjugal act: the unitive meaning and the procreative meaning. Indeed, by its intimate structure, the conjugal act, while most closely uniting husband and wife, capacitates them for the generation of new lives, according to laws inscribed in the very being of man and of woman. By safeguarding both

9. These include GIFT (gamete intrafallopian transfer), ZIFT (zygote intrafallopian transfer), and IVF (in vitro fertilization). They are similar in much of their basic processes. GIFT differs in that fertilization occurs in the body instead of in the lab. ZIFT and IVF differ slightly in terms of where in the woman's body the embryos are reinserted. For more discussion of the details of these technologies, see Scott B. Rae, *Brave New Families: Biblical Ethics and Reproductive Technologies* (Grand Rapids: Baker, 1996), chap. 6.

10. These would be cases of what is called "gestational surrogacy," in which the contracting couple contribute the genetic material, which is combined in the lab, and the embryos are implanted in the surrogate, who carries and gives birth to the child.

11. This is summarized from a more thorough exposition and critique of Catholic natural law and reproductive ethics in Rae, *Brave New Families,* chap. 2.

12. The *Instruction* is published in *Origins* 16, no. 40 (19 March 1987): 698-710. See note 1 in this chapter for further publication information on these two Vatican documents.

these essential aspects, the unitive and the procreative, the conjugal act preserves in its fullness the sense of true mutual love and its ordination towards man's most high calling to parenthood.[13]

The structure of the sex act is clearly bound up with God's creative purposes for man and woman in marriage. The intimate and unbreakable connection between the unitive and procreative purposes of sex was willed by God, is inherent to each sex act, and is necessary to give each sex act its fullness that God originally designed for it. According to this position, individual husbands and wives must not intentionally separate by any means the two divinely ordained and essential structural elements of sex in marriage: the unitive, which enables husband and wife to experience the oneness of marriage; and the procreative, which enables them to transmit life to the next generation, reflecting the creative hand of God. These two elements are rooted in the nature of human beings, and ultimately in the will of God, who placed that nature in them. Thus it is based on natural law because the teaching is grounded in that which is natural for human beings, which is ordained by God.

Donum Vitae addresses the reproductive revolution more specifically. The *Instruction* acknowledges that science and technology are a significant expression of the dominion that God originally entrusted to humankind at creation, of which medicine in general is a significant part. But moral principles from natural law must serve to limit technology appropriately.[14]

One of the fundamental values related to assisted reproduction is "the special nature of the transmission of human life in marriage." Here the *Instruction* reaffirms the essential teaching of *Humanae Vitae,* that all human procreation must take place in marriage and be connected to a specific sex act. The *Instruction* states that "from the moral point of view a truly responsible procreation vis-a-vis the unborn child must be the fruit of marriage. . . . The fidelity of the spouses in the unity of marriage involves reciprocal respect of their right to become a father and a mother only through each other. . . . in marriage and in its indissoluble unity [is] the only setting worthy of truly responsible procreation."[15] Therefore any reproductive interventions that involve third-party genetic or gestational contributors would not be allowed.[16]

13. Ibid., par. 12, p. 488.
14. *Instruction,* pp. 699-700.
15. *Instruction,* pp. 704-5.
16. The *Instruction* uses the term "heterologous artificial fertilization" to describe these. Technologies that use the genetic material of husband and wife are termed "homologous artificial fertilization."

The *Instruction* insists that these interventions violate the reciprocal commitment between the spouses in marriage, violate the right of the child, can hinder developing personal identity, and potentially damage the stability of the family for society.[17] The only reproductive technologies that are possible for faithful Catholic couples are those that use the genetic material of husband and wife. Artificial insemination by donor (AID), egg donation, and surrogate motherhood are not consistent with Catholic teaching.

The *Instruction* goes further and evaluates reproductive technologies that do not involve third-party contributors. It takes up the question, "What connection is required from the moral point of view between procreation and the conjugal act?" and answers that "The same doctrine concerning the link between the meanings of the conjugal act and between the goods of marriage throws light on the moral problem of homologous artificial fertilization (artificial insemination using the husband's sperm), *since it is never permitted to separate these different aspects to such a degree as positively to exclude either the procreative intention or the conjugal act*" (emphasis added). Thus the only morally legitimate way for procreation to occur is between husband and wife in marriage and as a result of a specific act of intercourse. The intrinsic nature of the act of sex is rendered incomplete by separating sexual relations from procreation. The *Instruction* puts it this way:

> From the moral point of view, procreation is deprived of its proper perfection when it is not desired as the fruit of the conjugal act, that is to say, of the specific act of the spouses' union. . . . The moral relevance of the link between the meaning of the conjugal act and the goods of marriage as well as the unity of the human being and the dignity of his origin, demand that the procreation of a human person be brought about as the fruit of the conjugal act specific to the love between spouses.[18]

Thus morally legitimate procreation must occur as the result of a specific sexual union in marriage. On in vitro fertilization, for example, the *Instruction* states that "the act of conjugal love is considered in the teaching of the Church as the only setting worthy of human procreation."[19] Therefore, in vitro fertilization, zygote intrafallopian transfer, embryo transfer, and artificial insemination are all judged to be morally problematic.[20] Virtually all repro-

---

17. *Instruction,* p. 705.
18. *Instruction,* p. 706.
19. *Instruction,* p. 707.
20. The *Instruction* does make an important distinction between a technology that *assists* normal intercourse and one that *replaces* it in the process of trying to conceive a

ductive technology according to the standard of practice is judged to be morally inappropriate.

The Scripture affirms the essential goodness of both the unitive and procreative aspects of sex, but there does not appear to be any biblical demand that the two aspects always be linked. The creation account establishes that the spheres of marriage and procreation be connected, but does not require that every time a couple has sexual relations it be open to procreation.

The Scripture affirms that sex has a variety of purposes, all of which are ordained only within the confines of marriage. For example, it clearly teaches that sex is one of the means by which a couple experiences the physical oneness and spiritual unity that is a part of the mystery of marriage (Gen. 2:24; Eph. 5:29-33). Second, sex was given for procreation. Third, it is designed for pleasure and is one of the ways a couple enjoy each other. Scripture views sex as good within marriage if it is an expression of a couple's love for each other. In fact, sexual pleasure between married persons is good even if pleasure is the only objective for any particular sexual act.

The Song of Solomon bears eloquent testimony to the high place Scripture gives to sexual pleasure. The royal couple in the Song revel in each other's love, exhibiting a depth of passion that most couples would like to reproduce in their own marriage. The imagery of sex as a meal of choice foods (4:13–5:1) indicates that pleasure was the objective of the couple on their wedding night. The way in which they describe each other's bodies in exquisite figures of speech (4:1-7; 6:4-9; 7:1-8) makes it clear that pleasure is the purpose for the sex recorded in the book. Interestingly, in the entire book there is not one mention of children or procreation. If the unitive and procreative purposes of sex must always go together, this is a most unusual omission. It seems to point to pleasure as an inherent and self-sufficient purpose of sex, apart from any procreative intention.

Similarly in I Corinthians 7, Paul speaks of sex as a source of physical release and enjoyment, since it is better to marry than to burn with passion (v. 9). Paul commands that husbands and wives come together for sex regularly so that they will not be tempted to look elsewhere for the pleasure of sex (vv. 2, 5; this seems to be the meaning of the phrase in v. 2, "because there is

---

child. Anything that assists intercourse is considered a part of God's wisdom that can be utilized in reproduction. The important aspect is that the unity of sex and procreation is maintained. What this means more specifically is that conception must occur according to its intended design. The movement of genetic materials may be assisted, but use of technology may not replace normal intercourse. For example, fertilization must always occur inside the body, and masturbation may not be used as a substitute for sex in order to collect sperm outside the body to be reinserted back into the woman.

so much immorality"). They are commanded not to deprive each other, presumably of the pleasure of sex (and perhaps also the source of physical release), except by mutual consent for temporary periods of prayer and contemplation (v. 5). Husbands and wives are enjoined to fulfill their conjugal (not necessarily procreative) duties to each other (vv. 3-4), and nowhere in this passage does it mention children. Rather, in this passage the purpose of giving pleasure to one's spouse appears to be the sole and sufficient reason for sexual relations. The Scripture does not recognize a necessary connection between the unitive and procreative purposes of sex. Thus, if it is biblically appropriate to separate the purposes for sex, and to separate the pleasure aspect from the procreative by using birth control, then it must be legitimate to separate procreation from sex by using some reproductive technologies.

A second criticism of the Catholic position is that the prohibition of medical technology to alleviate infertility is arbitrary and overly restrictive, particularly in light of the place of technology in God's economy. In view of technology as a legitimate exercise of human beings' dominion over creation, clearly sanctioned by the Catholic Church in these documents, it is odd and arbitrary that practically no technology is allowed to cure infertility. Since human beings are not only allowed but are entrusted with extensive dominion over most other areas of life, it seems inconsistent to deny them the same dominion over sex and procreation. This is particularly the case since reproductive technologies are medical technologies. Catholic teaching routinely allows for medical technology to intervene to restore malfunctioning organs and systems to their proper natural function. Many Catholic thinkers have difficulty understanding how reproductive technologies can be consistently excluded from legitimate medical treatment.[21] Not only does medicine intervene, but at times it substitutes for a failing bodily function. For example, dialysis substitutes for diseased kidney functions, ventilators substitute for diseased lungs, and pacemakers substitute for critical heart functions in the same way that some reproductive technologies substitute for diseased fertility functions. The technological developments that enable human beings to more effectively exercise dominion over the creation reflect a part of our cre-

---

21. See, for example, Edward Collins Vacek, S.J., "Catholic Natural Law and Reproductive Ethics," *Journal of Medicine and Philosophy* 17 (1992): 329-46. For a non-Catholic critique of the *Instruction* and a positive assessment of virtually all reproductive technologies, see the statement by the Ethics Committee of the American Fertility Society entitled "Ethical Considerations of the New Reproductive Technologies in Light of *Instruction on the Respect for Human Life in Its Origin and the Dignity of Procreation*," *Fertility and Sterility*, Supplement 1, vol. 49, no. 2 (February 1988), reprinted in *Ethical Issues in the New Reproductive Technologies*, pp. 8-20.

ative makeup that comes from our Creator. Professor Sidney Callahan speaks to the natural law aspects by suggesting that "the mastery of nature through technological problem solving is also completely natural to our rational species; indeed it is the glory of *homo sapiens*."[22] Thus the Catholic position that prohibits virtually all reproductive technological interventions does not seem to be warranted in view of biblical teaching on sex in marriage (which allows couples to separate the unitive and procreative elements of sex) and the theological notion of technology as a part of human beings' dominion over creation (i.e., excluding reproductive technology is arbitrary and inconsistent with the Catholic general acceptance of medical technology). There is no sound biblical reason to reject reproductive technologies per se.

However, rejection of the Catholic position on reproductive technologies does not mean accepting all reproductive interventions uncritically. There is a morally significant difference between those technologies that involve the genetic materials of husband and wife and those that require third-party contributors, of eggs, sperm, or womb. Technologies that can be used with the gametes of the married couple include intrauterine insemination (IUI), gamete intrafallopian transfer (GIFT), zygote intrafallopian transfer (ZIFT), IVF, and various types of sperm injection. Those that require a third-party contributor include donor insemination (DI), egg donation, and all types of surrogate motherhood. Within other guidelines set by theological principles, there is no good reason to reject technologies that employ the genes of a married couple. This seems consistent with biblical teaching about marriage, family, and procreation which limits procreation to the sphere of marriage. That is, God's design from creation is that children are to be procreated into a family that is built around heterosexual marriage.[23] Thus tech-

---

22. Sidney Callahan, "Lovemaking and Babymaking," *Commonweal* 114 (1987): 233-39, at 234.

23. This is spelled out in more detail in Rae, *Brave New Families*, chap. 1, entitled "Reproductive Technologies and a Theology of the Family." Here is a summary of the argument. In Gen. 1–2 there is a critical link between the man and woman in the context of marriage and the procreation of children. The institution of the family is clearly related to the command in Gen. 1:28 to "be fruitful and multiply." Though there are two creation accounts in Gen. 1–2, they are complementary and not contradictory. Gen. 1 provides the broad panoramic overview of creation. Gen. 2 views the most important aspects of creation, the creation of man and woman, their relationship to each other and to God, in more detail. Thus the account of the creation of man and woman that is described in Gen. 2:18-25 actually fits into the broader overview of Gen. 1. To be specific, it occurs after the divine initiative in 1:26 to create humankind and prior to the command to the newly formed couple in 1:28 to begin procreating and populating the earth. Thus the creation of humankind is described generally in 1:26 and specifically in the male and female of the

nologies in which only the genetic materials of the couple are required generally are not problematic.

Thus there does not appear to be any moral problem with using artificial insemination by husband (AIH), since this is a relatively simple procedure that gives the husband's sperm an additional impetus to fertilize the egg. It is often used in conjunction with fertility drugs, so the couple who uses this technology should be prepared for twins or triplets. The technologies that constitute the IVF family (GIFT, ZIFT and IVF), in which multiple ovulation is stimulated, eggs are surgically extracted and fertilized in the lab, and embryos are reinserted into the woman, are more complicated, and require appeal to other theological principles for moral parameters.[24] Though in GIFT fertilization occurs in the body, the normal procedure for all three in the IVF family is to fertilize all the eggs that are harvested and place the extra embryos in storage for future use if necessary. This is done primarily to minimize the burden to the couple, since egg retrieval is the most expensive and physically burdensome aspect of the entire process. If the couple conceive, especially multiples, then they no longer require the additional embryos that are in storage. In most infertility clinics these are routinely discarded when no longer needed. In rare cases they are donated to another infertile couple. As will be argued in chapters 4 and 5, discarding unwanted embryos is very problematic since the biblical teaching strongly suggests that personhood begins at conception. Unless the couple can insure that leftover embryos will not be discarded, these technologies violate an important theological parameter governing the use of this technology. The day when eggs can be stored is coming shortly, and embryo storage will not be as necessary. But to fertilize eggs

---

species in 2:18-25. The first command given to them that is recorded by Scripture is the command to reproduce in 1:28. Placing the more specific account of the creation of male and female and the subsequent institution of marriage back into the broader context of the creation in 1:26, the command to procreate is thus given to Adam and Eve in the context of their leaving, cleaving and becoming one flesh, that is, in the context of marriage. Though it is true that Adam and Eve are representative in a broader sense of the first male and female of the species, it is also true that this sets the precedent for heterosexual marriage and procreation within that setting. Though it clearly does not suggest that every male and female must be joined in marriage, it does indicate that marriage is to be between male and female, and only in marriage is procreation to occur. In other words, God has set up procreation to be restricted to heterosexual couples in marriage. There is continuity between God's creation of the family in Gen. 1–2 and the command to procreate within that context. This structure of the family seems to be basic to God's creative design, however extended the family became due to cultural and economic factors.

24. This is a summary of the moral problems with these procedures. They will be addressed in more detail in chapter 5.

that have been thawed out after being in storage requires sperm injection technology, which is considerably more expensive.[25] Given that reality, couples may still opt for the less expensive embryo storage as part of the process. If the couple is willing to take steps to insure that no embryos are discarded or damaged, then this family of technologies is morally appropriate.

Technologies that involve third-party contributors are more morally ambiguous. Egg and sperm donation are done routinely, and surrogate motherhood is a well-established practice in much of the world. The implications of relevant biblical passages have been the subject of considerable debate. It would appear at first glance that third-party contributors' involvement in procreation would violate the creation norm. But God allowed a variety of "violations" of the creation model in the Old Testament, from divorce to polygamy to surrogate motherhood. Of course, God's allowance of a practice does not constitute its sanction as a moral norm. But given the way the New Testament gives great weight to the order of creation, it would appear that the balance of Scripture tilts against legitimizing third-party contributors to procreation.[26] One should acknowledge the ongoing debate in this area within the Christian community and admit that the Scripture may not be clear enough to warrant a blanket prohibition of surrogate motherhood in particular.[27] However, it surely is a problem when single women want to use donor sperm to have their own child, apart from marriage and family relationships. This violates the creation norm for procreation, in that a child is not procreated into a stable heterosexual marriage, with both mother and father needed for child rearing. Intentionally creating "no-dad families" is problematic, particularly in today's culture in which the problems of children without a father figure are becoming more apparent.

Surrogate motherhood is morally problematic for other reasons besides the involvement of a third-party contributor. To explain why, a brief description of the process may prove instructive. Some of these arrangements depend on whether or not a fee is received and whether or not the surrogate mother contributes the egg as well as the womb. When the surrogate is hired for a fee, roughly $10,000-15,000 plus expenses, it is called commercial surrogacy. When she bears the child out of the goodness of her heart for no fee, it is

25. See Shari Roan, "Births from Thawed Eggs Reported," *Los Angeles Times,* 17 October 1997, pp. A1, 29-30.

26. For example, see Paul's argument against homosexuality in Rom. 1, or his argument dealing with women in the church in I Cor. 11 and I Tim. 2. In each of these texts, appeal to the norm of creation is considered sufficient to settle the debate at hand.

27. See Rae, *Brave New Families* (chap. 1), for more development of the biblical teaching on third-party contributors to procreation. See also Gary Stewart et al., *Sexuality and Reproductive Technology* (Grand Rapids: Kregel, 1998).

called altruistic surrogacy. As might be expected, the overwhelming majority of surrogacy situations are commercial, since most women would not bear a child they would not keep and raise without significant financial inducement. When the surrogate contributes the egg and gives birth to the child, she is said to be a genetic surrogate, since she is genetically related to the child she is carrying. She is simply inseminated with the sperm from the husband of the couple who has contracted her. The surrogate here is clearly the mother, since she provides all the relevant aspects of motherhood, both egg and gestational environment. When she does not contribute the egg, she is a gestational surrogate, since she is only providing the gestational environment for the child. In those cases, the woman who contracts the surrogate provides the egg and her husband's sperm is used to fertilize it in the lab through in vitro fertilization. The resulting embryo is placed in the uterus of the surrogate, and she gives birth to the child. There is considerable debate over who is the mother in these gestational surrogacy arrangements. There are numerous variables in this scenario, including the possible use of donor sperm and eggs and the fertilization of multiple eggs. In most surrogacy cases, however, the surrogate provides both the womb and the egg. She is simply inseminated with the sperm from the husband in the contracting couple.

Commercial surrogacy is problematic because it is the equivalent of baby selling. In most cases the surrogate receives a fee of $10,000 or more, in addition to expenses related to the pregnancy and delivery, in exchange for the child being turned over to the couple who has contracted and paid her. If the parties in a surrogacy arrangement were doing the same thing in an adoption situation, they would all be in violation of the law, since adoption laws prohibit the purchase and sale of children. Such a practice violates the Thirteenth Amendment to the Constitution, which outlawed slavery, for precisely the same reason: human beings, particularly the most vulnerable in the human community, should not be objects of barter. It is a fundamental assault on their dignity, and not only is it immoral, it should also be illegal. If the surrogate receives no money except expenses, then she is free of the charge of baby selling, but those cases are extremely rare and would fall under the same heading as other third-party procreative arrangements. If the surrogate does not contribute the egg but only provides the gestational environment for the child, then that also may be different, depending on how one assigns maternal rights in this scenario.[28] The vast majority of surrogacy cases involve baby

---

28. For more detail on the controversial practice of surrogate motherhood, both on the baby-selling aspect and the definition of the mother, see Scott B. Rae, *The Ethics of Commercial Surrogate Motherhood* (Westport, Conn.: Praeger, 1994).

selling, since the surrogate contributes the egg and receives a fee for delivery of the child.

There does not seem to be any reason to reject technology that is used to alleviate infertility, but there are moral parameters for appropriate use of such technology. Technologies that use the genes of a married couple are generally acceptable, as long as embryos are not discarded or damaged in the process. Technologies that require third-party contributors to procreation are more morally questionable — especially when the genetic link between parents and child is broken through the use of donor eggs or sperm — and probably should not be recommended. Surrogate motherhood in its most common form, in which the surrogate provides the egg, gives birth to the child, and receives a substantial fee for waiving her parental rights to the child, is both unethical and should be illegal since it constitutes the purchase and sale of children.

Human Cloning

Up until the past five years, human cloning was the subject of science fiction and even had an entry in the *Encyclopedia of Science Fiction.* From its beginning in Aldous Huxley's *Brave New World* to the mid-seventies novel by Ira Levin, and later a movie, *The Boys from Brazil,* in which a group of neo-Nazis attempt to clone a whole host of Hitlers, to the most recent example in the blockbuster movie *Jurassic Park,* cloning has never been viewed as something that society would actually have to face. It had always been something that was, at best, a distant, remote possibility. With the cloning of human embryos in 1993 and the cloning of an adult sheep in 1996, what was previously left to one's imagination is now becoming technologically feasible. Scientists are now able to clone or copy human embryos, and the technology to clone an adult human being may not be far off in the future. It is no longer strictly in the realm of science fiction.

When referring to human cloning, one should distinguish between cloning of embryos, which was originally done to assist infertile couples with treatments such as IVF, and cloning of adult human beings, also called somatic cell nuclear transfer, which to date has only been successful with animals. These are two different processes with overlapping ethical issues. Two different American government agencies have convened and issued reports on each of these different technologies. The National Institutes of Health convened the Embryo Research Panel in 1994 to outline the parameters for research on human embryos, some of which were created by the process of cloning.[29] In response to the successful cloning of an adult sheep in mid-1996, President Clinton convened the National Bioethics Advisory Commission (NBAC) to study and issue a report on this cloning procedure.[30]

Theologically based objections to both types of human cloning were quickly forthcoming soon after the technologies were announced. For example, the 8 November 1993 issue of *Time* magazine referred to in the introduction to this chapter was a vivid reminder that many people considered embryo cloning the equivalent of human beings taking a prerogative that belonged to God alone. It also called into question a fundamental Judeo-Christian assumption about human beings being unique creations of God, since that presumably unique genetic design was now capable of being copied outside of the body. Similar objections were raised by religious leaders when an adult sheep was cloned through nuclear transfer. Shortly after the announcement of the cloning of Dolly, the adult sheep cloned by researchers in Scotland, religious leaders from predominantly Roman Catholic and evangelical Protestant perspectives appeared in various media outlets and condemned the prospect of human cloning and sought government assistance in prohibiting the practice.[31] But other religious leaders, particularly those who testified before the NBAC, supported human cloning as a morally and theologically acceptable practice.[32] Debate over human cloning has been going on in theological circles for roughly the last twenty-five years.

Cloning of embryos in the lab does not appear to present any problems per se, since researchers are merely duplicating in the lab the natural

---

29. *Report of the Human Embryo Research Panel* (Washington, D.C.: National Institutes of Health, 27 September 1994). For commentary on this panel report and more discussion of embryo research and cloning, see Scott B. Rae, *Embryo and Fetal Research and Experimentation*, Crossroads Monograph Series on Faith and Public Policy, vol. 1, no. 15.

30. See note 3 above.

31. See, for example, Allen Verhey, who draws on the work of the late Paul Ramsey (*Fabricated Man: The Ethics of Genetic Control* [New Haven: Yale University Press, 1970]) in his two articles, "Cloning: Revisiting an Old Debate," *Kennedy Institute of Ethics Journal* 4, no. 3 (September 1994): 207-34, and "Playing God and Invoking a Perspective," *Journal of Medicine and Philosophy* 20 (1995): 347-64, and Gilbert Meilaender in his testimony before the NBAC panel. The testimony of theologians from a variety of traditions is included in chapter 3 of the NBAC report. Roman Catholic theologians who have opposed cloning include Richard A. McCormick, "Should We Clone Humans?" *Christian Century*, 17-24 November 1993, pp. 1148-49, and Lisa Cahill and Thomas Shannon in their testimony before the NBAC panel. Cloning is also opposed by the official Catholic document on reproductive technologies, *Donum Vitae*, cited earlier in this chapter.

32. For example, some Jewish theologians expressed openness to the NBAC panel about allowing nuclear transfer under some circumstances.

process that occurs in the body when identical twins or triplets are produced. The process was originally designed to help infertile couples maximize their chances at achieving pregnancy and minimize the expense and burden on the woman. This was done by cloning the original group of embryos and keeping them in storage for future use if necessary. There does not seem to be any morally significant difference between in vitro fertilization and embryo cloning. They are different aspects of a similar process. Of course, one can reject cloning and IVF both and be consistent. The primary ground for such a rejection is that both processes turn procreation into a production process, with the risk of children being objectified. That is, if procreation is done outside of the setting of sex in marriage, it cannot be the fruit of a couple's love. But the Scripture does not demand that the unitive and the procreative aspects of sex be combined in every case, as argued above. Further, children born out of IVF arrangements are desperately wanted children, whose parents welcome them as precious gifts for whom they have waited, often for many years. They are hardly objectified, and the fact that they were conceived through technologically assisted procedures rather than through natural sexual relations has no bearing on how the parents will love and accept those children. Though they are not born out of a specific act of sexual love between a married couple, it does not follow that these children are not born into a loving and caring family. Nor does it necessarily follow that their dignity is compromised by the process, since they are full persons with the image of God irrespective of the mode of conception. As argued above, there is no morally compelling reason to reject reproductive technologies such as IVF outright, and no reason to reject embryo cloning per se. To be sure, embryo cloning has the same moral dilemmas that IVF does, namely, the potential destruction of embryonic persons if the couple finishes conceiving its family and no longer has use for the embryos. The same restrictions that are used with IVF should apply to cloned embryos. This is also true for cloned embryos that are used for research purposes instead of helping to treat infertility.

Cloning for research purposes is highly problematic since all of the embryos used in the research are either fatally damaged during the research process or discarded after the research is finished. The degree to which the process of cloning damages the embryos in question raises serious problems with the process itself and may cast the entire practice in a negative light. But assuming that damage to embryos is avoided, either in the cloning process or after the couple is finished with procreation, there does not seem to be any inherent problem with such a technology.

However, the reason for cloning embryos, or the use to which cloned embryos will be put, is another question. Although the technology is per se acceptable, each potential application of it demands moral examination. Potential uses of cloned embryos include a form of "life insurance," or a way of "replacing" a child who has died prematurely. However, it is unlikely that parents will use a cloned embryo for this purpose, since it is not hard to imagine an identical twin born some years later as a daily painful reminder of the deceased child, actually cementing the parents in grief as they daily encounter this "replacement." Further, a child who is born and expected to substitute raises questions about how that child will be allowed to develop his or her own unique personal identity. Since environment as well as genetics significantly shape the person, this child will not be the same identical person, only a genetic duplicate of his or her deceased sibling. He or she will be a very different person developmentally.

A second potential use for cloned embryos is for a form of "health insurance," if an existing child is in need of compatible tissue or organs for transplant. Children have been conceived in the hope of producing an exact tissue match in some cases, and with cloning there would be no doubt. This practice raises serious questions about the donor's informed consent — at least if he or she was conceived for the purpose of making a bodily donation that entails at least a minimal risk of bodily harm. The problem is particularly severe if the risk is life threatening.

A third potential use, which would be entirely unacceptable, is cloning embryos for purchase and sale in the open market. It does not take much imagination to see the appeal of the genetic material of well-endowed athletes or models and the attraction of such a product on the open market. However, the supply for such embryos may actually far exceed the demand, since most parents place high value in procreation in the transmission of their genetic material, not someone else's. That is why infertile couples will go to great lengths to have a child of their own through assisted reproductive technology, rather than resort to adoption. There is great appeal in having one's own child, not someone else's. That is not to say that there will not be any demand for such well-endowed embryos, and in such a case the law should prohibit purchase and sale of human beings. At the least, the law should continue to prohibit sale of human organs and tissues, though embryos are clearly much more than "products of conception."

Cloning of mature adults, or somatic cell nuclear transfer, is what most people envision when the term "human cloning" is used. Its fascination is more with its novelty than with any particular use, and most who do not object to this kind of cloning only favor it in limited circumstances with rigid regulation to prevent abuses. Most people who object to cloning in this way see the benefits of medical technology in general but insist that use of this technology crosses moral limits and does not fit in the realm of responsible dominion over creation.[33]

Rather than copying embryos in the lab, as is done with embryo cloning, somatic cell nuclear transfer involves taking mature cells from the original and placing them in an egg that has had its nucleus removed — all other parts are kept intact — so that it can nourish the developing embryo. A few days later it is placed in the uterus of a surrogate mother, and if all goes properly it develops into a genetic twin of the original. This has only been accomplished to date in animals, but the procedure shows promise for application to human beings. There is, however, great debate concerning the time frame for such human application.

Virtually everyone in the bioethics community agrees that if somatic cell nuclear transfer cloning is successful in human beings, the child who is born from such a process will be a person who should be valued as would any other person, and should enjoy all the privileges of membership in the human community. There is no reason to think that a cloned person would not possess a soul or be made in the image of God, as would any other person who is procreated through normal sexual relations. How the soul would precisely be acquired is a different question, and is very difficult to say for sure.[34] The full personhood of cloned human beings makes it not only unethical but also unlikely that cloning would produce some sort of subhuman entities, who could perhaps be employed to perform mindless menial tasks that most people do not want to do, as was the case in the film *Blade Runner*.

As is the case with embryo cloning and other reproductive and genetic technologies, the ability to perform somatic cell nuclear transfer has come from God in the form of general revelation and common grace. Human beings could not have developed it were it not for God equipping them with the skills to unlock the creation and further responsible human dominion over

33. For examples of these positions, see the NBAC report, chaps. 3–4. A broad theological-ethical analysis of human cloning can also be found in John F. Kilner, "Human Cloning," in *The Reproduction Revolution: A Christian Appraisal,* ed. John F. Kilner et al. (Grand Rapids: Eerdmans/Paternoster, 1999).

34. For someone who holds to a creationist view of the transmission of the soul, this would not be a problem, since God directly creates a new soul each time a child is procreated. This is more of a problem for one who holds to a traducean view of the soul, that the soul is transmitted to the child through the parents. How one would explain the transmission of the soul to a cloned person from a traducean perspective is not clear. For more detail on this aspect of human cloning, see J. P. Moreland and Scott B. Rae, *On Human Persons: Metaphysical and Ethical Reflections* (Downers Grove, Ill.: InterVarsity, forthcoming).

what God has entrusted to human beings. Cloning technology is an extension of other types of reproductive technologies, and it is not an accident that human beings have somehow stumbled onto this technology, apart from God's common grace. As is true with all medical technologies, cloning possesses the potential for benefit or harm. Each potential use of cloning technology should be subject to moral assessment. It may be that there are no morally acceptable uses of this technology either now or in the foreseeable future. If that is the case, then there is no reason to go ahead with the technology and it is appropriate to enact legislation to prohibit it. Seeing technology in the light of God's general revelation should make one hesitant to suggest that cloning technology is inherently unethical. Many Catholic opponents of cloning hold that the process is per se immoral because it compromises the dignity and individuality of the "original" and the clone.[35] However, identical twins routinely "compromise" this notion of identity when they occur either naturally or through the use of mainstream reproductive technologies. In addition, there is more to a child's identity than simply genetics. Society should resist the notion that a person's identity is reducible to his or her genetic code, since what makes a person unique is far more than merely genetics. Identical twins or triplets are not the same persons because they develop differently and have different defining experiences in their lives.

Other than for curiosity and the narcissism of literally reproducing oneself genetically, one does wonder about the potential applications of cloning technology, particularly given the high cost of the process to any individual or couple who wanted to use it. Clearly inappropriate and immoral reasons for cloning would be to have cloned persons as organ donors, for eugenic purposes, for purchase and sale on the open market, or to produce clones with diminished autonomy, which would likely have to be done in conjunction with some sort of genetic technology. These are all immoral because the cloned person is just that, a person, and a person cannot be used for any of the above ends. It is unjustified to use persons as a source of biological spare parts, particularly if donation would result in their death. Producing a clone if an exact tissue match were necessary and could not be found anywhere else is less troublesome, but the problems with informed consent noted earlier remain. It is further immoral to buy and sell human beings or human genetic material on the open market, since human beings are not objects of barter. Eugenics has been consistently and justifiably condemned since the early days of this century, and cloning for eugenic purposes is not an appropriate use for this technology.

35. See NBAC, pp. 49-51.

Admittedly, some exceptional justifications seem more appealing at first glance than others. For instance, the rabbis who testified before the NBAC panel on cloning suggested that it might be justified to clone a person who is sterile, the last in his lineage whose predecessors were killed in the Holocaust.[36] Or take the person who has a life-threatening disease who needs a bone marrow transplant and no other tissue match can be found. In these cases parents have conceived a child in order to provide a tissue match, yet with cloning technology they could be sure there would be a perfect match. It is assumed that the parents would love and raise the child after the donation is made. Or consider the parents who both carry a recessive gene for a lethal genetic disorder. In order to avoid the risk of passing on the gene (the child has a one-in-four chance of inheriting both recessive genes), they opt for cloning when they discover that their other options include use of donor genetic materials; natural conception and selective abortion, which they oppose; or IVF and selective implantation of embryos, which they also oppose due to their view that personhood begins at conception. In these limited circumstances, cloning an adult as a means of procreating a child looks very appealing. However, these cases are so rare that, before using them alone as a basis for justifying the technology, we must be careful to take into consideration everything else that is at stake in opening the door to human cloning.

There are indeed some significant concerns about the technology per se that suggest that it should not be used, even for the above rare and justifiable reasons. One principal concern is the harm that will result to the embryo in the process. This was a major concern of the NBAC panel that prompted it to recommend that the technology as used to produce a child be prohibited.[37] When Scottish researchers cloned their now-famous sheep, Dolly, the technique failed in the overwhelming majority of attempts. Dolly was a single success accompanied by 277 failures, all of which resulted in the destruction of the embryo at some point in the process.[38] Other potential harms to parties in the process include hormonal manipulation in the egg donor, multiple miscarriages in the birth mother, and possible severe abnormalities in the child. The NBAC panel concluded, based on these harms, that

> Standard practice in biomedical science and clinical care would never allow the use of a medical drug or device on a human being on the basis of such a preliminary study and without much additional animal research. More-

36. NBAC, p. 55.
37. NBAC, p. 65.
38. NBAC, p. 65. See also Ian Wilmut et al., "Viable Offspring Derived from Fetal and Adult Mammalian Cells," *Nature* 385 (1997): 810-13.

over, when risks are taken with an innovative therapy, the justification lies in the prospect of treating an illness in a patient, whereas, here no patient is at risk until the innovation is employed. Thus, no conscientious physician or Institutional Review Board should approve attempts to use somatic cell nuclear transfer to create a child at this time.[39]

There would appear to be significant flaws in the technology that would preclude its use in human beings, at least at this time. The prospect of harm to all parties involved, particularly the child to be born, suggests that the couple or individual contemplating cloning should adhere to the same standards for the sanctity of unborn life that would be followed in other reproductive technologies. Since the embryo is a person from conception onward, the embryo is entitled to the same protections and rights to life as any other person.

A second concern has to do with the way procreation would be transformed by this technology. It is entirely possible that society would see cloned children as made rather than begotten, or produced rather than procreated.[40] It is possible that cloning could transform the way children are viewed — that is, as products of technology rather than gifts of God created in love.[41] These objections were raised in regard to IVF technology as well, but there is no reason why cloned children could not be seen in the same way as children from IVF, as loved and very much wanted children. If the purpose for cloning a child or adult suggested using the clone as a means rather than an end, then that use would be problematic, as opposed to the technology itself. A further and related concern is that with cloning and other technological developments in reproduction, it would be possible to procreate children entirely apart from not only marriage but also relationships. If and when human cloning is successful, men would no longer be necessary for procreation, since the mother could clone herself and carry her own clone. Add to that the advent of artificial wombs, and women would no longer be necessary to gestate and give birth to children. Catholic theologian Lisa Sowle Cahill, in her testimony before the NBAC panel, suggested that "At the extreme, cloning humans would not only free human reproduction from marital and male-female relationships, but would allow for the emancipation of human reproduction from *any* relationship."[42] This concern, in addition to the serious

---

39. NBAC, p. 65.

40. The phrase "made not begotten" is taken from the Anglican theologian Oliver O'Donovan in his work *Begotten or Made?* (Oxford: Clarendon, 1984).

41. NBAC, p. 53.

42. NBAC, p. 53. See also R. A. Mohler, "The Brave New World of Cloning: A Christian Worldview Perspective" (unpublished manuscript, March 1997).

potential for harm to the parties involved in the process, suggests that the harms of using cloning technology outweigh the few and rare justifiable uses. It is hard to imagine justifiably allocating resources for it, given the other pressing health care needs in society today.

Genetic Therapy and Engineering

Since the beginning of the genetic revolution, opponents have charged that genetic engineering was "playing God" with the building blocks of human life and should not be attempted. They argued that people should accept the roll of the genetic dice as from the hand of God, and not manipulate life at its biological core. As genetic technologies progress, researchers hold out the promise of curing genetic disorders by techniques such as gene splicing and gene surgery, both in adults and embryos. There is still some debate in the scientific community as to the time frame for application of genetic engineering technologies, and the moral discussion has been going on since the 1960s.

One should distinguish between somatic cell therapy, which corrects a genetic defect in the individual for that person only, and germ line therapy, which is a genetic alteration on a sex-linked chromosome, which thus passes on the modification to succeeding generations. In addition, there is a distinction between correction therapy, which corrects a genetic defect widely held to be harmful, and enhancement therapy, which takes existing traits and magnifies them or allows parents to select particular traits such as eye or hair color for their children. This could also be termed a distinction between therapeutic and eugenic genetic therapies. How to draw lines that separate morally acceptable uses from morally unacceptable uses is difficult, since there are not significant differences in the type of technology used. The difference is in the intent and purpose for using such a technology as well as the types of genes altered, whether somatic cells or germ line cells.

As is true with other medical technology, there is no reason not to welcome genetic interventions as a part of God's general revelation and common grace. Surely the skills that researchers possess to unlock the mysteries of the human genetic code come ultimately from God in his common grace. Genetic technology has the potential to cure patients suffering from genetic anomalies and thus help reverse the effects of the entrance of sin into the world. It clearly fits in the realm of medical technology that we can see as God's good gift to enable humankind to continue exercising dominion over the earth. As with other medical technologies, society and practitioners must distinguish between the technology per se and the appropriate uses of such technology.

The above assessment applies to somatic cell therapy, since the potential harms and benefits are restricted to the patient himself or herself. There is no reason why somatic cell therapy shouldn't be viewed as any other medical technology used to correct a medical problem. Up until a few years ago, genetic diseases were accepted as having no cure. With the prospect of genetic interventions to correct defective genes, there does not seem to be any morally significant difference between genetic therapy and other types of medical treatment. However, germ line therapy involves more risk to succeeding generations. Given the level of our understanding of the genetic code at this time and how recent germ line therapy has been developed, the potential risks of germ line therapy are a significant unknown. Researchers simply do not yet know if they are setting a process of inheritance in motion that will bring harm ultimately to the patient and to his or her succeeding generations. Because of unknowns and the fact that they cannot be reversed once put in place, it seems more prudent at this time to limit genetic therapies to somatic cell therapies until the risks of germ line therapies can be more clearly assessed. There does not seem to be any principled reason to reject germ line therapies once they are shown to be safe, if that indeed can be done.

The more difficult aspect of genetic therapies is how to draw the line between correction and enhancement, or eugenic therapies. What makes this difficult is that one's notion of a defect can be subjective. For example, someone who is diminutive in height might consider that a defect for which treatment, such as the human growth hormone, would be appropriate. Others may consider a certain hair or eye color to be a defect and desire genetic therapy to "treat" it. Parents might come to procreation with certain expectations for IQ or other traits and be tempted to select traits that accord best with their expectations. If correction therapy is appropriate, then why not enhancement therapy as well, especially given the similarity of the technology?

One theological principle that is an implication of what we've already suggested about medical technology is that humanity is called in the exercise of dominion over creation to resist the effects of the entrance of sin into the world. Similarly, throughout the Scripture God has called his people to fight the effects of sin in the world and to contest the conditions that are a consequence of sin. In other words, God's people are called to battle sin and attempt to alleviate its consequences. To use genetic technology to correct the gene for Down syndrome or Huntington's disease clearly fits within that mandate to resist sin and its effects. However, it cannot be said that being short (unless it is dwarfism), having a certain eye or hair color, or having an IQ that is only average (and not the result of any retardation) is the effect of the entrance of sin into the world. For example, cancer or heart disease is clearly the result of living in a fallen world. Having brown hair instead of blond is not. Theologian John Feinberg puts it this way: "if there is a condition in a human being (whether physical or psychological) and if there is something that genetic technology could do to address that problem, then use of this technology would be acceptable. In effect, we would be using this technology to fight sin and its consequences."[43] This would be an acceptable use of these technologies, consistent with the use of other medical technologies. If correcting human fallenness is not at issue, then an intervention is fostering a trait in a manner somewhat analogous to the process of cosmetic surgery.[44] Such intervention is particularly problematic morally when some people's standards are forced upon others, as would be the case in germ line or prenatal intervention.

Prenatal Genetic Testing

Prenatal genetic testing can be done through a variety of different technologies, ranging from routine and noninvasive ultrasound to invasive and sometimes risky amniocentesis and CVS (chorionic villi sampling) testing.[45] These technologies enable physicians to look into the womb and examine the genetic structure of tiny newborns and even smaller embryos. This technology too is an expression of God's general revelation. His wisdom revealed outside of Scripture has enabled human beings to develop the technology that identifies genetic diseases, which are the result of the entrance of sin into the world.[46] Thus, per

43. John S. Feinberg, "A Theological Basis for Genetic Interventions," in *Genetic Ethics: Do the Ends Justify the Genes?* ed. John F. Kilner et al. (Grand Rapids: Eerdmans/Paternoster, 1997), pp. 183-92, at 187.

44. Though cosmetic surgery can be seen as alleviating the effects of aging, another result of the Fall.

45. Amniocentesis involves drawing out some of the amniotic fluid from the pregnant woman's abdomen and examining some of the cells that the baby has sloughed off. It has a 1 to 2 percent risk of miscarriage. CVS is a similar test which also captures some of the fetus's cells but gets them from a different place in the woman's body. The chorionic villi make up the edges of the placenta, and they look like a cluster of small hairs that surround the sides of the placenta. The physician will obtain the chorionic villi either through the woman's abdomen, similar to amniocentesis, or through the cervix with a catheter. The advantage of this test is that it can be performed earlier in the pregnancy, around the tenth to twelfth week, during the first trimester of pregnancy.

46. That is not to say that any specific genetic disease is the result of a specific sin committed by one of the parents of the child in question. Far from it. Genetic diseases are the result of the general presence of sin in the world.

se, prenatal genetic testing does not appear to be wrong. That does not suggest necessarily that couples are morally obligated to use the available testing technology. But it is important that couples acknowledge that the womb is still "the secret place" over which God alone ultimately has control (Ps. 139:15). Further, they should realize that these tests are not infallible (all have some margin of error, greater for some than others) and some do involve a degree of risk both to the mother and the fetus. If the benefit of obtaining the information is greater than or proportionate to the risk incurred in the test, then utilizing genetic testing technology is morally appropriate. The amount of genetic information that is available to couples is increasing exponentially with the progress of the Human Genome Project, an international effort to map the entire human genetic code. Researchers have discovered hundreds of different genetic links and predispositions to a variety of diseases and inherited conditions. Many of these "links" are not causal, however, but merely indicate a higher risk for developing a particular disease. Genetic links for various types of cancers are examples of these genetic predispositions. Some genetic links, however, are 100-percent-certain connections. For example, if a person has the gene mutation for Huntington's disease, he or she will inevitably get the disease. There is an ever growing wealth of genetic information that is becoming available to couples seeking such information about their unborn child.

However, what couples do with the information gleaned from prenatal genetic testing is quite another matter. Though many genetic counselors insist that they operate with objectivity, it is widely assumed that if a couple receive bad news on their child's genetic test, they will end the pregnancy. Though genetic counselors are generally supportive to couples who are determined to continue their pregnancies, couples should realize that an abortion assumption is inherent in a good deal of prenatal genetic testing. Couples who use genetic testing technology normally do so for one of two reasons: either to decide to end the pregnancy should they discover the woman is carrying a genetically handicapped child, or to prepare themselves for the burden of caring for such a child. Though they will likely not admit it, at least in the West, some couples also use genetic testing technology for the purpose of gender selection. They will end the pregnancy if they discover that their child is not of the desired gender. This is more acute in parts of the Third World, where women have far fewer rights and female children are viewed as liabilities with bleak futures. In some of those countries, genetic testing is widely used for sex selection, a practice that is virtually universally condemned by the bioethics community.

Ending a pregnancy on the basis of genetic information received through one of the testing technologies is a misuse of these technologies, for a number of reasons. First, the couple must realize that these tests do have a margin of error. They are not infallible and should not be taken by the couple as error-free. The alpha-fetal protein blood test, which measures the amount of fetal protein in the mother's blood, indicating possible neural tube defects, is notorious for both false positives and negatives, often requiring involved follow-up testing and laying substantial anxiety on the couple awaiting the results. Even amniocentesis is not 100 percent reliable, and couples should be very careful about terminating a pregnancy based on tests that can be in error.

Second, even if the tests are accurate and indicate a genetic anomaly, the parents must know if the defective gene is causally linked to a specific disease or only gives the baby a higher risk of developing the disease. Normally parents only consider ending pregnancies for causal links, not predispositions. It would be unconscionable to end a pregnancy for a predisposition that only increases the risk factors for the child, especially if the disease for which the child is at risk is treatable, as is often the case.

Abortion for genetic anomaly is an inappropriate use of the genetic testing technology because the degree of deformity that the child will experience is difficult to predict. This assumes that the tests are entirely accurate and that there is a causal link between the defective gene and the inherited disease. For example, there are varying degrees of abnormality with Down syndrome. Those with mild cases often lead relatively normal lives and are virtually indistinguishable to the casual observer. Symptoms of some genetic diseases such as Huntington's disease do not appear until later in life. Until the symptoms develop, the person lives an entirely normal life, usually until sometime between the ages of thirty and forty.

Using genetic testing technology to help make a decision to end a pregnancy is a misuse of the technology because it is presumptuous to suggest that the lives of the genetically or otherwise disabled that would be aborted are not worth living. That is a value judgment, frequently used to disguise the real reason the child is being aborted, because of the burden on the parents. Though that should not be underestimated, the hardship on the parents does not justify ending the pregnancy, any more than the financial hardship of a poor woman justifies her ending her pregnancy. It is further presumptuous to suggest that the life of the genetically handicapped fetus is not worth living, for there is no inherent connection between disability and unhappiness. Nor is there any intrinsic link between disability and personal fulfillment.

The most important reason that ending a pregnancy based on genetic testing is a misuse of that technology is that, however genetically deformed, the developing child in utero is still a human person.[47] In fact, the handicapped are deemed more worthy of protection from discrimination, not less, because of their vulnerability due to the physical and mental challenges they face. The decision to end a pregnancy on the basis of genetic deformity alone is no different from eliminating adults simply because they are handicapped. If the fetus, irrespective of genetic defect, is a person, then the decision to abort based on such defect cannot be justified. Surely it is better to suffer the tragedy of accepting a child with genetic abnormalities than to inflict it on another person by abortion.[48]

Use of prenatal genetic testing technology is morally legitimate when used to get information about the child in utero in order to prepare the parents for care of this child and, if necessary, to prepare physicians for appropriate treatment of the child. To use the results to authorize and justify ending the pregnancy is not legitimate since the parents would be condemning the handicapped unborn to death simply on the basis of its genetic anomaly. The only way this can be justified is to assume that the fetus with inherited abnormalities is less than a fully human person, an assumption that cannot be

---

47. Some anomalies are so severe that they may seem inconsistent with the child being a person. For example, a child with anencephaly, perhaps the most severe abnormality with which a child can be born, will have no ability to do anything except maintain essential bodily functions. The child is born with only a brain stem, and has no cerebral part of the brain. Thus the child will have no sense of self-consciousness, no awareness of his or her environment, and no ability to interact or form any kind of human relationships. For many people, the decision to abort an anencephalic child is an easy one, and many medical professionals have concluded that anencephalics are not persons because they are so deformed. But simply because the child does not have the capacity to perform certain functions, it does not follow that the child is not a person. Functional definitions of personhood are both metaphysically inconsistent and socially potentially dangerous. Personhood is a matter of essence, not function. However, admitting that the anencephalic child is a person does not by itself mean that all treatment to save its life once born is appropriate. An anencephalic child is essentially born with a terminal illness. Most anencephalics die within the first month of life, though some do live for as long as a year. There is no obligation to treat a terminally ill patient when the treatment is futile, that is, when it would not improve the patient's condition and help restore him or her to health. Since the anencephalic child is, for the most part, imminently dying from birth, there is no obligation to offer aggressive medical treatment. Of course, for all dying patients there is the obligation to provide comfort and dignity care, that is, care that maintains their comfort and dignity while allowing the disease to take its natural course. Thus one does not have to deny personhood to the anencephalic child in order to justify not providing aggressive treatment.

48. Francis J. Beckwith, *Politically Correct Death: Answering the Arguments for Abortion Rights* (Grand Rapids: Baker, 1992). For more critique on this and the other justifications for abortion, his work is extremely helpful.

maintained. But if the handicapped unborn is indeed a person, then ending a pregnancy on the basis of the handicap is the most vicious form of discrimination.

Life-Sustaining Treatment

Treatments such as dialysis, ventilators, open-heart surgery, and cardio-pulmonary resuscitation are critical life-sustaining technologies that are employed every day to save lives and keep alive people suffering from life-threatening illness. In the majority of cases, use of these technologies is clearly a good thing, enabling people to live longer, and it is consistent with the theology of technology developed earlier in this chapter. But it has become increasingly obvious in the past few years that expensive life-sustaining technology is being overused. This has been a significant contributing factor in driving up the costs of health care and diverting health care resources to a smaller number of seriously ill patients at the expense of a larger number of people who need much less expensive care. For example, poor pregnant women are often unable to obtain proper prenatal care, and at times this results in their babies being born with illnesses that do require use of expensive technology. In addition, many children who could be vaccinated for childhood diseases are not because the resources are not available. Further, the rise of health care costs has driven many people out of the health care system altogether, leaving millions either uninsured or underinsured. To be sure, overuse of life-sustaining technology is not solely responsible for this state of affairs, but it is widely recognized as a significant contributor.

All of this raises the question of when application of life-sustaining technology is not appropriate. After all, doesn't this technology save lives and enable people to live longer? Isn't that a good thing? Of course, in a great many cases it is a good thing. People's lives are saved and they live longer and live productive lives as a result of the application of this technology. But it does not follow that it is always a good thing to have life prolonged, nor is it always a good thing to utilize life-sustaining medical technology.

There are at least three conditions under which use of life-sustaining technology may be inappropriate. The first is when a competent patient requests that these technologies not be used. For example, if a patient with terminal cancer and clearly only a few months to live decides that he or she has had enough of aggressive treatment and simply wants to be comfortable in his or her last days, that request should be honored. If the patient expresses those wishes in writing in some sort of advance directive and then becomes incompetent, family members should insure that the physicians and hospital follow that directive and no heroic measures be taken to prolong the patient's life. It may be that in rare situations a patient whose death is not imminent may also request that life-sustaining measures not be taken, such as a Jehovah's Witness or Christian Scientist whose religious views prohibit him or her from receiving such treatment. One could argue that those requests might be problematic due to the patient's obligation to family members to continue living, but in general, physicians and hospitals ought to follow those requests also, unless they obtain a court order to force the indicated treatments.

A second condition under which life-sustaining technology ought not be employed is when the burden of the treatment exceeds the benefit to a patient who is dying. Some treatments only prolong a difficult dying process. Even simple ones such as antibiotics for pneumonia in a dying patient may delay an inevitable death and make the last days more painful. Or with other types of patients, ventilator support and nasogastric feeding, both of which are highly invasive, may increase the patient's suffering at the end of life, making them more burdensome than beneficial. CPR may resuscitate the patient but also may leave him or her with broken ribs, punctured lungs, and possible brain damage if it takes too long to restore blood flow to the brain. If the net effect on the patient is an increase in the amount of harm done to him or her, without a proportionate or greater benefit, then application of such technology is highly problematic. In those cases neither physicians nor family should press for administering such treatment. Rather the patient should be kept comfortable and supported in his or her dying days. If family members are reluctant to authorize discontinuation of treatment, then the physicians are obligated to spell out the burden that the treatment brings to the patient. It is often difficult for family members, who normally do not witness administration of these burdensome treatments, to appreciate the burden they place on the patient. They only visit the patient during the best times, and are not usually in the room when physicians administer tests and procedures.

A third condition under which it is appropriate to discontinue or withhold life-sustaining technology is when such treatment is futile.[49] Physicians should not utilize expensive technology when it will not alter the inevitable downward course of a patient's terminal illness.

Medicine's dependence on sophisticated technology involves running the risk of what ethicist Daniel Callahan calls "technological brinkman-

---

49. This controversial notion of futile treatment will be addressed in more detail in chapter 7.

ship." He describes this way of thinking about life-sustaining technology as "a powerful clinical drive to push technology as far as possible to save life while, at the same time, preserving a decent quality of life. It is well recognized by now that, if medical technology is pushed too far, a person can be harmed, and that there is a line that should not be crossed. I define 'brinkmanship' as the gambling effort to go *as close to that line as possible* before the cessation or abatement of treatment."[50] The problem with this kind of gambling is that the line between living and dying is becoming more difficult to draw. As a result, the "appropriate" place at which to end treatment as futile is becoming more complex. Physicians can readily tell a patient when he or she has only a few days or weeks to live, but beyond that it is more complicated and dependent on more factors. A second problem is that this kind of thinking about technology assumes that physicians can manage death and dying with technology with a kind of precision that medicine has not shown to this point and may never be able to accomplish.[51] The result of medicine's dependence on technology at the end of life is, as Callahan puts it, "longer lives and worse health, longer illnesses and slower deaths, and longer aging and increased dementia."[52] A further result is the well-known indictment of hospitals and medical centers, that they are lonely, impersonal places in which to die. The focus on technology has diminished the importance of relationships, at times replacing them.[53] Though sophisticated medical technology is still the defining feature of hospital-based care, it may be that managed care will force a more balanced use of technology, though it is unlikely that managed care will encourage a renewed focus on relationships in the health care setting.[54]

50. Daniel Callahan, *The Troubled Dream of Life: Living with Mortality* (New York: Simon and Schuster, 1993), pp. 40-41.

51. Daniel Callahan, p. 41.

52. Daniel Callahan, p. 47.

53. Daniel Callahan, p. 41.

54. For example, it is becoming standard practice in many physicians' practices that receive a substantial portion of their patient population from HMOs to have a set of physicians who see patients in the office and a different set of physicians who are hospital based, disrupting the continuity of relationship with one's physician when hospitalized. For discussion of this, see Francis J. Beckwith, "The Physician as Gatekeeper," *Journal of Social Philosophy* (winter 1996).

Conclusion

Medical technology has clearly been a tremendous benefit to humanity and can be viewed in theological perspective as part of the common blessing of God. Medicine in general is a significant part of humankind's exercise of responsible dominion over God's creation, both a privilege and an obligation that God bestowed on humankind at creation. The tools necessary to develop this technology are part of God's general revelation. Medicine works to alleviate the effects of the entrance of sin into the world, namely, disease and the suffering that results from disease. Though medical technology has and will continue to conquer various diseases, it cannot conquer death. It can only delay it.

That is not to say that all medical technologies have morally appropriate uses, nor that all medical technologies should be used at all. Though the development of any given technology has come through application of God's wisdom revealed outside Scripture, any potential use of a medical technology must be subject to moral scrutiny. No technology that violates biblical principles should be utilized. The more controversial technologies, particularly reproductive and genetic technologies, all have more justifiable and less justifiable uses. Reproductive technologies, including cloning, must safeguard the lives of the unborn children they are attempting to produce. No reproductive technology that involves intentional destruction of preborn persons, or such destruction as part of the technological process, is morally appropriate. Genetic therapies that are sex linked (germ line therapies) are problematic at this time due to the vast amount of information that is still unknown about the human genetic code. Enhancement therapies are also problematic because they do not alleviate any condition that can be linked to the entrance of sin into the world. Life-sustaining treatment can be misused when it is applied against the wishes of a competent patient, when it brings greater burden than benefit, and when it is futile. We should beware of technological brinkmanship specifically and overreliance on technology in general, when it involves diminishing the interpersonal component of life.

CHAPTER 4

The Image of God and the
Sacredness of Human Life

M rs. B. was a popular top-level administrator at the local community
hospital when she suddenly had to be hospitalized for chest pains. She
needed open-heart surgery, which was successfully performed at the hospital
at which she was employed. During her recovery many of the medical and
nursing staff, who knew her personally, were concerned about her condition
and inquired of the nurses and physicians who were caring for her. Since she
was so well liked and since those making inquiries were genuinely concerned
for her welfare, nobody thought much about being fairly open about her diagnosis and prognosis. Staff physicians who were not caring for her but were
genuinely concerned about her could and did readily access her medical records on the hospital's computers. Within a day, virtually everyone in the hospital knew many of the details of her condition. Employees were overheard
talking about her in the elevator and in the hospital's cafeteria. They seemed
surprised when their supervisors reminded them about the need for confidentiality. Not surprisingly, Mrs. B., as the patient, was puzzled by and somewhat offended at the way in which her confidentiality had been violated. She
felt that her dignity had been compromised. Though there was no really dam-
aging information in her medical record, she wondered what would have
happened if there had been, such as mental health care or HIV-positive status. She resolved never again to be hospitalized at the institution at which she
was employed.

Mr. A. was a mid-level executive in the aerospace industry who had experienced a series of layoffs and, consequently, new employers over the past

decade. Every time he changed employers, he was forced to change health insurance plans. This meant that he was covered by a different HMO (health maintenance organization), with a different group of participating physicians. He and his family were growing increasingly frustrated at their inability to stay with the same group of physicians. Though things had improved a bit recently, he acknowledged that his wife and children had seen a wide variety of primary-care doctors, and even when they were in the same plan they were never altogether sure they would see the same physician regularly. They felt that they did not have a relationship with any particular primary-care physician, that none of their physicians really knew them and their history, and that they knew only what they could read in their medical record. With his wife having just been diagnosed with breast cancer, they needed a physician who would be *their* physician, whom they could count on seeing consistently and who could follow her treatment. They felt like nameless consumers of a product who were shuttled to any physician in the mega-physician group who could see them. They also wondered why it was virtually impossible to talk to the physician on the phone, and why all the physicians in the group seemed so rushed when they came in for an office visit. They seemed resigned to this kind of treatment, but were disappointed at the lack of any real relationship with the physicians who were caring for them. They felt like they were not treated as vulnerable, suffering patients, but rather as insurance customers. They felt like their dignity as persons and the compassionate care that the HMO said its member physicians would provide were being compromised.

At the root of the discussion on many issues in bioethics, a fundamental question is, what is a human person? For example, the debates over abortion, embryo research, fetal tissue transplantation, some reproductive technologies,[1] and end-of-life issues all must address these fundamental questions about what constitutes a human person and when in the process of development one possesses the constituent elements of personhood. In this chapter we will address these questions and attempt to lay a theological foundation for ethical decision making concerning human rights at both the beginning and ending edges of life.

The implications of this analysis extend to a variety of ethical issues. For example, concepts that are critical to good health care and a proper patient-

---

1. Specifically, the technologies that involve disposal of leftover embryos and/or selective termination of pregnancies that the couple does not want. These occur in technologies such as GIFT (gamete intrafallopian transfer), ZIFT (zygote intrafallopian transfer), and IVF (in vitro fertilization).

physician relationship come out of the view of a human person having fundamental dignity because he or she is created in the image of God. Principles such as informed consent for treatment, respect for patient confidentiality, and respect for cultural diversity are derived from the fundamental concept of human dignity. There is widespread agreement on this principle of dignity in bioethics. What is more controversial is the basis on which a person can hold that human beings possess fundamental dignity. Though the Scripture is not a metaphysical treatise on embryos and fetuses, theological considerations are extremely relevant to this discussion and set the parameters of a Christian position on these crucial issues. After setting out the theological foundations, we will then apply the conclusions to the issues of informed consent, confidentiality, and diversity, under the heading of "the patient-physician relationship." If it is true that human beings are made in God's image, this gives them inestimable worth and dignity. What do these notions suggest about the way persons should be treated when they become vulnerable because of disease or infirmity? When they become patients under the care of their physician, what should characterize the relationship between patient and physician? In both of the above cases, patient care was not consistent with the principle of respecting their dignity. In the case of Mrs. B., her rights to privacy and confidentiality were violated. In the case of Mr. A., he and his family did not have much of a relationship with any physician, through no particular fault of their own.

In chapter 5 we will suggest one way to work out this theological position philosophically, from a substance view of a person, and apply that analysis to issues such as abortion, embryo research, fetal tissue transplants, and end-of-life decisions.

Biblical and Theological Foundations

The sacredness of innocent human life is the foundational premise on which the proper theological view of the human person is based. The fifth commandment ("'You shall not murder,'" Exod. 20:13 NASB; Deut. 5:17) was intended to safeguard innocent human life. It was not likely intended as an absolute prohibition against the taking of life, since God allowed life to be taken both in warfare and in the exercise of capital punishment. Some would argue further that the taking of life is justified in situations of self-defense as well. But innocent human life cannot be taken without a corresponding penalty. This was considered a fundamental component of the community of God's people in the Old Testament, that they would protect life as a precious gift from God. Thus taking it was prohibited, with very strong sanctions applied to violators.

The reason innocent human life is sacred is because human beings are created in the image of God. From the beginning at creation, God said, "'Let Us make man in Our image, according to Our likeness. . . .' And God created man in His own image, in the image of God He created him; male and female He created them" (Gen. 1:26-27 NASB). God reiterated this same theme when humanity got a renewed start following the flood, when he said,

> "And surely I will require your lifeblood; from every beast I will require it. And from every man, from every man's brother I will require the life of man.
>
>> "Whoever sheds man's blood,
>> By man his blood shall be shed,
>> For in the image of God
>> He made man." (Gen. 9:5-6 NASB)

The sanctity of innocent human life is clearly rooted in the image of God in human beings. Human beings alone, not the animals, are said to be made in God's image.

The image of God in human beings makes for a clear species distinction between human beings and the animal kingdom. In the creation account, being created in God's image is what sets human beings apart on day six of creation from all of the rest of creation on days one through five. Though this view is roundly condemned in many circles as "speciesist," or as "human chauvinism,"[2] the clear intent of the creation narratives is to set humankind as male and female at the pinnacle of creation. The image of God in human beings is precisely what sets them apart.

Throughout the centuries there has been great debate over the precise meaning of the image of God in human beings. Among the suggested candidates are human beings' upright stature; rationality; combination of intellect, emotion, and will; dominion over creation; sexuality as male and female; and their moral nature and capacity to know God. These are capacities which a human being has and expresses to varying degrees. However, the creation account makes it clear that the image of God is not something that human beings possess, but rather something they are. It is a constitutive element of being human, something that we are made in. As theologian David Atkinson

---

2. See, for example, the work of Peter Singer et al. in *Embryo Experimentation: Ethical, Legal, and Social Issues* (Cambridge: Cambridge University Press, 1990).

puts it, "To be 'in the image of God,' then, is not primarily a matter of our capacity to do anything. It is a matter of the relationship to himself which God confers on us. . . . The image of God is both a status and a goal, a gift and a task."[3] Since the divine image has been tarnished by the entrance of sin into the world, the way human beings reflect God's image varies widely, not only among fetuses and embryos but also among newborns and even sinful adults. That is also to say that the goal and task of reflecting God's image is a part of our endowment as human beings with the status of being in God's image. The image of God is not a capacity we possess or lose, but rather a part of our essence. We are, or reflect, God's image, as opposed to possessing God's image in terms of certain capacities. Of course, the image of God will manifest itself in certain capacities and abilities. But that is not to say that those capacities define the image of God. Rather the capacities express God's image which is a part of the human essence. As ethicist Donal O'Mathuna summarizes it: "It is not that humans are the images of God because they have certain rational or spiritual capacities. It is because humans are images of God that spiritual and rational activity is part of what it means to be human."[4] Thus essence as being God's image, not capacity, is what gives a human being species membership and the right to life protection by the community.

On the surface, the notion of the image of God in human beings seems to beg the question of the moral status of embryos and fetuses. That is, it raises the question of whether or not the unborn is a person who is thus made in the image of God. If it is true that there is a continuity of personal identity between conception and adulthood (as we will argue more extensively in the following section on a substance view of a human being), then embryos do not differ qualitatively from adults, only developmentally. That is, as they develop, embryos and fetuses do not become something different from what they already are. Rather they mature into what they already are. This is the reason eggs and sperm are not entitled to the protection embryos receive. Sperm and egg, when combined, become something fundamentally different from what they were prior to conception.

The Scripture indicates that in human beings there is a continuity of personal identity from conception onward. An often cited text in the abortion debate, Psalm 139 strongly suggests that from conception to mature adult,

3. David Atkinson, "Some Theological Perspectives on the Human Embryo," in *Ethics and Embryos: The Warnock Report in Debate*, ed. Nigel M. de S. Cameron (Edinburgh: Rutherford House Books, 1987), pp. 43-57, at 47.

4. Donal O'Mathuna, "Abortion and the 'Image of God,'" in *Bioethics and the Future of Medicine: Toward a Christian Agenda*, ed. John F. Kilner et al. (Grand Rapids: Wm. B. Eerdmans Publishing Co., 1995), pp. 199-211, at 202.

King David was the same essential person. In this psalm David is addressing God both as a poet and a worshiper. He is coming to God in deep reverence and prayer, initiating a conversation with God and providing a reflection on that conversation in poetic form. In verses 1-6 the psalmist admits that nothing in his life has escaped the penetrating search of the living God. He is the object of God's thorough and ongoing knowledge, and he is known intimately by God. In verses 7-12 he attempts, probably hypothetically, to escape from God's knowledge of him. Such knowledge is threatening to him and he desires to get out from under it, but he admits that wherever he would flee, God would be there. This section is an eloquent statement of God's omnipresence. The critical part of the psalm comes in verses 13-18, in which the psalmist reflects on the way in which God has intricately created him. He describes the process with vivid figures of speech such as being knit or woven together in the womb. He marvels at the skill of God in fashioning the details of his being in the secret place of the womb. In verse 16 the psalmist describes himself as an "unformed substance," translated by the primary lexicon for the Old Testament as "embryo."[5] David sees the person who gives thanks and praise to God in verses 13-16 as the same person who was skillfully "woven together" in the womb and is known by God inside and out in verses 1-6. In other words, there is continuity of personal identity from the earliest point of development to a mature adult. That is the significance of Psalm 139 to the discussion of the nature of the human person. It is not solely that God painstakingly and intricately created David in the womb, but also that the person who was being created in the womb is the same person who is writing the psalm. This is not to downplay the significance of God's intricate special creation of human beings in the womb. In fact, God's special creation of human beings in the womb surely includes the notion of creation in his image. Thus, given the continuity of personal identity, it is not unreasonable to suggest that the divine image is present from the earliest points of embryonic life. That is not to say that it might not be anything more than a faint reflection of God's image. But neither is a newborn, or in some cases a severely morally depraved adult, any more than a faint reflection of God's image.

Other passages of Scripture also suggest this continuity of personal identity. For example, in Psalm 51:5 David states:

> Surely I was sinful at birth,
>   sinful from the time my mother conceived me. (NIV)

---

5. Francis Brown, S. R. Driver, and C. A. Briggs, *Hebrew and English Lexicon of the Old Testament*, 5th ed. (Oxford: Oxford University Press, 1977).

David here is confessing not only his specific sins of adultery with Bathsheba and the arranged murder of her husband, Uriah the Hittite (see II Sam. 11–12), but also his innate inclination to sin. This is a characteristic shared by all persons, and David's claim is that he possessed it from the point of conception. Thus an essential attribute of adult persons, an inclination to sin, is attributed to the unborn, underscoring the continuity of identity from conception to adulthood. The same sinful adult began as a sinful embryonic person in the womb.

In Job 10:8-11 the writer uses different figures of speech to describe God's intricate creation of him in the womb, but the point is similar to that made in Psalm 139: a continuity of personal identity from early embryonic life onward. Similarly, in Job 3:3 the writer uses the poetic form called synonymous parallelism to indicate the continuity between conception and birth. The passage states:

> "Let the day perish on which I was to be born,
> And the night which said, 'A boy is conceived.'" (NASB)

We should be careful about reading too much into the use of poetic parallelism, but the format is used to essentially restate the same point in different language. What the use of the parallelism may mean is that the writer regarded birth and conception as fundamentally synonymous, simply different language to state the same point. This is strengthened by the use of the term "boy" in the second half of the verse, which addresses Job's conception. This term for "boy" (Hebrew *geber*) is also used in other parts of the Old Testament to refer to a man and a husband, and thus a person. There seems to be a continuity of identity between conception and birth in the case of Job.

Some have cited Jeremiah 1:5 to indicate a similar point. Here the prophet quotes God in saying,

> "Before I formed you in the womb I knew you,
> And before you were born I consecrated you." (NASB)

Here the synonymous parallelism, if taken too far, would indicate something like preexistence and a separation between biological life and the person. But it may be that the passage points to a significance to what occurred in the womb because of Jeremiah's prophetic calling from before time.[6] One should be careful not to put too much weight on unclear texts such as this one.

One passage that appears to suggest a discontinuity between life in the

---

6. Atkinson, p. 50.

womb and life as an adult is the enigmatic section of the Mosaic Law in Exodus 21:22-25. It is a specific law designed to arbitrate a very specific case. The passage states: "'If men who are fighting hit a pregnant woman and she has a miscarriage, but there is no serious injury, the offender must be fined whatever the woman's husband demands and the court allows. But if there is serious injury (i.e. to the woman), you are to take life for life, eye for eye, tooth for tooth, hand for hand, burn for burn, wound for wound, bruise for bruise.'" Some contend that since the penalty for causing the death of the fetus is only a fine but the penalty for causing the death of the mother merits the death penalty, the fetus must not be deserving of the same level of protection as an adult person. It must have a different status, something less than the full personhood that merits the life-for-life penalty if taken. However, there is significant debate over the term translated "has a miscarriage." At best there is no scholarly consensus on the interpretation. The most likely translation is "she gives birth prematurely," implying that the birth is successful, only creating serious discomfort to the pregnant woman but not killing her or her child. The normal Hebrew word for miscarriage is *shakal,* which is not used here. Rather the term *yasa'* is used. It is normally used in connection with the live birth of one's child. The fact that the normal term for miscarriage is not used here and a term that has connotations to live birth is used suggests that the passage involves a woman who gives birth prematurely.[7] This would make more sense of the different penalties accruing to the guilty party. And it may be that the following phrase in verse 23, "if there is serious injury," would apply to either the woman or the child, so that if the woman actually did have a miscarriage, that would be punishable under the "life for life" scheme. Even if the correct translation is "she had a miscarriage," it would not necessarily follow that the unborn has less of a claim to personhood, since penalty and personhood are not necessarily related.[8] Though the interpretation of this text is debated, it surely does not justify intentionally taking embryonic or fetal life. At most, it might suggest that the continuity of personal identity is interrupted. But the most likely interpretation linguistically also makes the best sense theologically, given the Scripture's teaching about personal identity in Psalm 139 and other texts.

From the doctrine of the image of God and the continuity of personal identity from conception onward that is taught in Scripture, it would seem

---

7. For more on this text, see Umberto Cassuto, *Exodus* (Jerusalem: Magnes Press, 1967), p. 275, and Gleason Archer, *Encyclopedia of Bible Difficulties* (Grand Rapids: Zondervan, 1982), pp. 246-49.

8. Bruce K. Waltke, "Reflections from the Old Testament on Abortion," *Journal of the Evangelical Theological Society* 19 (1976): 3.

that the image of God, however faintly, is present in the earliest forms of embryonic life. To suggest that God is intricately involved in creating a human being from the earliest parts of embryonic life surely involves the idea that he is creating "in his image" from that point onward. Psalm 139 and the other passages cited can be seen as extended descriptions in figurative language of the statements in Genesis 1:27 when God created humankind in his image. Thus theologically it would seem that the divine image is present from the earliest moments of life, from conception onward. If the image of God is the constituent element of personhood, and it is present from the earliest point of embryonic life, then fetuses and embryos as well as newborns and adults are indeed full persons with the corresponding rights to life and full dignity that merit someone made in God's image.

A further implication of this view of God's image is that the person in the womb can make a valid claim to be a neighbor and thus has a moral claim to neighbor love.[9] A neighbor is not to be treated as a means but as an end in itself. It is not to be regarded as a product but as a person. Surely using embryos for research purposes and then discarding them or destroying them in the process is treating a neighbor as a means and not as an end in itself. Whether or not the neighbor can express certain capacities is irrelevant to its standing as a neighbor and its claim to neighbor love. The closer the proximity of the neighbor and the more dependent and vulnerable the neighbor is to us, the greater the claim on us for neighbor love.

A second theological doctrine that has implications for the concept of human personhood is the doctrine of the incarnation.[10] This is connected to the notion of the image of God in human beings and strengthens the point made above that the image of God is present from the earliest points of embryonic life. The great truth of the incarnation is that God became man in Jesus Christ, beginning with a virgin birth. However, the incarnation began not at the birth of Jesus, but rather at his miraculous conception. The significance of the virgin birth goes beyond simply the miraculous nature of Christ's conception. The full import of the virgin birth is that Christ took on human flesh not simply at birth, but earlier, at conception. As theologian Thomas Torrance has suggested, "The Lord Jesus assumed our human nature, gathering up all its stages and healing them in his own human life, including conception."[11]

The use in the Gospels of the term *brephos* for "baby" lends support to

9. Atkinson, p. 48.

10. I am indebted to Atkinson, pp. 54-55, for the insights in this section.

11. Thomas F. Torrance, *Test-Tube Babies* (Edinburgh: T. & T. Clark, 1984).

the significance of the incarnation for the personhood of embryos and fetuses. *Brephos* is used in classical Greek to refer to an embryo as well as a child. In Luke's Gospel the term is used to describe both the newborn baby Jesus and the baby Jesus in utero. For example, in Luke 1:41 the *brephos* leaped in Elizabeth's womb upon hearing the news that Mary was pregnant with Jesus. Similarly, in Luke 2:12, 16 the *brephos* is the newborn Jesus lying in the manger who was observed by the shepherds. Finally, in Luke 18:15 the term refers to infants and children who were being brought to Jesus. Thus there is continuity of identity again, between conception, birth, infants and children. The same term is used interchangeably to refer to the person at all of those stages.

Perhaps a more explicit reference to the significance of the incarnation comes from the visitation of Mary to Elizabeth in the early days of her pregnancy. In Luke 1:39-56 Mary visits Elizabeth only a few days after she had found out that she was pregnant with Jesus. The angel's announcement is recorded in Luke 1:26-38, and the passage indicates that Mary left in haste to visit Elizabeth and share this news with her. Allowing for travel time of roughly two weeks, when Mary arrives at Elizabeth's home she is in the very earliest stages of her pregnancy, with a fetus with a gestational age of less than three weeks. Upon arrival at Elizabeth's home, Mary is immediately recognized as the "mother of our Lord" (1:43). Even though she is carrying a very small, relatively undeveloped fetus, she is clearly recognized as a mother, and by implication Jesus is recognized as her son, a baby. Further, John the Baptist leaps in Elizabeth's womb, perhaps signifying his recognition of the significance of Jesus' conception and in utero development. What is clear is that all of the parties involved in this narrative, Mary, John, and Elizabeth, recognize that something very significant was occurring which was bound up with Mary being pregnant with the Messiah. The significance of the incarnation, though likely not grasped in its fullness, was nonetheless first recognized not at Jesus' birth, but far earlier, in the earliest stages following conception. That is, the incarnation was recognized to have begun months prior to Jesus' actual birth. From the earliest points of life in the womb, Mary and Elizabeth realize that the incarnation has begun. This lends support to the notion that the incarnation began with Jesus' conception, and that the Messiah took on human form in all of its stages, embryonic life included.

If this is true about the incarnate baby Jesus, this suggests that there is great value and significance to embryonic and fetal life. It also suggests that embryos and fetuses are capable of bearing the image of God, though not yet capable of reflecting it fully. If the incarnation began at conception, then that suggests that the image of God is resident in embryonic life, and that there was continuity of the messianic identity from the earliest points of pregnancy until he became a newborn and later a fully grown adult. If this is true of the Messiah becoming a man, then it must also be true of human beings in their normal conception. As ethicist Nigel Cameron states,

> For God to become man in embryo requires that man in embryo already bears the image (of God), and absolutely forbids the possibility that in the early stages of his biological life the divine image can be absent. On the contrary, for God to become man by the miraculous fertilising of one of Mary's ova, it is necessary that a fertilised ovum should be image-bearing already and of its own nature. Man the biological entity and man the creature must be one. The image (of God), with all that implies, must be present wherever this species is to be found.[12]

The combination of the doctrines of the image of God and the incarnation suggests that the image of God is resident from the earliest points of development, and thus embryos, fetuses, and newborn children are all full persons with the corresponding rights to life. The only distinction between embryos, fetuses, and adults is the stage of development. That is, they mature in what they already are. They do not develop into something different in different stages. These twin doctrines strongly suggest that the Scripture views personhood as something inherent to all human beings by virtue of being in the image of God, which is present from the earliest stages of development.

Further, the notion of God as the protector of the weak and powerless suggests that all vulnerable persons, particularly embryos and fetuses, are deserving of protection.[13] The Scripture indicates that the womb is a place of protection and at times uses the womb as a figure of speech to suggest God's protective supervision of people's lives. For example, in Psalm 139 God intricately fashions people in the womb. Even if there was not the continuity of personal identity referred to earlier, one should think very carefully before intentionally destroying the intricate creation that has begun at conception. Surely there is an obligation to protect what God has lovingly fashioned, particularly since the unborn bear the divine image and have standing as full persons. But the womb is described as a place of protection in Psalm 139 as well. For example, Psalm 139:15 uses the word *seter* ("secret place," NIV) in reference to the womb, and the most common use of the term *seter* is a hiding place or shelter, thus clearly implying a place in which God protects those

---

12. Nigel M. de S. Cameron, "The Christian Stake in the Warnock Debate," in *Embryos and Ethics*, pp. 1-13, at 13.

13. O'Mathuna, p. 207.

who take refuge there. Similarly in Isaiah 44, God reminds Israel of his formation of them in the womb so that they can be reminded of his current promise to protect them while in exile. Further, in Job 10:8-11 Job reflects on God's creation of him in the womb and finds it inconceivable that the same God who protected him in the womb would be destroying him in the present. God's involvement with human beings in the womb, whatever else it implies, is linked to protection, because of their vulnerability and because they bear the mark of God's creative hand. Since God's creativity begins at conception, it would seem that, in particular, embryos and fetuses are meriting of protection since they are at their most vulnerable in the womb.

Finally, the biblical notion of parenthood under God suggests that embryos and fetuses should be regarded as valued persons and should not be used as means or treated as products of conception.[14] From a Christian perspective, parents do not make children or reproduce, they beget them. That is, parents share in God's creative activity in procreation. Children are seen as a gift in Scripture (Ps. 127:3-5, for example) and are to be welcomed into the human community as neighbors and treated as the most vulnerable of the community, thus deserving of the highest degree of protection. Parenthood, whether planned or not, is seen as a calling to be involved with God in his creation of a child. Children are the result of God's creative love and are a blessing whether or not parents intended to conceive them. To see embryos and fetuses as only products of conception or parts of the pregnant woman's body which can be disposed of at will, is not consistent with such a view of parenthood. For example, the current emphasis in embryo research of treating embryos with profound respect but discarding them when finished suggests that embryos are being treated as mere means to a research end and as things that can be destroyed in the process of research or discarded when research is finished. If one accepts the biblical notion of a continuity of personal identity as well as this notion of parenthood as a calling to share in God's creative and loving action, then embryos must be accorded the same respect as full persons. Though they are developing into mature adult persons, they are no less persons simply because they are developing. Nor are they developing into something qualitatively different from what they already are.

14. Atkinson, pp. 55-56.

The Patient-Physician Relationship

Because of the dignity of the individual person made in God's image and the vulnerability of patients when they become ill and require invasive treatment, the patient-physician relationship must be structured to maintain the dignity of the patient. Physicians practice medicine under the obligations defined by a fiduciary relationship with their patients. Many of the professions have fiduciary relationships, such as lawyers, accountants, and therapists. In a fiduciary relationship the provider's job is to seek and safeguard the interests of the client. When the provider's interests conflict with the client's, the client's interests are to take precedence. The physician's goal is to safeguard the patient's interest in his or her health. When the physician's interests conflict with the patient's, generally the patient's interests take priority.[15]

Patients need this kind of relationship with their physicians because of the substantial differential in medical knowledge between patient and physician. This puts the physician in a position of significant power over the patient, and the physician is obligated to exercise that power for the benefit of the patient. Thus, for example, it is commonly regarded as unethical for physicians to administer treatment that is unnecessary or order tests and lab work that are unnecessary for determining the patient's diagnosis, even though it may profit the physician financially. Similarly, it is unethical for the physician to withhold medically appropriate treatment or tests if it would cost the physician in terms of his or her financial self-interest. Effective maintenance of the proper fiduciary relationship depends mostly on the physician, since he or she possesses the necessary information to keep the patient healthy.

The physician's role in the relationship also arises from the vulnerability of the patient. When people become ill, they become more vulnerable to a variety of coercive pressures. They are generally unable to shop around for medical care because obtaining care is urgent and time-constrained. That is what makes health care different from most other services sold on the open market, and why people consider at least a minimum level of health care to be a right as opposed to a commodity for market distribution. It is considered unethical for physicians to exploit the patient's vulnerability that comes with illness to gain personal advantage.[16]

15. One clear exception to this would be when the patient asks the physician to do something that he or she cannot do because of the dictates of conscience, informed by the physician's values. For example, the pro-life physician cannot be forced to perform abortions even though they are legal.

16. We are not suggesting that all pursuit of self-interest is problematic. Rather self-interest must be balanced generally by concern for the common good, or in this context,

There is more to the patient-physician relationship than what can be expressed by a fiduciary relationship. The patient is not just a client or customer, but a vulnerable person created in God's image with inherent dignity and with real health care needs. The physician provides not only the specific treatment needed by that patient, but does so in the context of a therapeutic relationship. Another way to put this is that the physician operates out of a covenant relationship with the patient.[17] That is, there is an aspect of the relationship that contributes to the healing process. This is readily evident in the mental health professions where the therapist uses the relationship of trust developed with the client to facilitate healing. The relationship is an integral part, by design, of the healing process. Perhaps to a somewhat lesser degree, the relationship of trust between patient and physician is important to the patient's healing. Since physicians treat people, not just diseases, good medical care is more than simply giving an accurate diagnosis and prescribing the appropriate course of treatment. It is done in the context of a relationship of caring, compassion, communication, and trust, in which the fundamental dignity of the individual patient is respected. Such a relationship is crucial not just for maintaining the physician's moral obligations but also for the healing of his or her patients. It is not an accident that most people speak of obtaining medical *care* when confronted by illness. They are not only seeking the right treatment, but they are seeking it within the context of a relationship with a physician who expresses care for them, has compassion in the administration of the treatment, and communicates in a clear and timely fashion with patients, and their families if necessary, about the diagnosis, prognosis, and treatment options.

In the traditional fee-for-service type of medical practice, giving this kind of attention to patients was more common and more in the physician's control. However, with the advent of managed care and particularly the payment option of capitation, in which a physician or physician group is paid a flat fee each month to take care of a specific population of patients, the model patient-physician relationship is more difficult to maintain. Managed care has put pressure on physicians to see more patients in less time, keep office

---

concern for one's patients. The fiduciary duty demands that when self-interest and the patient's interest conflict, that the patient's interest take priority. The Bible suggests that self-interest and the interests of others be kept in balance. For example, in Phil. 2:4 Paul teaches that we are not to look out for our own interests solely, but also for the interests of others. Notice that the passage never says that people should not look out for their own self-interest, only that they should not do that exclusively.

17. See William F. May, *The Physician's Covenant* (Louisville: Westminster/John Knox, 1983).

visits to a minimum time necessary to treat the patient, and limit the amount of time they can spend with patients on the telephone. Some HMOs that contract with physicians have specific guidelines about how much time the physician can spend with different types of patients, depending on the type of visit they need and whether or not they are new or returning patients. In addition, physicians have contractual arrangements with some insurance companies to offer their services for a substantial discount in exchange for being listed as a preferred provider, thus giving them access to an entire pool of potential patients who are covered by that particular insurance company. This discounted fee for service forces physicians to increase the number of patients they see on any given day in order to maintain their income level. Many physicians have reported that the time pressures they now face have compromised the physician-patient relationship as a result. In addition, with insurance coverage becoming increasingly dependent on one's employer, whenever the employer changes health plans for cost reasons, or when an employee changes jobs, the employee runs the risk of having to select another set of physicians who are contracted by the new insurance plan. This can threaten the continuity of the patient-physician relationship when a person must end a relationship with a physician and begin a new one because the person's new insurance plan does not include the former physician. Further, in many cases a family's insurance coverage is with a group of physicians, and there is no guarantee that the patient will be able to see the same physician on each visit. Maintaining a proper physician-patient relationship can be done, but it is a much greater challenge and takes more commitment on the part of the physician in today's managed care environment.[18]

Informed Consent

Respecting patient dignity involves a commitment to the notion of informed consent. Competent adults have the right to make their own decisions about treatment or experiments performed on their bodies. To be competent means

18. For more on the patient-physician relationship in the context of managed care, see Ezekiel Emanuel, "Preserving the Physician-Patient Relationship in the Era of Managed Care," *Journal of the American Medical Association* 273, no. 4 (25 January 1995): 323-29; David Orentlicher, "Managed Care and the Threat to the Patient-Physician Relationship," *Trends in Health Care, Law and Ethics* 10, no. 1/2 (winter/spring 1995): 19-24, Frank A. Chervenak and Laurence B. McCullough, "The Threat of the New Managed Practice of Medicine to Patient Autonomy," *Journal of Clinical Ethics* 6, no. 4 (winter 1995): 320-23.

to have decision-making capacity. Competence is normally considered compromised by unconsciousness, sedation, extreme pain, or mental impairment, whether temporary or permanent. People can slip in and out of competence, and incompetent patients thus require periodic reevaluation. Minors are generally not assumed to be competent, though the closer one gets to age eighteen the more competent he or she is considered.[19]

Informed consent is rooted in the rights of patients over their own bodies, a right grounded in the notion of individual dignity. If human beings are God's creations made in his image, then their dignity cannot be disregarded by physicians who think they are acting in the patient's best interest. This is also known as the right of personal autonomy, or the right of persons to decide before God what is best for their lives and for their bodies.[20] This right, and the moral principle of respecting human dignity underlying it, is considered so important in Western culture today that informed consent is required by law in most Western countries. That is, before administering any test or treatment, physicians are required to document that the patient has indicated understanding of what is about to happen to him or her and has freely consented to it. Except in rare situations, for a physician to administer a treatment, particularly an invasive one, without obtaining proper consent would be tantamount to battery, and the physician could be prosecuted.

Informed consent became institutionalized in health care as part of a broader movement to protect the rights of vulnerable patients when they submit to a physician for health care. This arose in response to a long history in medicine of paternalism, in which the doctor knew best and thus administered treatment with less regard for the patient's wishes than in today's culture of medical care.[21] This resulted in periodic abuses of patient rights, particularly at the end of life, when life-sustaining treatment was administered without regard to the patient's desires. A paternalistic approach to medical care still is widely practiced in parts of the non-Western world, but it is not

19. In a recent case that was the subject of most of the network newsmagazines, a seventeen-year-old boy suffering from liver disease elected to forgo the medication that was keeping him alive. He was tired of the severe side effects, which he felt were ruining his quality of life. He knew that refusing the medication would eventually cause his death, and made an informed choice to stop taking it. He lived roughly one more year free from the unpleasant side effects, and when asked whether or not he made the right choice, he clearly felt that refusal of medication was the right decision. Though only seventeen, he was treated as competent and his decisions were honored.

20. The troubling balance between autonomy and the common good, and between autonomy and beneficence, will be addressed in chapter 6.

21. For more on paternalism in medicine, see H. Tristram Engelhardt, Jr., *The Foundations of Bioethics,* 2nd ed. (New York: Oxford University Press, 1996), pp. 320-30.

considered as egregious an abuse of patient rights as in the West with its tradition of autonomy. However, irrespective of culture, treatment must not be provided when a competent patient does not give consent. Such patients have rights over their own bodies and should not be given invasive treatment they do not desire.

Genuine informed consent assumes that there has been clear and timely communication between the patient and the physician, which, as noted above, is more challenging in today's managed care environment. For a patient to give truly informed consent means that the patient must have a clear understanding of the diagnosis and prognosis; the treatment alternatives, including the alternative of no treatment; and the risks and benefits of the available alternatives. In many cases the diagnosis is simple and the plan of care is straightforward. Understanding it and giving consent is not complicated. But complex procedures, procedures that involve significant risk and/or questionable benefit, or decisions at the end of life about withdrawing or withholding treatment, are much more involved and take more time for the physician to properly communicate with patients and insure that they understand.

Nurses have a responsibility and an opportunity to help determine whether or not patients are adequately informed about the goals and plan of care. It is appropriate for nurses to interact with patients to insure that patients understand the diagnosis, treatment options, and risks and benefits of each option. If they observe that patients appear uninformed or misinformed about the treatment plan or appear not to have given consent, then it is appropriate for them to consult with colleagues for a second opinion, inform the attending physician of the facts that suggest defective informed consent, and document the facts and the response of the physician. If concerns about patient consent still persist, it is appropriate for them to inform their supervisor, and if still unresolved the issue may be taken to the medical department head, risk management, or the institution's ethics committee. If a treatment is about to be administered and it is evident that the patient has not given informed consent, nurses have the option, and perhaps even the obligation, to refuse to participate in the administration of that particular treatment.[22]

When patients are not competent, physicians turn to next of kin, or surrogate decision-makers (also called proxy decision-makers), for help in obtaining consent. In an advanced directive, in which persons make clear what

---

22. The role of nurses in informed consent is a growing one, and the guidelines suggested here are taken from formal guidelines developed by the Hawaii Nurses Association. They were published in *Ethical Currents*, no. 47 (fall 1996): 8, 10.

kinds of treatments they want should they become unable to speak for themselves, a person can designate a surrogate decision-maker, who is invested with decision-making authority for the patient. This is also called a durable power of attorney for health care (DPAHC). The surrogate is to make decisions for the patient using the principle of substituted judgment. That is, the surrogate substitutes his or her judgment for that of the patient, and attempts to represent the wishes of the patient for the physicians. The question for the surrogate to answer is, What do you think the patient would have wanted done under these circumstances? But the question frequently asked the surrogate is: "What do you want to do in this situation?" reflecting a desire for a decision so that the physician can get on with the treatment. That is the wrong question because it ignores the surrogate's role of representing the wishes of the patient. This assumes that the patient has had some conversation with the surrogate about treatment preferences, particularly if the patient is elderly or terminally ill and thus approaching the end of life. Generally, patients who designate a surrogate in a DPAHC also specify what kinds of care they desire at the end of life. Thus the surrogate's role is to insure that the patient's wishes, which have been expressed in writing in a living will (another name for an advance directive), are followed. If the living will is not well written, the surrogate may be called on to help interpret it, based on conversations the physician hopes the surrogate has had with the patient. Normally one's spouse is the surrogate; if one is unmarried or no longer married, adult children or siblings normally assume that role. Occasionally there is no consensus among family members about the decisions that need to be made, which creates a difficult situation in which one family member must be recognized as the principal decision-maker. With minor children it is assumed that the parents or guardians are the surrogates. In most cases the surrogate makes decisions in the best interests of the patient and accurately represents the patient's wishes. But occasionally that is not the case. For example, parents who are Jehovah's Witnesses or Christian Scientists sometimes do not authorize lifesaving treatments for their seriously ill children because of religious reasons.[23] In those cases hospitals seek to obtain a court order to force treatment, and in most cases are justified in so doing.

---

23. See the case in chapter 10 that concerns a Jehovah's Witness couple, in which the wife did not authorize a blood transfusion for her husband, who needed surgery for a subdural hematoma. Her refusal of treatment was followed by the hospital, and the patient subsequently died. Respecting religious beliefs is an important part of respecting dignity, but there are limits to which religious beliefs should be followed. For example, hospitals routinely go to court and win when parents withhold consent for treatment for a minor child.

An important part of informed consent is the informed refusal of treatment, which, in cases of truly informed and competent adults, physicians are obligated to respect. Specifically, this involves following a person's advance directive when it is appropriate to invoke it. Physician refusal to follow patients' advance directives is well documented, and constitutes an unethical breach of the covenant between patient and physician. In many of these cases the patient's competence is questionable and the family is dependent on the physician to make decisions. Family members do not aggressively represent the wishes of their loved one and allow themselves to be unduly influenced by the physician who does not want to let go of the patient or authorizes treatment to protect himself or herself from liability concerns. In some cases family members do not want to let go of a dying loved one, and they make decisions that are contrary to the patient's advance directive. In those cases, as difficult as it might be, the physician is obligated not to follow the wishes of the family, instead following the written wishes of the patient.

Informed consent is particularly important when patients are also research subjects. A good deal of medical research takes place in hospitals, especially teaching hospitals, and having available patients is essential for testing various procedures and pharmaceuticals. Normally medical research involves testing two groups, one of which undergoes the experimental treatment and the other, the control group, either having nothing done or following the normal course of treatment. Drug companies and other manufacturers of medical devices are anxious to test new products on human subjects, since animal testing, although helpful, is not generally a sufficient substitute for human subject testing. Informed consent for research is part of the protocol for any medical research involving human subjects and is regulated by the hospital's institutional review board (IRB), which reviews all research with human subjects to insure that it is conducted ethically. Informed consent for these subjects involves knowing the goal of the study and their role in it. They should be informed that the treatment they will receive is experimental and cannot be assured to have a positive outcome. They should further know that they might be in the control group and not actually receive the experimental product at all. They should know the nature of the test as well as the potential risks and benefits involved in their role in the study. To be sure, there are some things they cannot know without compromising the objectivity of the study, but research subjects should not be subjected to risks without their informed consent.

One egregious violation of research-subject informed consent came from the infamous Tuskegee syphilis experiments in the 1920s. Government researchers studied the effects of syphilis on black men and left the disease untreated in many of the men for years while giving them the impression that they were being treated for it. Thus they unknowingly spread the disease and did not seek treatment, since they understood that they were being treated as part of the research protocol. These experiments have been widely condemned as unethical since they subjected the research subjects to clear harm without their consent.

Confidentiality

Respecting patient dignity involves a commitment to maintaining confidentiality of the patient's medical information. This is considered a cornerstone of the physician-patient relationship because it creates the atmosphere of trust that is essential for a healthy and therapeutic covenant between patient and physician. Without the commitment to confidentiality, many fear that people would not seek out medical treatment as frequently. This is particularly true of people who suffer from socially stigmatized diseases such as AIDS and other sexually transmitted diseases. Confidentiality also encourages patients to be fully forthcoming about their symptoms and causes, without fear that any embarrassing information about them could become public. Thus it contributes significantly to the physician's ability to make accurate diagnoses and prescribe the proper courses of treatment, since he or she can be assured that the patient will disclose all relevant information about his or her condition. Confidentiality is also important because a person's medical information is deeply personal, and disclosure of it can be uncomfortable and embarrassing, as was the case with Mrs. B. in the introduction of this chapter. Mrs. B. felt that her dignity had been violated because many people now knew very personal things about her that she did not wish to be known. Confidentiality is part of the right to privacy as a basic human right, as an application of the principle of individual dignity.

Maintaining confidentiality was significantly easier prior to the widespread use of computers and the Internet for storing and transmitting medical records.[24] Very few people had access to a patient's medical information, and it was relatively easy for the physician and nurse(s) to hold that information close. Typically the only people who received access to a pa-

24. See recent discussions of this, including Greg Goth, "Record Roulette," *Los Angeles County Medical Association Physician* (11 August 1987): 28-31; and Kayhan P. Parsi, William J. Winslade, and Kevin Corcoran, "Does Confidentiality Have a Future? The Computer Based Patient Record and Managed Mental Health Care," *Trends in Health Care, Law and Ethics* 10, no. 1/2 (winter/spring 1995): 78-82.

tient's record were those who were either treating the patient or paying for the treatment, such as insurance companies. Family members could be informed with the patient's consent, and most patients did not, and still do not, object to family members knowing information about their diagnosis and prognosis. But with the advent of computerized medical records and transmission of them over electronic media such as the Internet, the number of people who can now access a particular patient's record has increased exponentially. In a large medical center, it is not uncommon for one hundred people or more to be able to easily access the patient's record, many of whom would not need to know that information. Some have suggested that the traditional notion of confidentiality in today's context is a meaningless concept and, in fact, no longer exists.[25] Siegler suggests that medical information be available only on a "need to know" basis, yet restricting access to such information can be difficult. For example, physicians affiliated at a local hospital can likely access the record of any patient in the hospital. So can their administrative assistants, who often have the physician's code or password to enter the computer system on the physician's behalf. Nothing prevents them from accessing other patients' information out of curiosity. Some computer systems do restrict access to some degree, but in many settings virtually any physician can enter a nursing station and access a patient's chart. It is not uncommon to hear hospital staff discussing a patient in the elevator or the hospital cafeteria, both violations of the patient's right to confidentiality.

In view of the fact that computers in medical centers have made information so much more accessible today, here are some guidelines for health care professionals when it comes to respecting patients' privacy and dignity in keeping information confidential. They should adhere to these guidelines, and patients and their families should also expect them to follow them.

1. Be aware of hospital policies with respect to confidentiality.
2. Communicate to patients and their families that they can expect confidentiality from those who hold their medical information.
3. When it becomes necessary to share patient information with outside parties, do so only with the explicit permission of the patient.
4. Discuss patient information with other health care professionals in private and on a "need to know" basis only.
5. If in doubt, treat information about the patient as confidential.

25. See, for example, Mark Siegler, "Confidentiality in Medicine: A Decrepit Concept," *New England Journal of Medicine* 307 (1982): 1518-21.

This area is a good example of the need for ongoing ethics education of those who have control over patients' medical information. To be sure, policies are helpful, and most hospitals have policies that aim to protect confidentiality. But enforcing them can be a challenge, and effective confidentiality involves education of staff and their ownership of how important confidentiality is.

The most difficult area with regard to confidentiality is determining when to override the patient's right to privacy and disclose confidential information. Consider the following case:[26]

A twenty-year-old Hispanic male was brought to a hospital emergency room, having suffered abdominal injuries due to gunshot wounds obtained in gang violence. He had no medical insurance, and his stay in the hospital was somewhat shorter than expected due to his good recovery. Physicians attending him felt that he could complete his recovery at home just as easily as in the hospital, and he was released after only a few days.

During his stay in the hospital, the patient admitted to his primary physician that he was HIV positive, having contracted the virus that causes AIDS. This was confirmed by a blood test administered while he was hospitalized.

When he was discharged from the hospital, the physician recommended that a professional nurse visit him regularly at home in order to change the bandages on his still substantial wounds and to insure that an infection did not develop. Since he had no health insurance, he was dependent on Medicaid, a government program that pays for necessary medical care for those who cannot afford it. However, Medicaid refused to pay for home nursing care since there was someone already in the home who was capable of providing the necessary care. That person was the patient's twenty-two-year-old sister, who was willing to take care of her brother until he was fully recovered. Their mother had died years ago, and the sister was accustomed to providing care for her younger siblings.

The patient had no objection to his sister providing this care, but he insisted that she not be told that he had tested HIV positive. Though he had always had a good relationship with his sister, she did not know that he was an active homosexual. His even greater fear was that his father would hear of his homosexual orientation and lifestyle.

The patient's physician is bound by his code of ethics, which places a very high priority on keeping confidentiality. Some would argue that the responsibility of confidentiality is even greater with HIV/AIDS because disclo-

---

26. This case is analyzed in more detail according to the ethical decision-making model outlined in chapter 10.

sure of someone's homosexuality normally carries devastating personal consequences for the individual who is forced "out of the closet."

On the other hand, the patient's sister is putting herself at risk by providing nursing care for him. Doesn't she have a right to know the risks to which she is subjecting herself, especially since she willingly volunteered to take care of her brother?

If you were the physician, what would you do in this case? Would you breach the norm of confidentiality to protect the patient's sister, or would you keep confidentiality in order to protect the patient from harm that would come to him from his other family members, especially his father?

When confidentiality conflicts with other obligations, such as to prevent harm, either to innocent third parties, as in this case, or to society in general, as is the case with infectious diseases,[27] or to oneself, health care professionals are faced with a difficult dilemma. Up until the mid-1970s, confidentiality was almost an absolute value, not only in medicine but also in the mental health and legal professions. Breaches of this practically sacred trust were rare and taken seriously by the respective professions. With the landmark *Tarasoff* case in California in 1976, confidentiality became less of an absolute.[28] Tatiana Tarasoff was a student at the University of California at Berkeley who eventually rejected the romantic advances of another student, who did not take kindly to such rejection, to say the least. He eventually saw a psychotherapist at the university, who learned of his intent to kill Tarasoff. The therapist informed campus security but did not inform Tarasoff, out of a commitment to maintain confidentiality. After she returned from an extended time away from the university, the student reestablished contact with her and eventually did kill her. Her family sued the therapist and the University of California for failing to warn them of the danger to their daughter. The court ruled in favor of the family, holding that a professional bound by confidentiality had an overriding duty to warn someone who was in significant and imminent jeopardy of either death or severe bodily harm. This has been most recently expanded to apply to AIDS patients, and physicians are generally allowed to notify spouses or lovers of AIDS patients of the HIV status of their partner. This is consistent with a long-standing policy of both contact tracing and noti-

---

27. The AMA Code of Ethics has had this caveat to confidentiality since 1912. See Leroy Walters, "The Principle of Medical Confidentiality," in *Contemporary Issues in Bioethics*, ed. Tom L. Beauchamp and LeRoy Walters (Encino, Calif.: Dickenson Publishing, 1978), pp. 170-73.

28. *Tarasoff v Regents of the University of California*, 131 California Reporter 14 (decided 1 July 1976).

fication of sexual partners and notification of public health authorities in other sexually transmitted diseases. Under the principle outlined by the court, the obligation to do no harm and to prevent harm when it is in one's power to do so overrides the obligation to maintain confidentiality. When applied to the case above, in which the sister is taking care of her recovering, HIV-infected brother, the physician has the obligation to disclose to the sister the risks of caring for her brother. To do so involves a justifiable breach of confidentiality. Overriding confidentiality could also be justified in cases when the public could be in danger if the physician does not disclose his or her patient's medical problem. For example, an airline pilot with a heart condition or a bus driver with failing eyesight should not expect that such conditions be kept confidential, since they have many lives for which they are responsible in the discharge of their jobs every day. Of course, one must weigh the degree of risk with the obligation of confidentiality. If there is minimal risk of the patient's condition ever affecting the lives of people in his or her care, then confidentiality should be upheld. But under *Tarasoff*, physicians and other health care professionals have the legal obligation to disclose patient information that would bring harm to innocent third parties.

Dignity and Cultural Diversity

Respecting the dignity of individual persons as made in God's image involves respecting the distinctives of their ethnic, religious, and cultural backgrounds. The recent emphasis on multiculturalism has rightly pointed out the need for greater sensitivity to a person's ethnicity, religion, and culture, and this has made its way into the arena of health care.[29] Since the physician-patient relationship is such an important part of good patient care, understanding and respecting the cultural distinctives of a patient population is essential to good care. It is also the appropriate treatment of a person as a human being, whether or not the person is a patient. Respecting diversity at its heart involves respect for the values of that person's culture and religion. To be sure, multiculturalism has increased appreciation for things like the art, literature, and music of other cultures. But those are pe-

---

29. See, for example, the series of books published by the Park Ridge Center for Faith, Health and Ethics that addresses how health care is viewed in various religious traditions. They bear titles like *Health Care in the Catholic Tradition*, for example, and include a variety of Christian and non-Christian religious traditions.

ripheral; though important, they are not central aspects of a culture. To take another culture seriously involves taking its values seriously and respecting those values as they inform the choices patients make about their health care.

This is not to suggest that to be culturally sensitive makes one a cultural relativist, where morality is determined by the cultural consensus.[30] There are clear moral absolutes that Scripture teaches, and thus there are limits on the degree to which anyone can accept the values of any particular culture. Most people realize that lines must be drawn somewhere, and that there must be some standards that transcend culture if society is to arbitrate competing cultural values. For example, there can be extreme examples of relativism under the guise of multiculturalism. An Arab-American family which had moved from the Middle East to California was confronted by the adult daughter's desire to choose her own husband, contrary to Middle Eastern practice, in which the parents of the bride and groom arrange the marriage. The girl's father insisted that her marriage be arranged in the traditional fashion. The girl refused, and when she announced her engagement to a man of her choosing, her father took the appropriate step to discipline his daughter according to his Middle Eastern background: he killed her. He was charged with murder, and in his defense his attorney argued that since this was acceptable in his Middle Eastern culture, that should be taken into account by the jury in deciding his guilt. In other words, it was a norm according to his culture, and the morality of his action should be determined by his cultural context. The jury rightly rejected this notion and held to an absolute standard in determining his guilt and prison sentence.[31] When the values of a patient's culture conflict with the physician's or medical center's values, respecting cultural diversity becomes difficult and creates complicated ethical issues.[32]

Though respecting diversity can create ethical dilemmas, generally physicians taking patients' values into account in the way they relate to patients is considered an important part of informed consent and good care. For example, it is well documented that attitudes toward death and dying and decision making at the end of life are very different for different ethnic groups. In one recent study investigators discovered that Koreans and Hispanics tend to work off of a model in which the family handles the decision

30. For an explanation and critique of cultural relativism, see Scott B. Rae, *Moral Choices: An Introduction to Ethics* (Grand Rapids: Zondervan, 1995), pp. 86-91.

31. This example is taken from Neal Gabler, "Moral Relativism? 'You Don't Get It,'" *Los Angeles Times*, 14 June 1992, p. M1.

32. Cases 2 and 3 in chapter 10 deal with conflicts created by attempts to take a patient's cultural values seriously.

making.[33] Blacks and whites work more off the classic patient autonomy model. The concept of patient autonomy can be somewhat foreign to Korean and Hispanic patients, and as a result they may appear passive in making treatment decisions and their families may appear overly aggressive in taking responsibility for those decisions.

The study further showed that in Korean and Hispanic groups, the family handles the burden of the patient's illness in order to protect the patient. This is one reason why families often insist that patients not be told their diagnosis. These families consider it their responsibility to do whatever is necessary to take burdens off the patient, who they believe is bearing enough of a burden in dealing with his or her illness. With blacks and whites the emphasis seems to be reversed. In these groups the patient in the midst of his or her illness does not want to be a burden to the family, and thus takes most of the decision-making responsibility personally.

In addition, with Koreans and Hispanics family loyalty is a very high value. For example, these groups usually want everything done for the patient so that the family can appear caring and compassionate for its loved one. Not to do everything for an ill family member would cause the family to lose face. Ironically, this may involve consenting to treatment that will actually increase the burden to the patient, precisely what the family is trying to prevent the patient from experiencing. Blacks and whites tend to be more individualistic, though there is usually concern not to be a burden to their families. Understanding these cultural distinctives can be very helpful to physicians and nurses as they attempt to provide optimal care for patients of different cultures. This is even more important in major metropolitan areas where there tends to be more ethnic diversity. In certain parts of the country it is not uncommon that the patient, physician, and nurses are all from different ethnic backgrounds, thus multiplying the possibilities for a conflict in values.

When such a conflict in values occurs, how should physicians and nurses respond? Consider the case of an elderly Hispanic widow who had been diagnosed with cancer that required chemotherapy as the preferred course of treatment. She had been in generally good health prior to the onset of her cancer. At the time of her admission she appeared to be fully competent and capable of making her own decisions. Her son and other family members were with her continually during her stay in the medical center.

33. See Leslie J. Blackhall et al., "Ethnicity and Attitudes toward Patient Autonomy," *Journal of the American Medical Association* 274, no. 10 (13 September 1995): 820-25, for a significant study of the attitudes of four major ethnic groups about decision making at the end of life. See also Jill Klessig, M.D., "The Effect of Values and Culture on Life-Support Decisions," *Western Journal of Medicine* 157 (September 1992): 316-22.

Since the patient did not speak any English, her oldest son took on the role of translator. He insisted that his mother not be told the details of her diagnosis and effectively prevented the physician and nurses from communicating with her any more than he wanted to get through. He was afraid that if she found out the whole truth of her diagnosis, she would give up hope and stop fighting to live. His insistence on withholding information from her also seemed to be based on a cultural value that emphasizes taking care of one's family and protecting it from harm. In addition, as the oldest male, he likely viewed himself as the head of the household and thus responsible for those in his care.[34] So he only translated the information that he felt was appropriate for her to hear.

Two principal ethical issues are raised by this case. The first concerns informed consent. The law requires informed consent when the patient is capable of making his or her own decisions. In fact, it would appear that the son was asking the medical center to violate the law by asking that key information about the patient's diagnosis be withheld. In addition, he was asking that the medical center violate the dignity of the patient by forcing physicians and nurses to treat her as if she were incompetent simply because she spoke a different language.

A second ethical issue revolves around confidentiality. The son, by virtue of being the translator, was putting himself in a position to gain access to confidential medical information on his mother. Her right to privacy was denied here by her son's insistence on being the translator. Confidentiality means that information about the patient belongs to the patient and is not to be released without his or her consent. Whether or not she would have objected to her son having access to that information is open to debate. But the benefit of the doubt should surely fall on the side of confidentiality.

In this case the values of the patient's culture can be protected while assuring informed consent and confidentiality. A substitute translator should be brought in and, through him or her, the physician should ask the patient, in her son's presence, if she wants to know her diagnosis and prognosis and make her own decisions or allow her son to have that information and make the decisions about her treatment for her. If the patient wants to work off a family decision-making model, that is her right, but it should be her in-

---

34. Often in more patriarchal cultures, the head of the household will view the patient's medical information as his property, not the patient's. Thus notions of confidentiality that are based on the patient's medical information belonging to the patient may be difficult to apply in some other cultures.

formed choice as well. In this case she wanted very badly to know her medical information and make her own decisions.

Or consider the case of the Jehovah's Witness who, for religious reasons, will not accept blood transfusions, thereby compromising many surgical procedures and, in some cases, actually leading to serious harm or death. To what degree should the physician respect the religious views of the Jehovah's Witness as the basis for providing care? Generally with competent adults, particularly if grounded with religiously based reasons, physicians should respect their choices, even if they result in harm coming to the patient. In most cases the law requires that those informed autonomous choices be respected, and courts are very hesitant to override informed choices made by competent adults, especially when based on religious reasons. One recent example concerned a pregnant woman whose obstetrician determined that her unborn child would die without a cesarean section delivery. The pregnant woman, who had a strong Pentecostal faith, believed that God would enable her to have a safe vaginal delivery. She insisted on refusing the C-section, and the hospital went to court to force her to undergo the C-section for the sake of the unborn child. Ironically the ACLU argued her case in court, and the court ruled in favor of the woman, who had a successful vaginal birth. This case is more difficult since it actually involves two patients, the pregnant woman and her unborn child.[35] With children, however, parents have the obligation to act in their best interests, and physicians and medical centers routinely go to court in order to obtain a court order to compel necessary medical treatment on minor children. For example, parents who are adherents of Christian Science, a sect that does not believe in any medical treatment, have been forced by court order to allow their children to undergo treatment that is clearly in the child's best medical interest.

Setting limits on how far one will accommodate the values of another culture is difficult but must be done. As a general guideline, the values of competent adults should be respected. If the physician or nurse cannot provide treatment according to the patient's values, then he or she has the right and the responsibility to turn over that patient's care to another physician or nurse who does not have the conflict of values. The medical center with which the physician affiliates also has the right to set some limits on how far it will accommodate a patient's cultural values. For example, Catholic hospitals routinely do not perform abortions, except when necessary to save the life of the mother, since they believe that the unborn child is a person from concep-

35. See Susan Mattingly, "The Maternal-Fetal Dyad: Exploring the Two-Patient Obstetric Model," *Hastings Center Report* 22 (1992): 16.

tion onward. Neither do they do nonmedically indicated sterilization procedures such as tubal ligations, nor would they ever participate in physician-assisted suicide should it become legal.

Conclusion

Both biblical testimony and theological reflection support the notion that human beings are persons from the point of conception onward, with the corresponding rights to life. Because persons are made in God's image and represent the pinnacle of creation, they possess inherent dignity. Thus they are to be treated as God's special creations who reflect his image. This view of a human being has significant implications for the physician-patient relationship. Specifically, this notion of a human person mandates a physician-patient relationship in which the physician exercises a fiduciary duty toward the patient, respects the need for fully informed consent prior to initiating treatment, maintains confidentiality of patient information, and respects the cultural and religious diversity of his or her patient population. This involves diligence about communication in order to obtain genuine informed consent for treatment as well as honoring patients' informed refusal of treatment; keeping their medical and personal information confidential, especially from those who could use it against them; and respecting their cultural and religious values when they conflict with the values of those who care for them. There are limits on how far one can accommodate those values, and caregivers also have the right to remove themselves from treating a patient if so doing would violate their values and consciences.

CHAPTER 5

The Personhood of the Patient

Introduction

Dave and Diane are considering technological assistance in conceiving a baby. One of the technologies they are looking at involves fertilizing as many of Diane's eggs with Dave's sperm as possible, implanting some of them and storing the rest in case they need them. When presented with this option, they asked the infertility specialist what happens to the fertilized eggs, or embryos, if they do not need them. They were told that they were simply discarded, and that most couples who had leftover embryos did this without a second thought. They wondered about the ethics of such a practice.

Or consider the couple who justifies a decision to have an abortion on the grounds that such a tiny entity as a fetus in the first trimester cannot possibly be a person with the same right to life as a newborn baby, school-age child, or grown adult. Perhaps the man and woman have received prenatal genetic testing results that indicate that their child has a genetic anomaly. They think that surely a fetus with a genetic defect such as theirs cannot be a person, and that they do not have the responsibility to continue a pregnancy knowing that they are likely condemning their child to a life of suffering.

Or think about the family who is caring for its elderly father who has Parkinson's disease. These family members have heard of wonderful new treatments that alleviate some of the symptoms of Parkinson's. These treatments involve the use of the neural tissue from electively aborted fetuses. They see the good end result, that their father will get better, but are disturbed at the means by which the treatment is obtained.

Or finally, consider the case of an elderly patient with end-stage cancer who has wasted away as the cancer has destroyed his body. The physician is afraid of regulatory scrutiny as well as of shortening his life, and thus will not prescribe enough pain medication to make him comfortable. Family members want the long and painful dying process for their loved one over so that they can grieve appropriately and get on with their lives. They talk about getting their physician to assist in suicide covertly, as they understand a growing number of physicians have done. They realize that it is against the law, but they justify it on the grounds that their loved one is so wasted away that to call him a person is not accurate. Rather he is, for the most part, only a body that medical technology is keeping alive. They suggest that the things that make life worth living, such as the capacity for relationships, awareness of one's surroundings, mental sharpness, and the capacity to realize life plans and goals, no longer are present in what is left of their father's life. They do not believe they are violating the fifth commandment, against murder, by requesting assistance in suicide because they do not believe their father is really a person any longer.

In this chapter we want to complement the theological foundation of personhood with one way to develop it philosophically, from the perspective of a substance view of a human person. By way of application we want to spell out the numerous implications of the principles of personhood developed here and in chapter 4.

This concept of a human person has significant implications for a variety of social policy issues in which the question of when personhood begins is central. We have already argued that personhood is a part of bearing the image of God and that, from the earliest points of pregnancy, the unborn in the womb are persons. There is a clear continuity of personal identity that is taught by Scripture and is consistent with philosophical reflection. If that is true, then much of what goes under the heading of research and experimentation is actually a form of medical killing and, as such, is prohibited by the Hippocratic oath and the fifth commandment. If our argument about personhood is sound, that makes virtually all killing of embryos and fetuses very problematic.[1] This has ramifications for the way medical researchers use embryos and fetuses as research subjects, for the way infertility specialists use some reproductive technologies, for the way obstetricians manage high-risk pregnancies and deal with the maternal-fetal relationship, and for the way physicians provide end-of-life care, both

---

1. The exception would be in the very rare cases in which continuing a pregnancy would cause a threat to the life of the mother.

in the area of assisted suicide and that of withdrawing medically provided nutrition and hydration.[2]

Philosophical Reflections on Personhood

Since the discussion of personhood undergirds so many issues in bioethics and is at the heart of many public policy issues, it is important to be able to articulate biblical teaching in a way that is persuasive to an increasingly secular culture, for which the Bible has little if any authority.[3] One way to do this involves insight from specific philosophical categories, which are consistent with the theological reflection and biblical teaching. These categories come from the area of philosophy known as metaphysics, and they provide a helpful way of working out the theological view that human beings are full persons because they reflect the image of God, from the earliest points of development.

A properly grounded philosophical view of human persons involves making a key distinction between two different types of entities, substances and property-things.[4] Living things such as plants, animals, and human beings are examples of substances, while inanimate objects such as cars and machinery are examples of property-things. The difference is that a substance has an internal essence which defines it and orders its change and development according to observable principles. A substance is an entity in which the whole is greater than the sum of its parts, and the whole contains the essence, or internal ordering principle, that gives it its unity and cohesiveness. A substance is more than the collection of its parts. By contrast, a property-thing is no more than an ordered aggregate of its parts. It is ordered, but the order is

---

2. We will address only one aspect of physician-assisted suicide here, the notion that the patient is no longer a person but only a physical body being maintained by life-support technology.

3. Taking a Christian bioethics to a secular culture will be the subject of chapter 9.

4. We are indebted to our colleague, John A. Mitchell, M.A., for his contribution to this section. This is a revision of an article he and Scott Rae co-authored, entitled "The Moral Status of Fetuses and Embryos," in *The Silent Subject: Reflections on the Unborn in Society*, ed. Brad Stetson (Westport, Conn.: Praeger, 1996). This notion of a person as a substance is part of a larger philosophical tradition that began with Aristotle and was systematically integrated with Christian theology by the Catholic philosopher/theologian Thomas Aquinas. The technical term for this notion of a human person is a Thomistic substance dualist view of a person. For a full treatment of this view, see J. P. Moreland and Scott B. Rae, *On Human Persons: Metaphysical and Ethical Reflections* (Downers Grove, Ill.: InterVarsity, forthcoming).

externally imposed and there is no internal defining essence or principle that directs its change and development. There is no internal essence that informs and unifies its parts and properties. It is merely a collection of parts, standing in external space and time relations that, in turn, give rise to a bundle of externally related properties that are determined by those parts.

The same is not true with a substance — for example, a dog. The properties of a dog are different from the properties of an automobile. The properties of the dog are grounded in, unified by, and emerge from the dog's essence. That is, a dog is the way it is because it possesses an internal essence that defines and orders its properties. Thus a dog is more than the external organization of its parts functioning in a given way. Its properties are deeply unified and related internally as part of the essential nature of "dogness." A dog is what it is apart from social convention, and its properties exist only in the context of a coherent, ontological whole. By contrast, a car has no essence beyond its parts. Those parts are bundled together to form a loosely unified whole. Since a car has no internal essence or nature, an ordering principle is externally imposed upon a set of parts to form a bundle of properties by human convention. In this case assembly line technicians put the parts of the car together according to a blueprint that engineers drafted. The order and structure of the car are imposed entirely from without, in contrast to a dog, whose order and structure emerge from within, from its nature. To possess an internal nature, then, is possible only for substances. Their essential nature informs their being and gives them the essential properties that are characteristic of their natural kind. All members of a given species express the same essential nature, though there are differences in what are called accidental properties, such as the color of a dog and whether or not the dog has spots.

So while substances possess an internal nature, property-things do not. There is no internal, ordering principle or force that is capable of grounding a car's unity, governing its change, nor guiding its movement toward any end. Instead there are only modifications caused by external forces, namely, engineers and mechanics who work on the car. Human beings designed and built the automobile by arranging its materials into a specific pattern that would allow the car to function according to their design. The materials that were used to manufacture a car had no inherent inclination to be so structured, and its parts are externally ordered, imposed by forces outside the car itself, namely, the assembly line workers who assembled the car. Each of the materials used to build the car could have been used to make a variety of other things, by arranging them in different designs. For example, the tires could be used for a variety of other vehicles, and the metal that makes up many of the engine parts could be used for countless other metal objects. It just so happened that the external forces, that is, the design of the engineers and assemblers, arranged these parts into a car. There was nothing intrinsic to the car that demanded that its parts be ordered as they are.

By contrast, a puppy matures into an adult dog and an acorn matures into an oak tree, according to their internal essence. This essence, or nature, directs the developmental process of the substance and establishes limits on the variations each substance may undergo and still exist. For example, the acorn will not grow into a dog and the dog will not become an oak tree. Consequently, a substance functions in light of what it is, and maintains its essence regardless of the degree to which its ultimate capacities are realized. While there are variations among the individual members of a class of substances, such as differences in features between a dalmatian and a golden retriever, and like differences in the stages of development, such variance does not affect the essential nature of their being. For it is the underlying essence of a thing, not its state of development at a given point, that constitutes what it is. A puppy is not of a different kind from an adult dog, nor is a sapling of a different kind from a full-grown oak tree. As a substance grows, it does not become more of its kind, but rather it matures according to its kind. The development and realization of its potential, or its capacities, are controlled by the substance's essential nature. The capacities for the acorn one day to develop a trunk, branches, and leaves are already embedded within the acorn, prior to their realization. Whether or not the acorn actually develops into a full-grown oak tree depends on conditions such as its environment and nutrients in the soil. That is, it has capacities that are currently latent and will be expressed if the conditions are right for their development. If they fail to develop, that is the fault of the conditions, not of the internal essence or nature. That is, these conditions are independent of the acorn's essential nature. If the conditions are right, it will develop according to its internal design. By contrast, the car has an external design imposed from without that is necessary for it to be assembled into a car.

One helpful distinction between substances and property-things follows from the above discussion. Specifically, substances maintain their ontological identity through change, while property-things do not. The reason for this is that a substance is more than the sum of its parts which are ordered by some external force. A person can lose a body part such as an appendix, or a dog can shed fur, or an oak tree can lose leaves, and its identity does not change. With each of these substances (persons, dogs, and oak trees) the whole is prior to the parts, and these parts have their order because of the internal nature of the substance. By contrast, a property-thing is a collection of its constituent parts. When it loses one of its parts, it technically becomes a different entity. Thus it cannot maintain its identity over time and through change, because there is no internal ordering essence or principle that grounds its unity. A property-thing becomes a different property-thing when its parts change. No single entity can endure through change. It can only undergo a series of changes that result in similar but ontologically different entities. Though we commonly speak of a car as still being a car if it loses a tire, technically that is not the case. We actually speak of cars as if they were ontologically the same as persons, as though they were both substances. Our common language about cars clearly does not reflect what is metaphysically true about them. Property-things have no enduring essences to ground their identity through change.

Thus it follows from this distinction that substances maintain their identity through change and property-things do not. To suggest that a human being is a substance, maintaining identity as change occurs, is consistent with the biblical teaching that human beings have continuity of personal identity as they develop from embryos/fetuses to adult human beings, as was the case with King David in Psalm 139.

The question that arises from this is, on what basis should a human being be called a substance and not a property-thing? We can briefly sketch four lines of argument suggesting that human beings are substances and not property-things.[5] First, every human organism is an ontological whole whose parts, properties, and capacities are related internally. To call someone a human being and thus have a "human" identity of bodily organs and structures of consciousness presupposes a whole (the human essence) of which these organs and structures are parts. Second, every human being exhibits behavior that is specific to the human species, such as rational thought and the use of language, strongly suggesting an essential nature that is common to all members of the human species. Third, we presuppose that persons have the same personal identity as they age, grow, and develop. This strongly suggests a substance view of a human person. For example, the fact that we have introspective awareness of ourselves, that we can reflect on our own life and being, suggests that we have absolute personal identity through time. Further and more importantly, the concept of moral responsibility that undergirds our criminal justice system supports the notion that human persons are substances that endure through change. If this were not the case, it would be impossible to hold someone morally or criminally responsible for any action. The reason is

5. We are grateful to our colleague, Dr. J. P. Moreland, for his insights regarding this issue. For a thorough defense of the idea that human beings are substances, see Moreland and Rae, *On Human Beings.*

that the "person" who committed the crime would ontologically be a different "person" at the time of the arrest, a different "person" at the time of trial, a different "person" at the time of sentencing, and a different "person" at the time he or she was sent to prison. For example, if human beings are property-things, then O. J. Simpson was a different entity at the beginning of his trial than he was at the time he was arrested for double murder. The same would be true for everyone who commits a crime or does something immoral. Our justice system and concept of moral responsibility presuppose a substance view of a human being that gives a person a constant identity through time and change.

The notion of a human being as a substance has great significance for the moral status of embryos and fetuses. Virtually everyone accepts that personhood begins at least at birth. The debate continues over the personhood of the unborn. Viewing human beings as substances that have continuity of personal identity through change strongly suggests that personhood begins at conception. If a human being is indeed a substance, then we could summarize the philosophical argument from substance for the personhood of the unborn, the most controversial of the aspects of personhood, like this. First, an adult human being is the result of the continuous process of growth that begins at conception. Second, from conception to adulthood there is no break in this development which is relevant to the moral status of personhood. Therefore one is a human being from the point of conception onward.[6] Few if any would deny that adult human beings are the result of a continuous process of development that begins at conception. Likewise, few if any would deny that the conclusion, that embryos and fetuses are persons from conception onward, follows from the two premises, that human beings are the result of a continuous growth process and that there is no morally relevant break in the process. The force of this argument clearly rests on the second premise, that there is no morally relevant break in the development from conception to adulthood. Since virtually everyone agrees that once a child is born, he or she is a full person with all the corresponding rights to life, we could state this premise more specifically like this: there is no morally relevant break in the process between conception and birth. Some disagree with this claim, however, and point to either "criteria for humanness" or "decisive moments" between conception and birth at which the fetus first acquires the status of human personhood.

The most common decisive moment is viability, that is, the point at which the fetus is able to live on its own outside the womb. Currently the av-

6. Richard Werner, "Abortion: The Moral Status of the Unborn," *Social Theory and Practice* 4 (spring 1975): 201-22.

erage fetus is viable at roughly twenty-four to twenty-six weeks of gestation, though some fetuses have survived as early as twenty weeks. Once this point is reached, some argue, the fetus acquires the status of personhood, by virtue of its ability to live on its own, though still dependent on medical technology but not dependent on a uterine environment.

"Viability" as a determinant of personhood is unhelpful, if for no other reason than because viability cannot be measured precisely. It varies from fetus to fetus, and medical technology is continually pushing viability back to earlier stages of pregnancy. Moreover, since viability continues to change, questions are raised about its reliability as an indicator of personhood. But proponents of viability argue that it is possible, at least in principle, that medicine will reach a lower limit, say at twenty weeks' gestation, and at this point there may be no reasonable prospect of pushing it back any earlier. Given this scenario, viability will be a more stable concept, and thus it is argued that it is more reliable as a determinant of personhood.

But what does viability actually measure about a fetus? The concept of viability is not a commentary on the essence of the fetus, but on the ability of medical technology to sustain life outside the womb. Viability relates only to the fetus's location and dependency, not to its essence or personhood. There is no inherent connection between the fetus's ability to survive outside the womb and its essential nature as a human being. Thus, while viability is a helpful measure of the progress in medical technology, it has no bearing on what kind of a thing the fetus is or is not.

Perhaps the next most commonly proposed decisive moment is brain development, or the point at which the brain of the fetus begins to function, at roughly forty-five days of pregnancy. The appeal of this decisive moment is the parallel with the definition of death, which is the cessation of all brain activity. Since the absence of brain activity is what measures death, or the loss of personhood, some argue, it is reasonable to take the beginning of brain activity as an indication that personhood has begun. This decisive moment, however, is unhelpful as well. The problem with the analogy to brain death is that the dead brain has no capacity to revive itself again. It is in an irreversible condition, but the fetus only temporarily lacks first-order brain function. Its electroencephalogram (EEG) is only temporarily flat, whereas the dead person has a permanently flat EEG. In addition, the embryo from the point of conception has all the necessary capacities to develop full brain activity. Until around forty-five days' gestation those capacities are not yet realized, but they are latent in the embryo. However, that a capacity is not expressed in the first order has no bearing on the essence of the fetus, since that capacity is only temporarily latent, not irreversibly lost. Thus there are significant differences between the fetus who lacks the first-order capacity for brain activity in the first four to five weeks of pregnancy and the dead person who lacks both the potentiality and the actuality for any brain activity whatsoever. Pointing to brain activity as the decisive moment for personhood, then, does not stand up to critical scrutiny.

A third suggested decisive moment is sentience, or the point at which the fetus is capable of experiencing sensations, particularly pain. The appeal of this point for the determination of personhood is that if the fetus cannot feel pain, then there is less of a problem with abortion, and it disarms many of the pro-life arguments that abortion is cruel to the fetus. As is the case with the other decisive moments, however, sentience has little inherent connection to the personhood of the fetus, since it confuses the experience of harm with the reality of harm. Simply because the fetus cannot feel pain or otherwise experience harm, it does not follow that it cannot be harmed. If a person is paralyzed from the waist down and cannot feel pain in his or her legs, that person is still harmed if someone amputates a leg. In addition, to take sentience as the determinant of personhood, one would also have to admit that the reversibly comatose person, the person in a persistent vegetative state (a person who has sustained a very serious head injury, leaving only the brain stem functioning), the momentarily unconscious person, and even the sleeping person are not persons. One might object that these people once did function with sentience and that the loss of sentience is only temporary. But once that objection is made, the objector is admitting that something else besides sentience is determinant of personhood, and thus sentience as a decisive moment cannot be sustained.

Another suggested decisive moment is quickening, or the first time that the mother feels the fetus move inside her womb. Historically this has been the first evidence of life to be detected clearly. This was obviously before the use of sophisticated medical technology such as ultrasound that can see the fetus from the early stages of pregnancy. Upon close examination, it becomes clear that quickening as a determinant of personhood is unacceptable because the essence of the fetus cannot be dependent on someone's awareness of it. This criterion confuses the nature of the fetus with what one can know about the fetus. In other words, this decisive moment confuses epistemology (knowledge/awareness of the fetus) with ontology (the nature or essence of the fetus). A similar confusion is involved in the use of the appearance of "humanness" of the fetus as a decisive moment for personhood. The appeal of this view is primarily emotional, in that, as the fetus comes to resemble a baby, one begins to associate it with the kind of being that one would normally consider a full human being (e.g., a newborn). But what the fetus looks like has no inherent relationship to what it is, and from the point of conception the fetus has all the capacities necessary to one day exemplify the physical characteristics of a post-uterine human being. The "human" appearance of the fetus, then, is an unhelpful criterion for human personhood.

A few assert that birth is the decisive moment at which the fetus acquires personhood. But this view is deeply problematic. It seems intuitively obvious that there is no essential difference between the fetus on the day prior to its birth and on the day after its birth. The only difference between the prebirth and postbirth fetus/newborn is its location. But as is the case with viability as the determinant of personhood, birth says nothing about what kind of thing the fetus is; it merely offers a commentary on its location and degree of dependence. But just because a person changes venues, it does not follow that there is any essential change in the person's nature as a person. Likewise, just because the unborn human substance changes its location, this does not change its essential nature as a fully human being.

A final suggested decisive moment is implantation, and proponents of this view offer at least three reasons in its defense. First, it is at implantation when the embryo establishes its presence in the womb by the "signals" or the hormones it produces. Second, since anywhere from 20 to 50 percent of the embryos spontaneously miscarry prior to implantation, some suggest that implantation is critical not only to the development of the embryo but also to its essence. Proponents also suggest that if we claim that a full human person exists before implantation, then we are morally obligated to save all the embryos (something that very few people actually hold). Third, twinning, or the production of twins, normally occurs prior to implantation, and, according to some, this suggests that individual human personhood does not begin until after implantation.

Though placing personhood at implantation would have little effect on the abortion question (since most induced abortions occur well after implantation), the ethical implications of this decisive moment are significant. First, if correct, it would make any birth control methods that prevent implantation, such as many forms of the birth control pill and the "abortion pill," RU-486, morally allowable, since an embryo that has yet to implant is not considered a person. Further, leftover embryos that are kept in storage in in vitro fertilization could be discarded or experimented with without any moral problem, since those embryos do not possess personhood. Further, all research on pre-implantation embryos could be justifiable.

Several things can be said against the arguments for implantation as a decisive moment. First, just because the embryo establishes its presence by the hormonal signals it produces, it does not follow that personhood is established at this point. The essence of the fetus is independent of another's awareness of its existence, whether that awareness includes its physical awareness, as in quickening, or chemical awareness in the production of specific hormones. Second, just because up to 50 percent of conceived embryos spontaneously miscarry, it does not follow that personhood comes at implantation, since the essential nature of the fetus is not dependent on the number of embryos that do or do not survive to implant. Moreover, even if the pre-implantation embryo is a full human person, as we contend, we are not morally obligated to save them all since there is no moral obligation to interfere in the embryo's natural death. Not interfering to prevent a spontaneous miscarriage is not the same thing as killing an embryo, just as removing life support on a terminally ill patient and allowing him or her to die is not the same thing as actively killing such a patient.[7] Third, just because twinning occurs prior to implantation, it does not follow that the original embryo was not a full human person before the split. In fact, it is equally possible that two persons existed prior to implantation and only individualized after that point. Thus implantation fails to serve as an ontologically decisive moment for personhood.

Given the apparent inadequacies of the above decisive moments, ethicists like Mary Ann Warren suggest that persons must meet one of five criteria: (1) consciousness, and in particular the ability to feel pain; (2) a developed capacity for reasoning; (3) self-motivated activity; (4) the capacity to communicate; (5) the presence of self-concepts.[8] To this list Joseph Fletcher adds (1) self-control, (2) a sense of the future and the past, (3) the ability to relate to others, and (4) curiosity.[9] Similarly, James Rachels draws a distinction between "biographical" and "biological" life,[10] placing the emphasis on the possession of lower-order capacities of persons. However, the entire project of defining personhood in functional terms fails because, as argued above, a thing is what it is, not what it does. Moreover, the absence of lower-order (expressed) functional capacities does not mean that the individual's ultimate

---

7. There is some debate on the parallel between killing and allowing to die in euthanasia. See, for example, James Rachels, *The End of Life* (New York: Oxford Press, 1986).

8. Mary Ann Warren, "On the Moral and Legal Status of Abortion," in *Morality in Practice*, ed. James A. Sterba (Belmont, Calif.: Wadsworth Publishing, 1980), pp. 144-45, quoted by W. F. Cooney, "The Fallacy of All Person-Denying Arguments for Abortion," *Journal of Applied Philosophy* 8, no. 2 (1991): 163.

9. Joseph Fletcher, "Indicators of Humanhood: A Tentative Profile," *Hastings Center Report* 2 (1972), cited by Scott B. Rae, "Views of Human Nature at the Edges of Life," in *Christian Perspectives on Being Human: An Integrative Approach*, ed. J. P. Moreland and David Ciocchi (Grand Rapids: Baker, 1993), p. 239.

10. Rachels, *The End of Life*, p. 5.

capacities to express those abilities are absent. Instead, philosopher J. P. More-land suggests that "Higher order capacities are realized by the development of lower order capacities under [them]. . . . When a substance has a defect (e.g., a child is born color blind), it does not lose its ultimate capacities. Rather, it lacks some lower order capacity it needs for the ultimate capacity to be developed."[11] Thus, applied to the unborn, from the assertion that the unborn, defective or otherwise, may[12] be incapable of first-order human person skills like reasoning, communication, willing, desiring, self-reflection, aspiring, etc., it does not follow that they are not human persons. For these capacities still exist within the individual human substance as ultimate capacities constituting its essence. Therefore, even if these criteria were among the legitimate identifiers of personhood, every human substance, born and unborn, would qualify as a human person, since a human being is a substance with all the ultimate capacities for fully expressed personhood, including those listed by Warren, Fletcher, and Rachels.

The inadequacies of functional criteria for personhood are clearly evident if we try to practice them consistently. Consider the person under general anesthesia. That person is clearly not conscious, has no expressed capacity for reason, is incapable of self-motivated activity, cannot possibly communicate, has no concept of himself or herself, and cannot remember the past or aspire for the future. According to the functionalist view, he or she is not a full person — but this is absurd. In response, it may be argued that in that state, he or she is a person who is only temporarily dysfunctional. But this claim is not available without appealing to something outside of functional criteria. To argue that the person before anesthesia remains a person while under anesthesia, we must point to what that person is, irrespective of his or her functional capacities. To insist that the person remains a person because he or she had once expressed capacities of consciousness begs the question, since this merely reasserts the functional premise as a defense against the substance view of a human person.

Finally, if essential personhood is determined by function, it follows that essential personhood is a degreed property. After all, some will realize more of their capacities to reason, feel pain, self-reflect, etc., than others.

11. J. P. Moreland, "Wennberg, Personhood, and the Right to Die," *Faith and Philosophy* 12 (January 1995): 6, 7.

12. Much of this argument boils down to epistemological, not metaphysical, issues. Our ability to reliably ascertain the functional abilities of the unborn is hardly exhaustive. The budding field of prenatal psychology, experimental though it may be, points to the fact that much of the cognitive/self-awareness capabilities of the unborn remain unexplored.

Moreover, it is undeniable that the first several years of normal life outside the womb include an increasing expression of human capacities. Likewise, the last several years of life may include a decreasing expression of human capacities. Consequently, if the functionalist view is correct, the possession of personhood could be expressed by a bell curve, in which a human being moves toward full personhood in the first years of life, reaches full personhood at a given point, and then gradually loses personhood until the end of life. Presumably, the commensurate rights of persons would increase, stabilize, and decrease in the process. Without appealing to something other than function, it is difficult to resist this counterintuitive conclusion. Indeed, intellectual honesty has driven many to embrace this end, and the slope is ever so slippery. Bioethicists Helga Kuhse and Peter Singer comment on the ontological status of newborns: "When we kill a newborn, there is no person whose life has begun. When I think of myself as the person I am now, I realize that I did not come into existence until sometime after my birth. . . . It is the beginning of the life of the person, rather than of the physical organism, that is crucial so far as the right to life is concerned."[13]

While their intellectual consistency in applying their notion of personhood evenly in ethical issues is admirable, their chilling consistency reveals the danger of defining human personhood in functional terms. Not only are the unborn and newborns less than persons, apparently all of us are subject to graded personhood and the commensurate rights therein.

No Medical Killing

Treating patients as persons made in God's image and with inestimable value means that they must not be killed in the process of medical research or treatment of others. Since human beings are persons from the point of conception onward, they are entitled to the right to develop into fully mature adults. Thus physicians and medical centers committed to this notion of a human person cannot be involved in abortion or physician-assisted suicide. They must understand that patients at the end of life do not lose their personhood as they lose the capacities to live a full life. They need to treat both the pregnant woman and

---

13. Kuhse and Singer, *Should the Baby Live?* (New York: Oxford Press, 1985), p. 133. It is quickly apparent that Kuhse and Singer equivocate on the question of personal identity. After all, if *I* do not exist until sometime after *my* birth, in what sense is the birth *mine?* The only way for "*my* birth" to be more than a linguistic convention is to admit that "I" existed before I was born, or at least at the time of my birth. But if this is the case, Kuhse and Singer's attempt to define personhood in terms of function fails.

the unborn child as obstetric patients. They should not support embryo research or experimental treatments using the tissue from electively aborted fetuses. They cannot endorse the myriad of assisted reproductive options available for infertile couples without some moral parameters.

Abortion

For the person who holds that personhood begins at conception, clearly abortion, except in the very rare cases in which the mother's life is in grave, imminent jeopardy, is the equivalent of killing an innocent person, and cannot be justified. Health care professionals who hold this view of personhood cannot morally justify being involved in performing abortions. Nor can they support the right to choose to end the life of an unborn child. Abortion is simply a form of medical killing based on the desire of the mother not to be pregnant any longer. Once it is accepted that the unborn is a person, there cannot be any justification for taking its life in the womb, apart from those rare situations in which the mother's life is in real danger. All of the arguments for a pro-choice position are difficult to maintain, since they all beg the question by assuming that the unborn is not a person.[14] For example, the commonly cited argument that abortion is justifiable because the fetus is part of the woman's body and she has the right to do with her own body as she chooses, assumes that the unborn is not a person. But if the unborn is a person, then that argument is in essence that a woman has the right to arbitrary execution of her unborn child. The argument depends on the assumption that the unborn is not a person, which is at the heart of the debate.

This is similar to other arguments for abortion rights, such as that abortion should be allowed in cases of genetic deformity or cases of extreme poverty. These two arguments assume that the unborn is not a person, for if it is, then these arguments would be asserting that there is no morally significant difference between abortion for poverty and eliminating the poor, or between abortion for genetic deformity and eliminating all the genetically disabled adults. Of course, such arguments are absurd, and the pro-choice advocate would respond that we would not eliminate the poor and the genetically dis-

14. Some pro-choice advocates grant that the unborn is a person and justify abortion on other grounds, such as the priority of the rights of the mother over the rights of the child. This seems difficult to maintain since historically, when life and liberty have conflicted, life has taken precedence. Others hold that abortion is immoral but should not be legislated. See Scott B. Rae, ed., *Abortion: Private Morality and Public Policy, Three Christian Views* (Grand Rapids: Zondervan, forthcoming).

abled because they are persons with the corresponding right to life. But that makes their assumption clear about the unborn, an assumption that we have argued cannot be upheld. Other arguments further beg the question, such as the argument that denying abortions to poor women would be an unjustifiable form of discrimination, since wealthy women can travel to other countries and procure abortions there. But this assumes that the right to abortion is something to which everyone should have access, such that denial of it constitutes discrimination. But that is the issue under discussion — whether or not it should be a right accessible to all women.[15]

Embryo Research

Research on embryos and fetuses marks another stage in the long line of social policy repercussions that came out of the 1973 *Roe v. Wade* Supreme Court decision that allowed for abortion on demand. The current debate over the use of embryos in research began in August 1993, when the National Institutes of Health (NIH) requested a broad-based panel to suggest guidelines for research and experimentation on pre-implantation human embryos.[16] The request was granted in September 1993, and in February 1994 the Embryo Research Panel was convened by the NIH for the purpose of developing ethically and legally appropriate guidelines for the controversial area of embryo research. The report of the panel was finalized and released in late September 1994, and President Clinton approved most of the funding recommendations.

Two primary purposes for embryo research provided the initial impetus for the panel's recommendations. First, there was a desire to improve the success rates of in vitro fertilization and other treatments for infertility. Experimentation on pre-implantation embryos promises to help medical researchers and infertility practitioners understand more fully why roughly 75 percent of all embryos implanted in infertility treatments fail to result in a pregnancy. A second and broader purpose was to better understand the process of embryonic development so that miscarriages could be prevented and early stages of pregnancy be better managed, so that chromosomal abnormalities could be better understood, and so that cell lines could be developed to produce fetal tissue for

15. For more detail on the various pro-choice arguments, see Francis J. Beckwith, *Politically Correct Death: Answering the Arguments for Abortion Rights* (Grand Rapids: Baker, 1993).

16. The account of the background to the current debate is taken from National Institutes of Health Human Embryo Research Panel, *Report of the Human Embryo Research Panel* (Washington, D.C.: National Institutes of Health, 27 September 1994), pp. 14-18.

use in treatments. A third rationale for this research comes from the newly discovered ability to isolate stem cells from embryos. This is a key first step toward manufacturing human tissue and possibly even organs from stem cells.

The panel was asked to make three different types of recommendations: areas of research that are acceptable for federal funding, areas that are not acceptable for federal funding, and areas that warrant additional review.[17] The panel concluded that research on embryos left over from in vitro fertilization and on embryos created in vitro is acceptable for funding if a compelling case for the benefit of the research could be made. It further concluded that the development of cell lines to produce various types of fetal tissue for transplantation was also acceptable for funding. The panel suggested that research on embryos not occur after roughly fourteen days' development, or after the appearance of the primitive streak, the time at which the cells begin to differentiate into various types of tissues. The panel grounded its recommendations in the promise of benefit of the research, the lower moral status of the embryo vis-à-vis fetuses and children, and ongoing ethical and scientific review of the research that federal funding would enable.

The panel further recommended that the following areas constituted types of research not acceptable for federal funding:

1. Research on embryos beyond twenty-one days' development
2. Research involving fetal eggs with transfer to another woman's uterus
3. Cloning of embryos with transfer to the uterus
4. Attempted gestation of human embryos in animals

These considerations were grounded in the potential harmful consequences for children and adults, respect due the pre-implantation human embryo, concern for public opinion about controversial research, and concern for the meaning of parenthood and procreation.

A third category of recommendations was those that merited further review and reflection. These include research on embryos between fourteen and twenty-one days' development, cloning of embryos without transfer to a uterus, research on fetal eggs without transfer, and development of tissue cell lines from embryos deliberately created for such purposes.

The panel devoted one entire chapter of its report to the moral status of the pre-implantation embryo. That section constitutes the heart of the panel's views on embryo research and experimentation, and reflects the views

17. This summary is taken from "What Research? Which Embryos?" *Hastings Center Report* 25 (January-February 1995): 36.

of many in the culture and scientific community on the nature of the embryo. In it panelists argued for what they called a "pluralistic approach" in which the personhood of the embryo is approached from a variety of criteria, not simply a single criterion for establishing its personhood. The panel rightly rejected grounding personhood in criteria such as sentience, or the ability to experience sensations, the beginning of brain function, and certain basic cognitive functions such as self-consciousness. It also unfortunately rejected the view that personhood begins at conception, suggesting that such a view involves defining personhood based on genetic identity.

A pluralistic approach does not rely on any single criterion for personhood but rather takes a number of considerations into account, such as "genetic uniqueness, potentiality for full development, sentience, brain activity, cognitive development, capacity for survival outside the womb, and degree of relational presence." The panel argued that while "none of these qualities is by itself sufficient to establish personhood, their developing presence in an entity increases its moral status until, at some point [which was left unspecified], full and equal protectability is required."[18] With the formation of what is called the primitive streak (the first elements of the spinal column and nervous system) at fourteen days' development, the embryo makes a significant step forward in its organization and differentiation, thus meriting an increased level of protection. For this reason the panel recommended that research on the embryo be essentially limited to the time period prior to the appearance of the primitive streak. It held that the embryo be entitled to "profound respect, but this respect does not necessarily encompass the legal and moral rights attributed to persons."[19] Thus the pluralistic approach "accords some moral weight to the preimplantation embryo but does not rule out justified research."[20] Unfortunately, in the report the important question of how one weights the consideration given to the embryo against the potential benefits of embryo research is not addressed, leading some to conclude that the weight given to the embryo is merely symbolic, not substantial, and shouldn't be allowed to stand in the way of research.[21] This is even more striking given the report's omission of any realized benefits of the research that has been going on in other countries for some time. Some have concluded that this appears to be a "free ride for research, whose potential benefits are treated with the kind of credulity not seen since the days when the golden calf was worshipped."[22] In addition, the panel seems to have missed the obvious problem of

18. Human Embryo Research Panel, p. 49.

19. Human Embryo Research Panel, pp. 49-50.

20. Human Embryo Research Panel, p. 51.

21. John A. Robertson, "Symbolic Issues in Embryo Research," *Hastings Center Report* 25 (January-February 1995): 37-38.

how to have "profound respect" for something that will be discarded after research on it has been completed. Daniel Callahan of the Hastings Center comments that "I have always felt a nagging uneasiness at trying to rationalize killing something for which I claim to have profound respect."[23]

This pluralistic approach appears to be at the heart of the panel's desire to approach the public policy aspects of embryo research independent of any particular worldview. In justifying its pluralistic view, it states that "Public policy employs reasoning that is understandable in terms that are independent of a particular religious, theological or philosophical perspective, and it requires weighing of arguments in light of the best available information and scientific evidence."[24] Interestingly, the panel appeared to place philosophical traditions in the same category as religious convictions, both under the umbrella of private perspectives and thus not suitable for public policy. This would seem to leave the panel with at least an implicit commitment to empiricism as its starting place, given its emphasis on the available scientific evidence on the moral status of the embryo. But personhood is not a scientific concept, it is a philosophical one that is by definition worldview-dependent. The panel's deliberate omission of philosophical considerations seems particularly problematic here. In addition, it actually was not followed by the panel itself. Callahan suggests that "The report has in fact adopted a particular philosophical viewpoint on the purpose of law, on the imperative of scientific research and on the moral status of the fetus. If the Panel did not notice that, just about everyone else will."[25] Research on embryos that will result in their destruction, either through the research process or by being discarded after the process is finished, is very problematic for the person who holds that personhood begins at conception. It would be difficult to see how a person who holds such a view of personhood could support or participate in embryo research because it involves the deliberate destruction of embryonic persons for the debatable benefits of such research.

Fetal Tissue Research and Transplantation

There is currently great excitement in the medical community about the prospects of fetal tissue transplantation. The use of fetal tissue is actually part of a long-established tradition of using fetal cells in research. However, in the

22. Daniel Callahan, "The Puzzle of Profound Respect," *Hastings Center Report* 25 (January-February 1995): 39.

23. Callahan, p. 39.

24. Human Embryo Research Panel, pp. 50-51.

25. Callahan, p. 40.

early use of fetal cells the source was only spontaneous abortions and ectopic pregnancies, not elective abortions done for birth control purposes. Fetal tissue is a good source of transplant material due to its potential for growth, its ability to differentiate, and its ability to integrate into the recipient. It is also less subject to rejection in the transplant process.[26] In addition, it is currently in high supply.

There are many different potential uses of fetal tissue for transplants, but the focus to date has been on the treatment of Parkinson's disease and diabetes. The state of fetal tissue transplant technology can best be characterized as still "experimental," though with progress being made each year.[27] Should the technology be perfected, it shows promise for application to a number of other degenerative diseases such as Alzheimer's disease, Huntington's chorea, and spinal cord or other neural injuries. In addition, the use of fetal liver cells shows promise for treating bone marrow diseases and blood disorders, and fetal pancreatic cells have been shown to help treat diabetes.[28] Should the technology develop as anticipated, the amount of tissue would fall far short of the demand.[29]

In the aftermath of *Roe v. Wade,* the federal government established regulations to limit the scope of experimentation on the fetus. In 1974 the Department of Health, Education and Welfare created the National Commission for the Protection of Human Subjects of Biomedical and Behavioral Research. The regulations recommended by this commission were adopted the following year. Experiments on the live fetus are permitted only if the research is of benefit to the fetus and if there is minimal risk to it. The regulations further state that any experiments with dead fetuses be done in accordance with state law. Most states permit the use of tissue from dead fetuses under the provisions of the Uniform Anatomical Gift Act (UAGA), which allows next of kin to donate the tissue, similar to organ donation from cadavers.[30]

The current discussion on this issue began in October 1987 with an

26. A helpful summary of the scientific advantages of fetal tissue for some of these transplants is found in Robert Auerbach and Harold R. Wolfe, *Report of the Human Fetal Tissue Transplantation Research Panel,* vol. 2, pp. D28-D31.

27. Henry T. Greely et al., "The Ethical Use of Human Fetal Tissue in Medicine," *New England Journal of Medicine* 320 (20 April 1989): 1093.

28. Kathleen Nolan, "Genug ist Genug: A Fetus Is Not a Kidney," *Hastings Center Report* 18 (December 1988): 13.

29. James Bopp and James Burtchaell, "Fetal Tissue Transplantation: The Fetus as Medical Commodity," *This World* 26 (summer 1989): 67-68.

30. John A. Robertson, "Rights, Symbolism and Public Policy in Fetal Tissue Transplants," *Hastings Center Report* 18 (December 1988): 5.

NIH request for federal funding to transplant fetal neural tissue into the brain of a Parkinson's patient. In March 1988 the NIH convened a twenty-one-member panel to study the issue. The panel published its findings and made the following recommendations as parameters for research it considered ethically acceptable:[31]

1. The decision to abort must be made prior to discussion of the use of the tissue.
2. Anonymity is to be maintained between donor and recipient.
3. Timing and method of abortion are not to be influenced by the possibility of tissue use.
4. Consent of the pregnant woman is necessary and sufficient unless the husband objects.
5. No financial or other incentives are to be given to the woman who aborts and thus "donates" the tissue.

In considering the ethical issues, it should be clear from our biblical and philosophical analysis that the fetus is a person with full attendant rights. This makes the use of fetal tissue from elective abortions problematic since an evil means, the deliberate taking of the life of the fetus, is used to accomplish a good end, alleviation of suffering of patients with diseases for whom the tissue can be helpful. Some would argue that the tissue will be available in any case, since abortion is legal and people will continue to have surgical abortions. Therefore, why not put the tissue to some good use rather than simply discarding it? Those who argue for this position insist that the abortion and the donation of tissue can be morally separated, and that one can oppose abortion and still favor use of tissue from aborted fetuses.

Here are some of the arguments against use of fetal tissue from induced, elective abortions.

1. *Fetal tissue transplants are* not *parallel to adult organ transplants.* Advocates of fetal tissue transplants either assume or explicitly invoke the framework of UAGA (Uniform Anatomical Gift Act). The UAGA has governed adult organ transplants for some time, and recently, with the rise of fetal tissue transplant technology, the law was expanded to include the fetus as an organ donor. The primary part of the UAGA framework is the parallel between the dead fetus and the adult cadaver as an organ donor. For example, in

---

31. Consultants to the Advisory Committee to the Director, National Institutes of Health, *Report of the Human Fetal Tissue Transplantation Research Panel* (December 1988), vol. 2, p. A25.

a article in *Christianity Today,* Dr. Billy Arant, Jr., of the University of Texas Southwestern Medical Center, makes this parallel when he compares the debate on fetal tissue transplants to the earlier debate on organ donations in general: "The ethical and moral concerns raised during the early years when human organ transplantation was considered experimental were not very different from the ones heard today regarding the use of fetal tissue." Later he asks, "Where, then, is the difference in using tissue obtained from human fetuses to restore health or extend life, especially if the tissue is obtained from fetuses aborted spontaneously — which will occur unpredictably in many pregnancies just as accidental deaths provide a source of donor organs?"[32] Accidental death is precisely the parallel that is appropriate, and there is no moral difficulty with using the tissue from spontaneous abortions.

However, most fetal tissue used in transplants comes from induced, not spontaneous, abortions. There are enormous differences between fetal tissue transplants from induced abortions and adult organ transplantations from accidental deaths that render this parallel invalid. The use of the tissue from induced abortion is inconsistent with the UAGA framework, since the death of the fetus is intentionally caused, not accidental. Though a small amount of fetal tissue from miscarriages and ectopic pregnancies is useful for transplants, the great majority of fetal tissue usually becomes available when pregnant women agree to end their pregnancy intentionally, thus killing developing fetuses. This is hardly the same situation as when organs are recovered from people killed in tragic accidents. LeRoy Walters, in charge of ethical and legal issues for the NIH panel, said in 1974, when only experimentation with the fetus, not the tissue transplants, was being deliberated: "Ought one to make experimental use of the products of an abortion system, when one would object on ethical grounds to many or most of the abortions performed within that system? If a particular hospital became the beneficiary of an organized homicide system which provided a fresh supply of cadavers, one would be justified in raising questions about the moral appropriateness of the hospital's continuing cooperation with the suppliers."[33] Another parallel might be a banker who regards the drug trade as morally wrong, yet agrees to accept drug money at his bank in order to finance low-income housing for the community. This banker would be involved in complicity with the drug trade, even though he is not involved with the actual sale of narcotics. Use of the tis-

32. Dr. Billy S. Arant, Jr., "Why the Government Should Lift the Moratorium," *Christianity Today,* 19 November 1990, p. 28.

33. LeRoy Walters, "Ethical Issues in Experimentation on the Human Fetus," *Journal of Religious Ethics* 2 (spring 1974): 41, 48.

sue in cases of elective abortion involves a morally unacceptable complicity with the evil of taking the life of an innocent unborn child. Though the tissue can be put to good use, its use is morally tainted as a consequence of being obtained through elective abortion.

The parallel between adult organ donors and fetal tissue transplants is undermined by the fact that valid consent is impossible. To date, fetal tissue transplants are treated as any other organ transplants under the UAGA, thus requiring consent of next of kin. However, the mother cannot give morally legitimate consent, since she authorized the termination of the pregnancy. According to the normal understanding of proxy consent, her role assumes that she is acting in the best interest of the unborn child. Yet she is also the one who has authorized the termination of the pregnancy. The late ethicist Paul Ramsey concluded that it is morally outrageous and a charade to give the woman who aborts any right to proxy consent for the donation of or experimentation on the aborted fetus's body parts.[34] James Bopp and Father James Burtchaell conclude in their dissent from the NIH panel report: "We can think of no sound precedent for putting a living human into the power of such an estranged person, not for his or her own welfare, but for the 'interests' of the one in power."[35]

One may object to the need for consent in the first place, if the fetus is not recognized as a person. Yet the fetus is a person, which explains why fetal tissue is so valuable: precisely because it is human. Biologically the fetus is much more than an organ or a piece of tissue. It is a developing human being with potential for full maturity and thus full membership in the moral community from the time of conception. Clearly, if abortion is taking innocent human life, use of fetal tissue for experiments and treatment is ethically troubling, since it is doing evil to accomplish good. The notion of the fetus as the source of biological "spare parts" is uncomfortably reminiscent of Huxley's *Brave New World*.[36]

A more significant conceptual problem is encountered when one considers that the fetus is simultaneously both a donation and a donor. It is difficult to see how the fetus can be called a donor under the UAGA in parallel to an adult organ donor, if the features that give the fetus personhood are discounted. The fetus is a victim rather than a willing donor. When the donation

---

34. Paul Ramsey, *The Ethics of Fetal Research* (New Haven: Yale University Press, 1975), p. 89.

35. Bopp and Burtchaell, p. 59.

36. Stuart A. Newman, "Statement on Proposed Uses of Human Fetal Tissue," in *Report of the Human Fetal Tissue Transplantation Research Panel*, vol. 2, p. D207. This is even more the case now that researchers can isolate the stem cells from embryos.

of fetal tissue is described as a gift from the fetus as a donor, only miscarriages and ectopic pregnancies can stand on a moral basis, since these fetuses were only unable, and not unwelcome, to join the human community.[37] This is not a parallel to surrogate motherhood, where the mother is viewed as the donor and the tissue as the donation. Kathleen Nolan summarizes the alternative to rejecting the UAGA framework for fetal tissue transplants:

> If we reject the framework of the UAGA, we seem doomed to accept arguments that implicitly or explicitly equate fetuses with things or beings that they are not — among them kidneys, tumors and discarded surgical specimens. Yet biologically, the fetus is not a tissue or an organ but a body, and morally, the fetus is a developing being and potential member of the human community. Fetal remains accordingly ought to evoke emotions and protections beyond those given tumorous tissue or unwanted organs.[38]

2. *Most of the proposed restrictions governing the use of fetal tissue are unenforceable.* For example, given the increasing public awareness of the medical technology and the growing benefits that will occur, keeping the two distinct acts of consent (for the abortion and for the tissue donation) separate is virtually impossible. All of the proposed guidelines treat this as one of the nonnegotiable aspects of the transplants. It is difficult to imagine that, given separate consent forms, coercion to donate the tissue would not enter in, in view of the potential transplant benefits, the likely scarcity of available tissue as the technology develops, and the vulnerability of the women in anticipating an abortion.

In addition, given the potentially lucrative market for the transplants, keeping *financial inducements* from entering in would be difficult, and impossible to enforce. The fetal tissue industry has the potential to become very big business. Abortion clinics stand to reap a substantial increase in revenue simply from the small amount (on average, twenty-five dollars per organ, multiplied by the hundreds of thousands of abortions performed annually) that the nonprofit acquisition organizations offer. The financial incentives to "recruit" fetal tissue donors would be significant. There are numerous noncash inducements that are difficult to detect and impossible to adequately police that would be especially appealing to poor and minority women. For example, the clinic could offer a "discount" on the abortion procedure itself or promise to provide future medical care for a specified time period following the donation of the tissue. With the anticipated prof-

37. Nolan, p. 18.
38. Nolan, p. 16.

itability of the industry once the technology can alleviate a larger number of diseases, there will be increasing pressures to "share the wealth" being produced by these transplants.

A recent California court decision may set a precedent that will make it more difficult to prevent women from obtaining compensation for the donation of fetal tissue. In *Moore v. Regents of the University of California,* an appeals court reversed a lower court decision, ruling that a person does have a property interest in his own cells.[39] In treatment for leukemia, doctors at the UCLA Medical Center removed the spleen of a Mr. Moore and discovered that they could manufacture a cell line from that tissue that was effective in slowing certain types of leukemia. The medical center then sought out a commercial arrangement with a pharmaceutical company to market the cell line. When asked for his consent, Moore refused and sued the university for his share of any profit resulting from the cell line. Though the court did not rule on his right to compensation, it did hold that individuals have a property interest in their own cells, and thus a right to control what becomes of their tissues. One can see how this could open the door not only to financial inducements but to a right to compensation for fetal tissue donation.

This potentially lucrative market will make it increasingly difficult to enforce another of the proponents' guidelines: the separation of the transplant physician/researcher and the one who performs the abortion. This is a key distinction for proponents of the transplants, even for those who are against abortion in most cases, who assume that the morality of abortion and fetal tissue transplants can be separated. Yet clearly, the means as well as the ends have moral significance. For the best medical results there must be an institutional, symbiotic relationship with the abortion industry, thereby making the separation of abortion and tissue procurement very difficult. This partnership may also make it more complicated to isolate the timing and method of abortion from what is necessary to procure the best possible tissue. Mahowald and associates already propose that pregnancies be prolonged and the method of abortion be modified, if necessary, in order to procure the most fresh, and thus the most useful, tissue.[40] In addition, some acknowledge the legitimate possibility that tissue be removed from live, nonviable fetuses.

3. *The use of fetal tissue from elective abortions will serve to enhance abor-*

---

39. *Moore v Regents of the University of California,* California Court of Appeal, 249 Cal. Rptr. 494 (1988). Review granted by California Supreme Court, 252 Cal. Rptr. 816 (10 November 1988).

40. Mary Mahowald et al., "The Ethical Options in Transplanting Fetal Tissue," *Hastings Center Report* 18 (1988): 7-15.

tion's image, or at least make it morally neutral. At a minimum, the possibility of donating tissue will relieve some of the guilt that many women feel when electing abortion, thus alleviating some of the ambivalence that usually accompanies it. The routine retrieval of the tissue would no doubt make the death of the unborn child seem less tragic. Nolan puts it this way: "Enhancing abortion's image could thus be expected to undermine efforts to make it as little needed and little used a procedure as possible."[41] Though it is true that the use of tissue for research has not increased the incidence of abortion, its use for transplants produces concrete benefits rather than research possibilities and statistical lives, thus making it more likely that the potential for use of the tissue will increase the incidence of surgical abortion.

Studies show great ambivalence toward abortion among the women considering it.[42] There is usually intense anxiety during the final twenty-four hours before the abortion is performed. Studies of pregnant women choosing abortion show that between 33 and 40 percent change their mind at least once, and around 30 percent do not finally make up their mind until just prior to the procedure. Thus it is likely that the prospect of solace over the guilt that usually accompanies abortion will enter into the complex set of factors that are involved in the decision to abort. The possibility of "redeeming abortion" throws a powerful human motivation into the already complex situation that will have an effect on those 33 to 40 percent who change their minds during the process. Bopp and Burtchaell, in their dissent from the NIH panel report, state: "It is willful fantasy to imagine that young pregnant women estranged from their families and their sexual partners, and torn by the knowledge that they are with child, will not be powerfully relieved at the prospect that the sad act of violence they are reluctant to accept can now have redemptive value."[43]

4. *Fetal tissue transplants from elective abortions have substantial potential for abuse.* There are possibilities for abuse about which even the more moderate advocates are wary. Already there have been people not simply willing but eager to conceive just to donate the tissue.[44] Fetal tissue is currently being used to make cosmetics in Sweden, and fetal kidneys from Brazil and India are being sold in Germany to physicians for transplant.[45] It is true that

41. Nolan, p. 17.

42. Michael Bracken, Lorraine Klerman, and Mary Ann Bracken, "Abortion, Adoption or Motherhood: An Empirical Study of Decision-Making during Pregnancy," *American Journal of Obstetrics and Gynecology* 130 (1978): 256-57.

43. Bopp and Burtchaell, p. 67.

44. Tamar Lewin, "Medical Use of Fetal Tissue Spurs New Abortion Debate," *New York Times,* 16 August 1987, p. 1.

most advocates recommend some laws or voluntary guidelines to keep such abuses from taking place. These may be adequate for the short run, but there are no guarantees that these kinds of abuses can be prevented in the long run as the process becomes more acceptable. It is naive to think that the long-run pressure can be resisted, given the powerful incentives to donate the tissue that the advances in medical science promise to provide. In addition, with the likely introduction of RU-486 into the marketplace, the incidence of surgical abortion should decrease substantially, restricting the available supply of fetal tissue, while at the same time the demand is exploding due to the advance of technology. In that case it is difficult to see how the tissue can be obtained without many of the inducements that proponents of the tissue use suggest are unethical. The only way to secure adequate tissue for treatment and research will be either to pay for it, thus creating a market for fetal tissue, or allow pregnant women to abort and designate the recipient of the tissue. This would lead to the likely scenario in which women are conceiving for the purpose of becoming pregnant, aborting, and donating the tissue for a specific recipient, a scenario that most advocates of the tissue use insist is unethical.

Technologically Assisted Reproduction

For the person who believes that personhood begins at conception, some types of reproductive technologies have potential moral difficulties. The procedures involved are in the in vitro fertilization family of technologies. They include GIFT (gamete intrafallopian transfer), ZIFT (zygote intrafallopian transfer), and IVF (in vitro fertilization). These procedures involve surgical retrieval of as many of the woman's eggs as possible, after she has been stimulated hormonally to produce as many as she can. They are either fertilized with the husband's sperm in the lab and some of the resulting embryos (usually four) inserted in the woman's body (IVF and ZIFT), or the eggs are reinserted into the woman's body along with the husband's sperm so that fertilization can occur in the body (GIFT). In IVF and ZIFT leftover embryos are stored in the lab for future use should the woman not become pregnant. In GIFT the remaining eggs are fertilized in the lab and kept in storage if necessary for future use should pregnancy not occur. Using the leftover embryos for future implantation attempts dramatically cuts the cost of the procedures and reduces the physical toll on the woman. Since roughly three out of four

45. Debra McKenzie, "Embryos to Lipsticks?" *New Scientist,* 10 October 1985, p. 21; "Third World Kidneys for Sale," *New Scientist,* 28 March 1985, p. 7.

attempts at assisted reproductive technology fail, having a backup mechanism in these leftover embryos is important.

The reason this is a problem is that embryos are persons, deserving of full human rights. They are not potential persons, a concept that itself is problematic. Either one is a person or one is not a person. What one normally means by this imprecise use of that term is that the embryo (and fetus also) is a person with the potential to become a full-grown adult. It is better to say that the embryo is a "person with potential."

In GIFT, ZIFT and IVF leftover embryos are usually discarded. In some cases they are used for experimentation, and if the couple consents they may be donated to other infertile couples. Donations like this would be seen as the practical equivalent of adoption. The couple would simply put embryos, not newborn babies, up for "adoption." Embryo donation is not anywhere near as complicated as formal adoption, and the infertile couple gets the experience of carrying and delivering their child.

The normal practice of discarding embryos is problematic for couples who hold that personhood begins at conception. Throwing away embryos that a couple does not plan to use is no different morally from abortion at any point during the pregnancy. Only the location of the unborn child and its stage of development are different. Since the embryo has all the capacities to develop into a fully grown adult from the point of conception, needing only the proper environment in which to develop, then the point at which it is destroyed and discarded is irrelevant. A person with a unique genetic endowment and with full potential to become a fully grown adult human being has been destroyed. Some have further lamented the fact that human embryos are being treated as the equivalent of "industrial waste," a by-product of the procedure that is thrown out when no longer needed.[46]

Not only are some complicated moral problems raised by having leftover embryos, there are some legal problems that would have tested the wisdom of Solomon. What happens to embryos when they are orphaned, that is, when the parents die or divorce, is very difficult and complicated to determine.[47]

What is a couple to do with leftover embryos that have been preserved

---

46. Roger Rosenblatt, *Time*, 14 February 1983, p. 90.

47. In the case of the orphaned embryos, see George P. Smith, "Australia's Frozen 'Orphan' Embryos: A Medical, Legal and Ethical Dilemma," *Journal of Family Law* 24, no. 1 (1985-86): 26-41. See also Donald DeMarco, *Biotechnology and the Assault on Parenthood* (San Francisco: Ignatius Press, 1991), pp. 104-5. In the case of the parents divorcing and the determination of "custody" of the embryos, see *Davis v Davis*, 1990 Tenn. App. LEXIS 642 (13 September 1990). For further reading on the *Davis* case, see George J. Annas,

in storage? The most obvious alternative to discarding the embryos would be for the couple to insist that the clinic freeze and store the woman's eggs prior to fertilization in the lab. That way eggs, not embryos, are being stored. The couple has eggs left over to use again in the future, avoiding the entire process of egg retrieval, while at the same time not destroying and discarding embryonic human persons. Unfortunately, storing eggs is not a viable alternative medically at this point in the development of these various technologies. The success rate at thawing eggs is so low that virtually no infertility clinic offers it as an alternative to infertile couples.

A second alternative that some couples have contemplated is not intentionally discarding the embryos, but allowing them to die a natural death in the lab. They reason that it is parallel to a miscarriage, only it happens in the lab and not in the body. Those who suggest this alternative insist that they are simply allowing something to happen in the lab that happens frequently in the body. They argue that the location in which it occurs, either the body or the lab, should not make a morally significant difference. Thus they would say that allowing them to die a natural death is more akin to a miscarriage than to an intentional abortion.

However, there is a morally significant difference besides location between a miscarriage and allowing embryos in storage to die natural deaths. Most miscarriages cannot be prevented. In many cases no one fully understands why they occur. Of course, some can be traced to deformities in the fetus or problems in the woman's reproductive system. But a great many miscarriages are random, spontaneous occurrences. However, the destruction of embryos in storage in a lab is easily prevented. Simply thaw and implant them, either in the woman in the original couple whose genes contributed to the embryo or with a couple who is seeking an embryo donor. In medicine in general, it is certainly justifiable to allow someone to die a natural death when it cannot be prevented, that is, when further treatment is futile. But to allow someone to die from an easily preventable disease or condition is morally very problematic, and people who allow others to die natural deaths in this way are doing the moral equivalent of killing them. There does not seem to be any morally significant difference between discarding embryos when they are

---

"Crazy-Making: Embryos and Gestational Mothers," *Hastings Center Report* 21 (January-February 1991): 35-38, and Alexander Morgan Capron, "Parenthood and Frozen Embryos: More Than Property and Privacy," *Hastings Center Report* 22 (September October 1992): 32-33. See the summary discussion of these two cases in Scott B. Rae, *Brave New Families: Biblical Ethics and Reproductive Technologies* (Grand Rapids: Baker, 1996), pp. 132-34.

no longer needed and allowing them to be discarded when they can no longer be thawed successfully.[48]

A third alternative is to give the embryos away to another infertile couple. Donating the embryos is certainly a possibility that is morally different from discarding them, but most couples are uncomfortable with the idea of donating their embryos to another couple that they have never met and will never meet or see again. This is because embryo donation is done anonymously in many cases to prevent the donors from attempting to locate the child and intrude on his or her stable family life. The notion of another couple, not to mention one they do not know, raising a child that is the combination of their genetic materials and may even look like one or the other of them, is very unsettling. As one person who was contemplating embryo donation put it, "I don't want my progeny running around all over the country without my knowledge!!" This uncomfortable feeling is often more intense when a husband and wife realize that they have not one but a number of embryos in storage, all of which would need to be donated to a variety of other couples to keep from having to destroy them. Even though donation does not involve discarding the leftover embryos, and is more ethically acceptable, it is difficult to accept emotionally for many couples.

The most prudent course for couples to follow and for their physicians to encourage in these procedures is to avoid having leftover embryos as best they can. This can and does happen by chance, that is, if couples actually use all the embryos that are produced in the lab through their sperm and eggs. But it can also happen through wise planning. A couple can inform the clinic of their views concerning when personhood begins, and tell the clinic they do not want any leftover embryos after they are finished doing business there. When beginning the procedure, a couple should insist that the clinic is to fertilize a sufficient number of eggs for only one round of embryo implants. That is, the number of eggs to be fertilized depends on the number of embryos that the couple wants implanted at any one time. This would usually mean that anywhere from four to six eggs would be retrieved. Four embryos are usually implanted, and often some of the eggs do not fertilize in the lab, so it may be prudent to allow for some attrition in the process. But to be perfectly safe the couple should insist that all the eggs that are harvested be fertilized and implanted. This will mean that fewer eggs will be retrieved and fer-

---

48. The latest consensus on how long embryos can remain in storage is roughly five years. However, in January 1998 an embryo which had been in storage for seven and a half years was successfully thawed and implanted, resulting in a live birth. This is the longest time period in which an embryo had been stored and thawed with the outcome being a live birth.

tilized, and should all the implanted embryos fail to develop, or the eggs retrieved fail to be fertilized, then the couple would be faced with another cycle of egg retrieval and fertilization in the lab. This will likely increase the cost significantly should the couple elect to continue trying to become pregnant with one of these procedures. Many couples will not be comfortable with these restraints that could drive up the costs of achieving pregnancy, and in an effort to keep the costs down, go ahead and harvest and fertilize as many eggs as they can retrieve, and keep embryos in storage. But for couples who hold that human personhood begins at conception, that is morally problematic, since if they are not implanted, they will likely be discarded. Since the physicians cannot predict how many eggs they will successfully retrieve or how many will fertilize, it may not be technologically feasible to operate within these limits. If it is inevitable that a couple will have leftover embryos, and if the couple is unwilling to donate those that remain, then this raises serious questions about the moral acceptability of these techniques. If personhood begins at conception and if location of the embryos is not relevant to their personhood, then discarding leftover embryos is problematic. The couple should be prepared either to work within limits that will likely not produce leftovers, donate those that remain after they achieve pregnancy, or have the remaining embryos implanted themselves. The couple should think this through in advance, since the difficulties in having leftover embryos are magnified when the couple does not realize the problem until after the embryos are already in storage.

A second and even more troubling ethical issue in these techniques results not from the failure of the embryo implants but from their success. Multiple pregnancies are not uncommon with these technologies. Some couples are clearly distressed with multiple pregnancies, because they did not want as many children as the woman is carrying. In some cases more embryos will implant than the woman can safely carry to term. When either of these occur, clinics will suggest what is called a "reduction" in the number of pregnancies the woman is carrying. It is also called "selective termination." The clinic normally does not perform the reduction but will refer the couple to a practitioner in the local area who can decrease the number of pregnancies without risk to the remaining ones.

For a couple who holds that personhood begins at conception, these "reductions" are very problematic. There is no morally significant difference between these "reductions" and abortion for unwanted pregnancies. Reductions are particularly egregious because the embryos were deliberately implanted in the woman. The couple consented to the implants, knowing from the start that each one might "take" and develop in the uterus. There is a degree of intentionality in these techniques that is not a part of abortions with unplanned pregnancies. Embryonic life is deliberately, not accidentally, created in the lab and intentionally implanted in the woman. This makes pregnancy reduction in these cases seem more callous and less respectful of developing personhood than with ordinary abortions. To deliberately create human life, implant it in the uterus where it can grow, and then terminate it if it "takes" because the couple does not want that many children, is very troubling when it comes to society's respect for the life it is intentionally creating.

A close friend recalls going through GIFT and conceiving triplets, after already having one child. This gave the couple a total of four children, clearly more than they had anticipated and originally wanted. Having this many children would significantly stretch them financially. The temptation to undergo a reduction was strong. But they continued all of the pregnancies, and even though it was physically very taxing on the woman (she was in a wheelchair for the last three months until delivery, and delivered over a month early) and very stressful to have three newborns at the same time, they are glad they made the decision they did. After the triplets were born, one of the man's colleagues at work was in the middle of IVF with his wife. This couple too had conceived triplets, and were seriously contemplating a reduction. The two men talked, and the man whose wife had successfully had triplets explained that he and his wife were offered the same opportunity by their clinic. But after the children were born, in thinking back on that, he saw his children's faces, not just clinically detached embryos. He admitted that it was difficult to imagine which one of the three children would have been terminated in the reduction, or how that choice would have been made. These were persons growing in his wife's uterus. The colleague admitted later that they had decided to continue all three pregnancies. These are simply agonizing decisions even for couples who hold that abortion is justifiable. They are decisions that can be avoided with proper planning.

In some cases a reduction is proposed to safeguard the lives and health of the other fetuses the woman is carrying. For example, if by carrying four fetuses as long as she can she runs the risk of delivering prematurely, this may seriously compromise the health and even the life of the children who have been delivered early. If such a reduction is truly medically indicated because the presence of an additional fetus is seriously jeopardizing the others, then it may be appropriate to reduce the number of pregnancies that the woman is carrying. One must be careful not to expand the notion of medically indicated to also encompass the emotional and financial health of the family. In some cases the idea that a reduction is required medically may mask the parents' desire to decrease the number of babies that will be born. If there are genuine medical reasons for a reduction, then it is appropriate by extension of the principle that it is justifiable to reduce to save the mother's life.

The way to avoid the agonizing dilemma created by the prospect of a pregnancy reduction is to limit the number of embryos that are implanted from the start. The couple should insist that the number of embryos being implanted only be as many as they are willing to raise if all of them success-fully implant. In addition, they should not implant more embryos than the woman can safely carry to term should all of them successfully implant. This will likely decrease the probability of achieving a pregnancy, but couples who enter into these procedures should be aware of the potential for multiple pregnancies.

Physician-Assisted Suicide

The notion of personhood is important in the debate over the morality of physician-assisted suicide. The long-standing tradition in medicine and the law of prohibiting assistance in suicide comes from the fifth commandment ("Thou shalt not murder"). Physicians assisting in suicide were commonly seen to be violating the Hippocratic oath, which prohibited them from killing their patients, even with motives of mercy. Recent advocates of assisted sui-cide have suggested that assisting the terminally ill in suicide does not violate the norm that prohibits killing of innocent persons, because the terminally ill for whom death is imminent are in reality no longer persons, simply bodies which medicine is maintaining through life-support technology.

This case is made most persuasively by philosopher James Rachels.[49] He distinguishes between biological and biographical life and insists that only those with biographical life are persons for whom it is a problem if they are killed. For Rachels, biographical life is the sum total of one's goals, dreams, as-pirations, accomplishments, and human relationships. It consists of those things that form the narrative of one's life and the essence of one's person-hood. In Rachels's view modern medicine has enabled one to exist biologi-

---

49. See his work *The End of Life* and the summary of his position in "Active and Pas-sive Euthanasia," *New England Journal of Medicine* 292 (9 January 1975): 78-80. For a thoughtful and more extended critique of Rachels than we can offer here, see J. P. More-land, "James Rachels and the Active Euthanasia Debate," *Journal of the Evangelical Theolog-ical Society* 31 (March 1988): 81-94, and Moreland, "Review of *The End of Life*," *Thomist* 53 (October 1989): 714-22. A summary of these is presented in Scott B. Rae, *Moral Choices: An Introduction to Ethics* (Grand Rapids: Zondervan, 1995), chap. 8, and Rae, "Views of Human Nature," pp. 235-61.

cally while the person's biographical life has ended, as would be the case with the terminally ill for whom death is imminent and with certain classes of severely handicapped newborns. That is, corporeal existence continues, but the person has died. Since biographical life is what gives persons their distinctive value, Rachels reasons that when that has been lost, what is essential about personhood has been lost, or has died. Thus he suggests that concerns about killing persons in assisted suicide are minimized, which removes the major criticism of assisted suicide.

He uses a case well known in bioethics circles, Dax's case, to illustrate his point. Dax Cowart was a strong, athletic man in his early twenties when he and his father were severely burned by an explosion in an underground gas line. His father was killed and Dax was burned over 90 percent of his body, causing loss of sight and hearing, speech impairment, and loss of a good deal of use of his hands. Following the explosion, Dax begged a passerby to shoot him and end his suffering, but the passerby refused and instead took him to a hospital, where Dax began the long process of painful burn therapy. Repeatedly he asked his physicians to stop the treatment and allow him to die, which they did not do. He also requested assistance in suicide and was refused, and as a result awkwardly attempted it himself and failed. Rachels suggests that Dax lost much if not all of his capacity for biographical life in the accident. Those priorities that were most important to him were now impossible for him to pursue. Thus he should not only have been allowed to refuse treatment, he should have been granted his wish for assistance in suicide, and it would not have been killing a person, since his biographical life had died in the explosion.[50]

Dax's case, however, is probably not the best one to illustrate this distinction between biographical and biological life. The reason is that in his recovery from burn treatment, he recovered his biographical life. He got married, went to law school, and set up a legal practice in his hometown, with a focus on protecting the rights of patients wishing to refuse medical treatment. The irony of this case is that Dax not only regained his biographical life, but one of its significant goals revolves around this very distinction between biological and biographical life. Yet Dax's own experience of recovering his biographical life indicates that this distinction (between biological and

50. In retrospect, it does seem that Dax's refusal of treatment should have been honored, not because he was no longer a person but because it constituted an informed refusal of treatment, which was his right. The reason it was not honored was likely because the physicians saw it as not in his best interest, and perhaps because they considered him incompetent to make decisions because of the level of pain he was experiencing.

biographical life) cannot be consistently maintained, and calls into question its use for justifying assistance in suicide.

In response to the biological-biographical life distinction, biographical life, far from rendering biological life irrelevant, rather presupposes it. The substance view of a human being outlined in this chapter is very helpful here. The capacity to have a biographical life is grounded in the person being of a specific kind, a human being. A human being has an essence that is capable of constructing those necessary elements of a biographical life. That is, a person has certain qualities necessary for biographical life because a person is a substance and not a property-thing. The possibility of a full, coherent biographical life is grounded in biological life, both of which are part of the essence of being human. Personhood is not lost when the ability to exercise its capacities is lost, any more than losing the use of an arm is the same thing as having it amputated.

A second criticism of this distinction is that it leads to a subjective view of the value of biographical life. For Rachels, it seems that biographical life is meaningful independent of any normative standards of validity. That is, one's biographical life is meaningful simply by virtue of being one's own. But surely some biographical lives are dehumanizing and inconsistent with being genuinely human. For example, take the person whose life goal was to be the most effective administrator of torture in his country, or one of the Nazi executioners whose aspirations revolved around the extermination of Jews. We would certainly insist that biographical lives constructed around those aspirations would be inconsistent with membership in the human community and that they would devalue someone's life rather than give it value.

A third criticism extends this point. If biographical life is that which gives life its value, and when it is gone essentially only body can be said to exist, then what prevents society from stripping the "person" of all remaining rights? This presumes that one can identify the point at which one loses biographical life, a difficult if not impossible task. No criteria have been proposed for determining when biographical life has been lost, short of permanent unconsciousness or a persistent vegetative state, and it appears that one simply has an intuitive sense as to when this happens. The difficulty in determining when biographical life has been lost surely suggests that it cannot be used as a justification for assisted suicide.

If biographical life is the basis for giving life its value and thus all other rights, when it is lost, what would prevent the family from burying the person and treating the person like a corpse, assuming proper respect for the dead is given? That would seem to be justifiable and consistent with biographical life being lost. Could physicians take organs from that "person" while still alive but having lost biographical life, assuming consent of next of kin? It would appear that they could. Can there be experimentation on the person, again with appropriate proxy consent? If the essentials of one's life are lost and one's rights are tied up with biographical life and that is lost, there does not seem to be any consistent way of preventing any of these scenarios, as long as they are done with proper respect for the dead. One could argue that if rights have been lost with biographical life, we should not be as concerned about proper consent for assistance in suicide as we are. Non-voluntary euthanasia becoming is a justifiably a great concern to the advocates of euthanasia, yet if biographical life has been lost and that is the basis for personhood, why is consent so important? If this is no longer a person, and there is no concern about killing a non-person, what is so important about securing consent for euthanasia? This distinction between biographical life and biological life cannot be maintained consistently and is not compatible with the substance view of a human being taught by Scripture.

Some have applied the distinction between biological life and biographical life (or between a human being and a person) to patients in a persistent vegetative state (PVS), usually the result of a traumatic head injury. That is, the higher brain functions are gone but the brain stem, which controls the involuntary functions, is still intact and working. People can live in a PVS for many years but need to be fed through medical means. This raises the issue of whether it is morally justifiable to remove feeding tubes from PVS patients. Many people view medically provided nutrition and hydration as medical treatment that can be refused by a patient's surrogate decision-maker if there is clear and convincing evidence that such was the patient's wishes.[51]

Some commentators in the Christian community have adopted a form of Rachels's dichotomy between biographical and biological life as a way of justifying removing nutrition and hydration from patients in a PVS. For example, one Christian philosopher put it like this:

> When an individual becomes permanently unconscious, the *person* has passed out of existence, even if biological life continues. There cannot be a person where there is neither the capacity for having mental states nor even

---

51. This was the conclusion of the Supreme Court in the landmark *Cruzan* decision and is the majority view among the bioethics community. See *Cruzan v Missouri Department of Health*, 110 S. Ct. 2481 (1990). For a different view, see Gilbert Meilaender, "On Removing Food and Water: Against the Stream," *Hastings Center Report* 14 (December 1984): 11-13.

the potentiality for developing that capacity (as with infants). For persons are beings who have the capacity (potentially or actually) to think, will, affirm moral and spiritual ideals, love and hate, desire hope, plan and so forth. . . . where no such capacities exist *at all* due to permanent loss of consciousness, there we no longer have an individual who commands the special respect due a person, because we no longer have a person.[52]

As was the case with Rachels, this distinction between a person and a body is not consistent with the view of a human being as a substance and a continuity of personal identity from conception onward. The substance notion of a person suggests that personhood is part of a person's essence and is not dependent on that person's ability to perform particular functions. Simply because someone does not possess the capacity to exercise all the attributes of personhood, it does not follow that he or she does not possess personhood at all. An entity losing its function does not mean that the entity itself no longer exists, only that it cannot function, or perform all of its functions. If through neurological damage one lost the ability to use one's leg, that is one thing. It is quite another to insist that it is the same thing as losing the leg. Even if one had never had the use of the leg from birth and will never again have the use of it, that is not the same thing as having it amputated. Because patients in a PVS cannot exercise any of the functions of personhood, it does not follow that they do not possess the essence of personhood. The capacity to function is grounded in the essence of being a person made in God's image. That is the point of the substance view of a human person that is emphasized in Scripture. The testimony of Scripture, as Catholic ethicist Richard Sparks puts it, is "that one's value is not wholly or even primarily ability-related . . . , one's basic significance does not depend on the amount of functional abilities one has been endowed with nor how well one exercises those talents."[53]

Conclusion

If, as we have suggested, all patients are persons irrespective of their stage of development, then those who practice medicine, particularly the more invasive kind, owe them respect for their dignity as persons made in God's image,

52. Robert N. Wennberg, *Terminal Choices: Euthanasia, Suicide, and the Right to Die* (Grand Rapids: Wm. B. Eerdmans Publishing Co., 1989), pp. 159-60.
53. Richard C. Sparks, *To Treat or Not to Treat? Bioethics and the Handicapped Newborn* (New York: Paulist Press, 1988), pp. 256-57.

and thus with incalculable value. If personhood extends to the earliest stages of pregnancy, then abortion is extremely problematic unless the mother's life is in imminent danger. Experimenting on embryos and using the tissue of fetuses obtained from elective abortions are also problematic since persons cannot be the subject of nontherapeutic experiments without their consent, and surely experiments which take the life of the person in the process cannot be morally legitimate. Further, reproductive technologies which leave embryos to be discarded after the infertility procedures are finished, or which involve selective termination of pregnancies after embryos are implanted in the woman's body, are the moral equivalent of abortion. Though these technologies can still be used, the couple must implant all the embryos, either themselves or by way of donation to another infertile couple. The couple should insist that the clinic help them minimize the number of leftover embryos, even if that makes the procedures more expensive. Finally, the terminally ill are persons until the point of their death. Personhood is not a degreed property, and it cannot be lost prior to one's death. The distinction between biological life and biographical life cannot be maintained, and cannot be used as a justification for physician-assisted suicide or euthanasia.

CHAPTER 6

Autonomy and the Common Good

Introduction: Autonomy Abused?

To introduce this chapter we will present a number of scenarios, each involving hypothetical physicians who attend a number of different patients. These physicians must make difficult decisions about respecting the wishes of each particular patient. In each scenario the doctor is faced with a conflict between the right of the patient to choose the course of treatment for himself or herself, including the option of no treatment, and the physician's obligation under the Hippocratic oath, and as a Christian, to beneficence, or the obligation to bring a benefit to these patients. The conflict in these cases is magnified because, by following the wishes of the patients, the doctors will be allowing harm to come to them, violating one of the first principles of medical ethics, "do no harm."

The first case involves a neurosurgeon.[1] His patient is the victim of a hit-and-run accident in which, while riding a bicycle without a helmet, he was hit by an automobile. Although the collision occurred at low speed, it nevertheless threw him from the bicycle and caused him to hit his head on the pavement. Upon examination of the patient, the neurosurgeon discovers that he is suffering from a subdural hematoma, or bleeding causing pressure on his brain. This condition, though serious, is correctable through surgery, but if it is left untreated it will lead to the patient's death. The course of care in surgery sometimes involves blood transfusion. Most patients who have the

---

1. This scenario is a summary of case 3 in chapter 10. It is developed in more detail and analyzed according to a model for bioethical decision making in that chapter.

surgery do very well and recover completely, which the doctor determines would also be the likely outcome in this case.

However, while attempting to obtain consent for the surgery from the patient's wife, the neurosurgeon explains the procedure and mentions that it might involve a blood transfusion. He reassures her that this is not unusual but is a normal part of the surgery, and is no cause for alarm. She is agreeable to everything he is proposing, but when he mentions the blood transfusion she resists, indicating that both she and her husband are of the Jehovah's Witness religion. She informs the neurosurgeon that the couple's religious beliefs prohibit her from consenting to blood transfusion for her husband. The doctor indicates that her husband will die without the surgery, and may die on the operating table without blood being available for transfusion. He further learns that she has a two-year-old child and is in the early stages of pregnancy with her second child. He is very uncomfortable with the idea that his patient will die without this surgery, leaving his wife a widow with two young children. Does he respect the patient's autonomy, as relayed to him by the patient's wife, whose judgment is substituting for his? Or does he override the patient's autonomy and seek a court order to force the surgery on him without his consent, since doing so will prevent harm?

A second scenario deals with an obstetrician who serves in a clinic in a part of a city populated predominantly by the underinsured and uninsured. She sees three particular patients on one day, all of whom have conflicts between autonomy and beneficence. The first is a pregnant woman who admits to her that she is a drug user. The obstetrician knows that the drug use of the mother puts the unborn child at great risk for a variety of birth defects. She encourages the drug user to get into a drug treatment program not only for her benefit but also for the benefit of her unborn child. But the drug user steadfastly refuses, and insists that she can handle her life just fine. The doctor has strong suspicions that she will use drugs regularly during her pregnancy and considers what she could do to force her into a treatment program, for her own good and for her unborn child's good.

A second patient is much like the first, only the physician suspects from her drug use and history of sexual contact that she might have contracted the HIV virus. She has been reading in the medical literature about some recent tests that indicate that the drug AZT is very effective in preventing the spread of the virus to the fetus. She informs the patient of that fact and strongly suggests that she be tested for HIV, and if she tests positive, that she begin taking AZT immediately. However, to her surprise, the drug user refuses to be tested. She has no interest in finding out if she is HIV positive, believing AZT has some side effects that she does not want to experience. The obstetrician's frustration is evident, because she knows that the law does not allow her to override the patient's autonomy and force her to be tested, but she dislikes having to sit by and watch her possibly endanger her developing fetus.

Her third patient is a woman she has been seeing in her private practice. She is in labor and on her way to the hospital. When the doctor arrives and examines her, she discovers to her dismay that the baby is in distress and needs to be delivered immediately by cesarean section. However, the woman refuses to consent to the C-section, instead choosing to trust God to deliver her baby naturally. The doctor recalls reading in the paper some time ago about a woman whose Pentecostal beliefs motivated her to similarly refuse a C-section, and in that case the woman did deliver naturally and successfully.[2] But the obstetrician really thinks it is in everyone's best interests to have a C-section performed immediately. Should she seek a court order to force the C-section? Should she override her patient's autonomy and do what she thinks is in everyone's best interests?

The third scenario involves a pediatrician. He is beside himself because one of his friends has asked his opinion about what to do about the friend's neighbor's two-year-old child. The child has a high fever and is very lethargic, which in a small child suggests meningitis, an infection of the lining of the brain which, when left untreated, leads to serious brain damage and eventually death. The pediatrician offers to see the child and makes a home visit, but when he suggests that the child needs to be hospitalized, he is stunned when the parents refuse, citing their Christian Science beliefs in prayer and other nonmedical means of healing. They steadfastly refuse to take the child for any medical treatment, which prompts the doctor to consider requesting a court order to compel treatment for the child, overriding the autonomy of the parents as rightful guardians of the child.

A fourth scenario deals with an oncologist whose patient is an eighty-one-year-old man who is in seriously declining health due to cancer that started in the stomach and has spread throughout his body. Various complications have arisen from the surgery and treatments, and in the oncologist's view, all further treatment is futile and should be stopped. The patient is also suffering from Alzheimer's disease and is lucid at times and disoriented at other times. The doctor has questions about this man's ability to make all his medical decisions for himself. The man has designated his oldest daughter to

2. This case occurred in Chicago in late 1993. Interestingly, the hospital tried to get a court order to force the woman to undergo the C-section, and the ACLU defended the pregnant woman on the grounds that her First Amendment rights to freedom of religion were being violated. The court ruled in the woman's favor.

make decisions for him if he is not able to, and she is determined to fight the cancer until "God takes him." She will not hear of stopping treatment and will not even discuss a "do not resuscitate" order with the oncologist. Even if her father must be fed by medical means and use a ventilator to breathe, she wants everything done for him for as long as possible. The doctor makes every effort to convince her that such a treatment plan is futile, and in her judgment is more burdensome than beneficial. She even invites the daughter to observe the tests and treatments that her father is receiving, thinking that if she sees what he is enduring, she will authorize stopping treatment. The oncologist could also appeal directly to the father, but he is becoming increasingly disoriented and she simply cannot be sure that he is competent to make his own decisions. The oncologist has already taken it to the hospital's ethics committee, which agrees with her judgment, but the hospital has no policy on futile treatment, so the institution cannot help her out of this dilemma. Should she override the daughter's autonomy to speak for her father and only provide comfort care, discontinuing further aggressive treatment? Should she attempt to transfer the patient to another physician who will provide the treatment the daughter desires, knowing that most of her colleagues with whom she has spoken about this case agree with her and would be unlikely to accept a transfer?

All of the above scenarios involve a conflict between the wishes of the patient or surrogate decision-maker and what the physician believes is in the patient's best interest. In the language of the bioethics tradition, it is a conflict between autonomy and beneficence.[3] In the past, it was more common for the physician to act with beneficence toward patients, even if it meant overriding their wishes. This was commonly known as paternalism, and was an accepted part of medical practice for most of medicine's history. The reason for this should be obvious: physicians knew much more about the human body and medicine than their patients, and as a result, physicians expected that their judgment of what was in the patient's best interests would not be challenged. This led to many abuses in which patients often had little say in the course of treatment they received or were not adequately informed about the treatment options. For example, in the widely publicized Dax's case, Dax Cowart was administered painful burn therapy despite his repeated protestations over the months of treatment that he wished to be left alone and allowed to die.[4]

---

3. For further discussion of these key principles in bioethics, see Tom Beauchamp and James Childress, *Principles of Biomedical Ethics,* 4th ed. (New York: Oxford University Press, 1995). See our discussion of Beauchamp and Childress's approach in chapter 2.

4. Lonnie Kliever, *Dax's Case* (Dallas: Southern Methodist University Press, 1989).

But beginning in the 1960s, coinciding with the advent of bioethics as a discipline, patients' rights were more aggressively asserted. Paternalism was balanced by a recognition of the decision-making authority of the individual patient. A bill of rights for patients was adopted, and today virtually every hospital in the West displays it prominently at the admissions desk. Patients are empowered to say no to treatments they do not want, and informed consent to treatment is the law in medical practice. That is, patients have the right to be informed of the diagnosis, the risks and benefits of treatment, and alternatives, among them the right to no treatment. This is particularly important since there is so much ethnic and cultural diversity today that, within limits, physicians must respect the cultural distinctives of their patients when it comes to medical treatment.

However, it is now widely recognized that patient autonomy has gone out of control. This is part of a larger social perspective that recognizes that individuals are exercising their rights as absolutes, with declining consideration of their corresponding responsibilities and the common good.[5] In medicine, autonomy is out of control when patients can demand and expect that treatment will be provided them irrespective of their condition, prognosis, or ability to pay. It is further "run amok"[6] when patients can determine the criteria that define death for them, presumably in conjunction with their cultural or religious beliefs.[7] It is out of control when patients' advance directives can indicate that they want everything done for them without regard to their condition, chances for recovery, or long-term survival or cost.[8] It is out of control when what the physician deems good for the patient is determined by the patient's desires. One patient advocate puts it like this: "A commitment to individualism allows us to define the interests that the patient would choose as those that his attending health professionals should pursue because of the [physician's] fiduciary role."[9]

---

5. See, for example, the work of Harvard Law School professor Mary Ann Glendon in her book *Rights Talk: The Impoverishment of Political Discourse* (New York: Free Press, 1991); see also the widely read work by sociologist Robert N. Bellah et al., *Habits of the Heart: Individualism and Commitment in American Life* (Berkeley: University of California Press, 1985), and Willard Gaylin and Bruce Jennings, *The Perversion of Autonomy* (New York: Free Press, 1996).

6. This term was coined by Daniel Callahan in his article in reference to euthanasia, "Self Determination Run Amok," *Hastings Center Report* 22 (March-April 1992).

7. Robert Truog and James Facider, "Is It Reasonable to Reject the Diagnosis of Brain Death?" *Journal of Clinical Ethics* (spring 1992).

8. Leonard J. Weber, "The Patient as Citizen," *Health Progress* (June 1993): 12-15, at 13.

9. Henry Perkins, "Another Ethicist Looks at Mr. B's Case: Commentary on an Ethical Dilemma," *Journal of Clinical Ethics* (summer 1990): 127, cited in "The Patient as Citizen," p. 15.

Others suggest that the demand for physician-assisted suicide is autonomy run amok.[10] Both the Second and Ninth Circuit Court of Appeals grounded their approval of assisted suicide in the logical extension of autonomy from the *Roe v. Wade* decision legalizing abortion, an extension which was rejected by the U.S. Supreme Court. Many pro-life advocates have consistently argued that legalized abortion is the ultimate abuse of a woman's autonomy since the exercise of it allows her to end the life of her unborn child simply because she chooses to.

Western Tradition of Autonomy

How did we in Western culture get to a place where personal autonomy is subject to such abuse, where notions of the common good are so subordinate to the exercise of personal liberty? Columbia University psychiatrist Willard Gaylin and political philosopher Bruce Jennings suggest that "autonomy now preempts civility, altruism, paternalism, beneficence, community, mutual aid and other moral values that essentially tell a person to set aside his own interests in favor of the interests of other people or the good of something larger than himself."[11] The emphasis on personal autonomy is one of the primary components of liberal democracy, and, as is the case with the Western democratic system, the stress on autonomy is of relatively recent origin.

Autonomy literally means "self-law," from the Greek *auto* (self) and *nomos* (law), and refers to the freedom that a person has to order his or her life according to his or her own desires and values. It involves independence, self-reliance, and what is called "negative liberty," sometimes referred to as negative rights, or the right to be left alone to pursue life as one sees fit. In medicine it came to refer to the rights of patients to make their own decisions about their lives and treatments, as opposed to the paternalistic prerogative of physicians to make those decisions for them.

The current emphasis on autonomy and freedom has its roots in the political philosophy that arose out of the Enlightenment period. These concepts originated as a response to conditions in medieval Europe, instituted by oppressive monarchies, which denied people many of the rights that are commonly recognized today, and out of a static view of the world, in which everyone had an appointed place in that order, making social mobility and the exercise of freedom difficult if not impossible.

The Reformers laid the groundwork for massive social change by institut-

---

10. This is the point of the article by Callahan, "Self-Determination Run Amok."
11. Gaylin and Jennings, p. 58.

ing changes in the way individuals were viewed from a theological perspective. As opposed to the medieval Catholic view in which one's relationship with God was mediated by the church and the priesthood, Luther and Calvin emphasized the notion of the believer-priest. They held that individuals stood alone before God, with no intermediaries except Christ himself. Salvation was thus not mediated through any institution or person, but an individual believer could know and relate to God directly. The notion of the individual standing alone before God was one of the primary ideological starting points for liberal democracy with its emphasis on the rights of the individual. Out of the concept of the believer-priest came the stress on the high place given to individual conscience. If believers could relate directly to God without any mediating persons or institutions, then God could form their consciences directly, particularly if they had access to the Bible in their own language, another emphasis of the Reformation. Thus individuals stood directly before God with freedom of conscience, which gave birth to the idea of religious liberty. It was not long before the concept of religious liberty was expanded to include political liberty in the form of liberal democracy and economic liberty in the form of free-market capitalism. Many of the people who came to the United States came in order to experience religious freedom, and the social order they constituted embodied both political and economic liberty, which the Founding Fathers saw as consistent with religious liberty.

The medieval view of the world was also under attack from those outside the religious sphere. The theological view of the world was strongly challenged, and human beings, not God, became the measure of all things. At roughly the same time as the Reformation, thinkers in the Enlightenment period were putting forward ideas of humanism, natural rights, and the social contract, all of which were foundational ideas for individual liberty and liberal democracy. Thinkers like Thomas Hobbes, John Locke, and Jean-Jacques Rousseau put forth the ideas that led to many of the political revolutions of the 1600s and 1700s. These ideas also had a seminal influence on the formation of liberal democracy in the United States. Hobbes emphasized that individuals had natural rights, which existed apart from any religious revelation or authority. He further emphasized that individuals enter society by choice, not by nature or by the predetermined will of God. Thus social mobility became a real possibility for people who had previously been stuck in their predetermined place in society. This led to the notion of the consent of the governed, that if individuals entered society by choice, not by predetermination, then it followed that they would choose who would govern them. Government was by consent of the people, not by decree, heredity, or blessing of the church. This was later formalized and expanded by Rousseau in his notion of the social contract.

For Locke, a Christian who was profoundly influenced by the Calvinists in Scotland and France, with whom he studied, natural rights were ultimately theologically grounded. Since rights are natural, from creation, people must consent to give up some freedoms in order to be governed. The state is limited by his notion of the right to property. Property, according to Locke, was the best guarantor of liberty since it marked out a sphere into which the state could not intervene. Property was grounded theologically, in the creation mandate, with humanity seen as co-creator with God, unlocking the creation. It was also grounded in his view of human nature. Locke held the view that a person has a right over his or her own body. Thus the labor of a person's body can produce goods to which the person is entitled as fruit of his or her labor. This was an important concept in the rise of capitalism as an economic system, an outgrowth of the emphasis on individual liberty.

These notions of individual liberty and autonomy were critical in the formation of capitalism as an economic system. Adam Smith, the moral philosopher, popularized the idea that the "invisible hand" of the market guided the individual pursuit of economic self-interest toward the common good. It was the first time in which wealth was systematically created and profit was not considered an evil, but a good to be pursued. Smith held that individuals exercising their freedom to pursue their self-interest would also benefit the common good by making products and providing services that were needed by the community, thereby bringing them a profit and enhancing their economic self-interest. Smith's concept of the market benefiting the common good, combined with the Reformers' expanded concept of one's calling from God to include "secular" work, provided the ideological engines that helped drive capitalism. As the sociologist Max Weber argued in his classic work *The Protestant Ethic and the Spirit of Capitalism,* once capitalism became entrenched as an economic system in the West, the theological underpinning became less important, thus separating individual liberty from its theological roots.

Most of the thinkers who provided the concepts for individual liberty were also concerned about maintaining social order once people understood and exercised their freedom. The Founding Fathers in the United States were aware that liberal democracy could only work for a religious and moral people, that is, for people who had the internal resources to enable them to limit their pursuit of their own interests and who realized that liberty meant the freedom to do what was right, not the freedom to do whatever one wanted. Adam Smith was very clear that the invisible hand of the market operated when individuals pursued "enlightened self-interest," or self-interest that was capable of being restrained, in his view by Judeo-Christian moral values. Though there were examples of extreme individualism on the American frontier and cutthroat capitalism in the cities, generally as democracy developed in the West, order was maintained by the internal constraints of the Judeo-Christian moral system. Even though people may not have believed all the elements of the theological system undergirding society, they largely held to its moral values as necessary conditions for society to function in a healthy way. Thus for most of the years of the democratic experiment in the West, individual liberty was constrained by a Judeo-Christian moral consensus, and many of the excesses were checked by religious values. For example, around the turn of the twentieth century in the United States, when capitalism became abusive to worker rights and welfare, religious leaders stepped in and called for curbs on the pursuit of profit, and moved government to act to protect those who were thrown out of work by the business cycles. They were very influential in limiting child labor, improving working conditions, and establishing living wages for workers.

However, in recent years, with the unraveling of the Judeo-Christian moral consensus, individualism has become corrosive in its effect on society. Individuals have lost the concern for the common good that was rooted in the value system that until roughly the 1960s was widely shared in the culture. We have become increasingly concerned about individual rights, and freedom has come to mean the liberty to do whatever one desires, as long as no tangible harm comes to clearly identified others. We have become increasingly dependent on the courts to settle disputes over rights and have become easily the most litigious society the world has ever known.

Numerous commentators have noticed the corrosive effect of unrestrained liberty on the society at large. They have called for a renewed emphasis on the community of which one is a part and a new commitment to restraining one's pursuit of self-interest and contributing to the common good. This has become known as the "communitarian" movement, and it is a part of a growing number of people who are concerned about the destructive effect of individual rights and autonomy in society today.[12]

---

12. Though not all of these would call themselves communitarians, the commentators who are concerned about the corrosive effect of individualism include theologian Stanley Hauerwas, *A Community of Character* (Notre Dame, Ind.: Notre Dame Press, 1981); Glendon, *Rights Talk;* Robert Hughes, *Culture of Complaint: The Fraying of America* (New York: Oxford University Press, 1993); Jean Bethke Elshtain, *Democracy on Trial* (New York: Basic Books, 1995); Philip K. Howard, *The Death of Common Sense: How Law Is Suffocating America* (New York: Random House, 1994); Gertrude Himmelfarb, *The Demoralization of Society: From Victorian Virtues to Modern Values* (New York: Knopf, 1995); Ar-

Autonomy and Community in Biblical Perspective

How are we to evaluate the Western tradition of autonomy from the perspective of Scripture? What resources can the Christian theological tradition bring to help temper the corrosive effects of autonomy and individualism today? The notion of autonomy arose in part out of a reaction to the theological understanding of a human person that was a part of the medieval view of the world. In this view, human beings were not autonomous at all. They were subject to a sovereign God who had ordered their place in society. Christianity gave the average person in the Middle Ages the perspective and resources to accept his or her place in God's order. Furthermore, human beings were morally and spiritually accountable to God for their actions, decisions, and motives. The judgment day that awaited each person was a significant motivation to do right and avoid sin. The church at times misused its theology in an oppressive way, keeping people from flourishing. With the decline in the theological view of the world that began with the Enlightenment, people eagerly threw off the shackles of the church and discarded its theology as outdated and not in keeping with the modern world. The Reformation contributed to the demise of the medieval Catholic worldview with its reform of Christian theology. One of the most basic points of emphasis, beyond the *solas* (*sola fide*, or faith alone for salvation; *sola gratia*, or grace alone for salvation; and *sola Scriptura*, or Scripture alone as the authority for faith and life), was the doctrine of the believer-priest. Later proponents of autonomy jettisoned the Reformers' theology and developed a secular form of autonomy quite foreign to the Reformers' concept of the individual believer before God. The human person became autonomous without reference to God, free to make his or her own decisions apart from the moral standards of the Bible, and free to order his or her life apart from accountability to God and direction from God. In other words, the human being became "the measure of all things" and exercised his or her newfound right of self-determination. The human being was the master of his or her own fate without regard for God and the church.

In one sense, to speak of autonomy for the Christian is something of an oxymoron, since the Christian lives all of life under God's sovereign direction.[13] The Christian is constrained by the moral parameters of God's Word

---

thur M. Schlesinger, *The Disuniting of America* (New York: Norton, 1992); Amitai Etzioni, *The Spirit of Community* (New York: Crown Publishers, 1993). The seminal communitarian critique of individualistic autonomy is still Bellah et al., *Habits of the Heart.*

13. For further development on the issue of autonomy in medicine from this theological perspective, see John H. Frame, *Medical Ethics* (Phillipsburg, N.J.: Presbyterian and Reformed Publishing Co., 1988).

and the activity of the Holy Spirit in guidance and direction. Though the Reformers liberated human beings from the static view of the world that characterized the Middle Ages, they were very clear about the believer's place under the sovereignty of God. From the perspective of Scripture, the believer does not have ownership of himself or herself, but belongs to God, having been purchased by the death of Christ (I Cor. 6:19-20). As a result, the believer is not free to do whatever he or she pleases, but rather, is free to do what is right. The New Testament is filled with admonitions to temper one's Christian freedom with love and responsibility to others and the community. The apostle Paul makes it clear that the believer is not to abuse his or her freedom from the demands of the law for salvation, but is to use that freedom in order to pursue love, not his or her own selfish desires (Gal. 5:13-14). One's freedom is not to be used as a pretext for doing evil, but rather believers are to live life as slaves, hardly an imagery that would promote unconstrained autonomy (I Pet. 2:15-16). Numerous places in the New Testament call the believer to a life of servanthood, using the term for "bondservant" or "slave," which is figurative of the most constrained person in all the ancient world. Paul admonished the church to restrain even the exercise of legitimate Christian freedom in the moral gray areas out of regard for the brother or sister of weaker conscience (Rom. 14:1-23; I Cor. 8:9). Paul modeled this voluntary restraint of freedom in his own ministry when he gave up his right to earn his living from his preaching and church planting in order that the common good, the cause of the gospel, might be advanced (I Cor. 9:14-18). He imposed numerous restraints on his freedom and autonomy in order to more effectively serve the church and advance the gospel (9:19). Individual believers were to follow this model, giving up their freedom in order to be subject to one another in the life of the church (Eph. 5:21). Thus it would not be an understatement to insist that the Scripture knows little of independent men and women and thus cannot provide a model for people who are searching for what these kinds of people look like. The reason is that they were too committed to a community of committed relationships, which took priority over the exercise of one's individual autonomy.[14]

This emphasis on community has its roots in the Old Testament, particularly in the way the Mosaic Law structured the society of ancient Israel. God's intent in the Law was not only to give individuals moral and spiritual direction but also to outline how he desired Israel to function in society as "one nation under God." One of God's primary intentions in the Law of Mo-

---

14. For further discussion of this, see Stephen B. Clark, *Man and Woman in Christ* (Ann Arbor, Mich.: Servant Books, 1980).

ses was thus to create an ideal society which could corporately bear witness to the reality of God to Israel's neighbors.[15] This is one of the aspects of God's command to Israel to be a "kingdom of priests and a holy nation" (Exod. 19:6 NASB). The civil law of Moses helped create structures that embodied and reinforced the kinds of community obligations that would no doubt appear onerous today in our culture of individualism and autonomy.

For example, the laws concerning the ownership and transfer of real estate reflected this notion of community and interdependence. Since most people made their living from agriculture, ownership of land was critical to the ability of a man to support himself and his family. If someone was cut off from the land of his or her family, he or she was left with virtually no means of sustenance. Insuring that people had access to land was thus critical for prosperity and social order. The way in which real estate ownership and transfer was governed was essential to people in the community living together in peace and well being.

The civil law had a variety of clauses that were designed to protect those who were economically vulnerable by giving them access to real estate and a continual renewal of opportunity to make a living. The law made it clear that God owned the land and was entrusting it to Israel to use for their benefit and holding them responsible for its proper use as stewards (Lev. 25:23). As a consequence, real estate could not be permanently bought or sold, only leased. There was no notion of the rugged individual who owned property outright. Nor was there the option to accumulate large portions of land for oneself. Rather, extended families, or clans, were to settle the land and use it as stewards of God's gift to them.

In this context of God's ownership of the land, the year of Jubilee and the law of redemption are set. The Jubilee (Lev. 25:8-17) required that every fiftieth year, all land was to revert back to the family that had originally owned it; land transfers that occurred in the meantime were only temporary transfers. The lease price of the land was set according to the proximity to the Jubilee. The closer to the Jubilee, the less the price, since the purchaser was buying the opportunity to grow crops on the land, not the land per se. The purpose of the Jubilee was to prevent the poor from permanently losing access to the necessary property for making a living. The Jubilee provided a regular redistribution of opportunity for growing the food necessary to keep oneself and one's family sustained. Individual freedom to do with one's land

15. For more on this aspect of Old Testament theology, see Christopher J. H. Wright, *An Eye for an Eye: The Place of Old Testament Theology Today* (Downers Grove, Ill.: InterVarsity, 1983).

what one wished was limited by the obligation of the Jubilee. One could not permanently sell it, nor could one accumulate an inordinate amount of real estate. Property rights, with real estate being the most important property asset, were significantly limited by the tradition of the Jubilee. In addition, at the Jubilee all slaves were to be released and all debts were to be forgiven, further restricting the ability of individuals to do what they desired with their property. The purpose for these latter clauses was similar to that which dealt with the land: to give regular renewal of opportunity for a new start economically. The law of the Jubilee was structured to limit personal freedom to dispose of property in order to benefit the community. In other words, the common good of the community took precedence over individual rights of property and ownership, notions considered central to the modern ethos of autonomy.

A more immediate help for the economically vulnerable than the Jubilee, and a more burdensome limit on freedom in the area of real estate, came with the law of redemption (Lev. 25:23-34). The law states that if someone became so poor that he must sell his land in order to survive, the nearest next of kin had the legal and moral responsibility to buy the land back from the purchaser and return it to his poor relative, thus giving the latter a fresh start and a new opportunity to make a living. To be sure, the next of kin who redeemed the land would do what he could to insure his family member's prosperity so that he would not need to repeat the sacrifice of redeeming the land. In addition, if the seller of the land became able to repurchase the property he sold, the buyer was obligated by law to sell it back to him at a fair market value, depending on the proximity to the Jubilee. If the seller could not buy it back himself, and did not have a relative to redeem it for him, then it would revert back to him at the Jubilee. The civil law similarly called for redemption of slaves, in cases in which people became so poor they had to sell themselves into slavery, with the same procedure as the redemption of property (Lev. 25:47-55). Other means of insuring the common good and taking care of the poor included the law of gleaning, in which the owner of a field was required by law to leave the outer areas of the field unharvested in order that the poor could come and take for their sustenance (Lev. 19:9-10). Further, one could not charge usury (Exod. 22:25; Lev. 25:35-37), and one was responsible for taking care of immigrants and was not to exploit them (Deut. 10:19). The community was responsible for the most vulnerable among them, including the childless widow. In these cases the law mandated that the nearest next of kin marry the widow and raise up a child who would carry on the lineage of her deceased husband, and support them, in many cases, at substantial cost to the next of kin (Deut. 25:5-10; Ruth 3–4).[16] These laws were designed to protect the vulnerable and insure that the community was properly cared for, and meant great sacrifice to those who had the means to perform the various responsibilities. These were substantial limits on one's autonomy for the benefit of the community, mandated by the civil law of Moses. They illustrate the way in which personal autonomy was limited by the law to benefit the common good.

What was mandated by law in the Old Testament was done voluntarily in the New Testament. The early church voluntarily accepted great limits on personal freedom in order to benefit the early Christian community. For example, in the early parts of the book of Acts, the early church held its goods in common, distributing them to whoever among them had need (Acts 2:42-47; 4:32-37). This may have been only temporary because of the church's belief that the Lord would return shortly. But it illustrates the way in which the individuals in the early church put their own freedom aside in order to give attention to the common good. The Epistles consistently urge self-sacrifice for the good of others, both within and outside the believing community (Rom. 15:1-2; Phil. 2:4; Gal. 5:13). For the Christian, autonomy is at best a constrained pursuit, to be limited by concern for the community and the common good, and ultimately limited by the sovereignty of God.

Autonomy in Medicine Today

There is little doubt that autonomy reigns supreme in medicine today. It arose as a necessary and justifiable response to decades of paternalism. During that time, physicians took the attitude of "doctor knows best" and patients rarely questioned it because of the differential in knowledge between physician and patient. When added to a legacy of aggressive treatment and conquering disease as well as the dramatic developments in medical technology that can extend life, it was very difficult for patients to say no to physicians who thought they knew best and had an impressive technological arsenal at their disposal. Today autonomy is generally the most heavily weighted principle in bioethics.[17] When the

16. The cost to the next of kin, called the "kinsman-redeemer," could be substantial. In the book of Ruth, Boaz is not the nearest relative. The closest relative to Ruth was unwilling to undertake his responsibility as kinsman-redeemer, and refused. Thus the responsibility fell to the next in line, who was Boaz (Ruth 4).

17. See the discussion of the system of Childress and Beauchamp in chapter 2. They suggest that when autonomy and beneficence conflict, the autonomy of competent adults should take precedence.

autonomy of a competent adult comes into conflict with virtually any other principle in bioethics, particularly beneficence, autonomy virtually always takes priority. Autonomy has become the trump card in bioethical dilemmas, and the law supports this in the overwhelming majority of cases. The law protects competent individuals from being subject to medical treatment they do not want, and physicians can be prosecuted for battery for violating this law, except with minor children, in which physicians can attempt to obtain a court order to override the surrogate decision-maker's decision. This has produced some puzzling scenarios in which individuals are making decisions that are clearly not in their best interest, or in the best interests of those who are dependent on them, such as children and, sometimes, unborn children.

Take, for example, the scenarios presented in the introduction to this chapter. Without making conclusive judgments on each case, an argument could be made in each that autonomy is being abused, and that the choice being made is immoral. In the case of the Jehovah's Witness refusing a blood transfusion, one could argue that his wife's refusal will, at worst, cause the patient's death, and at best, has put the neurosurgeon in the very difficult position of having to operate without a key component for the patient's recovery and perhaps his survival through surgery. Though the refusal does come from religious beliefs — and in the couple's belief system and in their view, the patient's eternal destiny is at stake — it could be argued that he has a responsibility to the family he would be leaving behind. A similar argument can be made for the Christian Science parents who are exercising their religious freedom by refusing ordinary treatment for their seriously ill child. Here the courts have generally allowed physicians to override parental choice and force treatment on minor children when it is clear that the parents' exercise of their autonomy in deciding the course of treatment for their children is not in the children's best interest. When the exercise of one's liberty brings clear harm to others, particularly those who are entrusted to that person's care, such as a child who is entrusted to parental care, beneficence toward the other generally takes precedence over autonomy and is supported by the courts. Again, one should be careful to use the force of law to override someone's religious beliefs, but when the exercise of those beliefs causes clear harm — in this case it costs a child his or her life — then one can make a good case that autonomy is being abused and should be subordinate to the principle of non-maleficence, or "do no harm."

Much the same argument can be made that a pregnant woman should voluntarily give up some autonomy and liberty in order to safeguard the development of her unborn child. Most pregnant women care deeply about the welfare of their unborn children and would readily relinquish some freedoms such as drinking and smoking in order to give them the best chance for a healthy start in life. Many feel similarly about drug testing and treatment as well as HIV testing and AZT therapy, all of which are proven to be beneficial to unborn children. One can make a strong case that failure to take such steps is immoral and that the principle of liberty/autonomy should be subordinate to the principle of "do no harm." The same holds true for a more tragic situation, when a pregnant woman refuses an emergency cesarean section deemed necessary to save the unborn child's life or prevent serious injury to the unborn child. Even though the decision to refuse the C-section may be grounded in religious views, one can make a good case that the pregnant woman should consent to the C-section for the sake of preventing harm to her unborn child. Not to so do would be an abuse of autonomy, particularly since the degree of harm expected to come to the unborn child far exceeds the harm to the mother from the C-section.[18] Most pregnant women do whatever is necessary for their unborn children. But when the behavior of the pregnant woman conflicts with the welfare of her unborn child, one can make the case that she has the moral obligation to place the welfare of her unborn child ahead of her autonomy to live her life as she chooses.

In the case of the terminally ill patient whose family wants everything done, this is an example of family members speaking for the patient and exercising their autonomy by requesting continued aggressive treatment when it is clear that it is futile. One can make the case that this too is an abuse of autonomy. Though it is understandable that family members want to do everything for a seriously ill relative, one can argue that autonomy is being abused when they request treatment that will not reverse the course of a terminal illness. This is particularly the case when the family requests treatment for which it has no insurance or for which Medicare will only partially reimburse the physicians and hospital. Another complication is the fact that these pa-

---

18. Interestingly, in the 1993 case of the Pentecostal pregnant woman in Chicago (see n. 2 above), the ACLU defended the pregnant woman's autonomy and right to make the decision to refuse the C-section. Her choice was defended precisely in terms of autonomy, that it was her body and thus her right to have done to her body what she saw fit. There is a great deal of debate on the issue of forced C-sections. See Susan S. Mattingly, "The Maternal-Fetal Dyad: Exploring the Two-Patient Obstetric Model," *Hastings Center Report* 22 (January-February 1992): 13-18; George J. Annas, "Forced Cesareans: The Most Unkindest Cut of All," *Hastings Center Report* 12 (June 1982): 16-17, 45; Carol A. Tauer, "Lives at Stake," *Health Progress* (September 1992): 18-27; Veronika E. B. Holder et al., "Court-Ordered Obstetrical Interventions," *New England Journal of Medicine* 316, no. 19 (7 May 1987): 1192-96; Ronna Jurow and Richard H. Paul, "Cesarean Delivery for Fetal Distress without Maternal Consent," *Obstetrics and Gynecology* 63, no. 4 (April 1984): 596-99.

tients occupy ICU beds and utilize scarce resources needed by patients with better prognoses.

Whether or not the law should compel any of these people to limit their autonomy is a different and more complicated question. To date, the courts have generally reinforced the notion of autonomy as the trump card in many medical decisions, and as a result many physicians are understandably afraid to make decisions that go against the wishes of their patient or the patient's family. For example, physicians often order treatment they deem futile if the family is insistent in its request for it. In addition, they often continue treatment such as ventilator support that they judge to be futile and feel should be withdrawn, because the family requests it. They fear that the family will sue them if they do not provide or continue the treatment that the family thinks is appropriate for its loved one, and in some cases the courts have ruled for the family when these suits have been brought.[19] This legal threat can be very intimidating to physicians and hospitals, particularly since patients and families do sometimes win these suits. Only recently have the courts begun to rule for the physicians in these cases of futile treatment. One should be hesitant to use the force of the law to coerce people to limit their autonomy in these situations, but surely one can make the case that, morally, these exercises of autonomy are misguided. Though it is true that the law is used routinely to coerce individuals to limit their autonomy, one should be careful to use the law in this way in medicine when dealing with competent adults as patients. One reason is the long legacy of paternalism in medicine, which denied many patients' rights in the past and still exists today in the numerous cases in which patients' advance directives are ignored. A further reason is that if people do not have confidence that their wishes about treatment will be honored, they will likely be hesitant to see a physician for treatment. In cases in which competent adults are making informed choices that do not harm others, their choices should be respected and the law should protect those choices.

For example, though painful to those involved, the law should protect the choice of a Jehovah's Witness to refuse blood transfusions for surgery that could save his life, since that choice comes from deeply rooted religious be-

---

19. See the well-known *Wanglie* case in Minnesota, in which an elderly woman was on a ventilator for roughly fourteen months, and after repeated efforts by the hospital to withdraw treatment, the court ruled for the family. By contrast, in the *Gilgunn* case in Massachusetts the court ruled for the physicians in their right to determine when treatment is futile. For more on these cases see Steven H. Miles, "Informed Demand for Non-Beneficial Treatment," *New England Journal of Medicine* 325 (1991): 512-15 (on the *Wanglie* case), and Alexander Morgan Capron, "Abandoning a Waning Life," *Hastings Center Report* 25 (July-August 1995): 24-26 (on the *Gilgunn* case).

liefs and he is the primary one harmed. What makes that case difficult is that his choice indirectly harmed his surviving family. Though it could be argued that it was an immoral choice, it nonetheless should be allowed and respected. However, given the consequences for the family, the hospital could not be faulted for pursuing a court order, one it would be unlikely to obtain. But when clear harm comes to others as a result of a patient making his or her autonomous choices, the law should limit such choices. This is consistent with the role of the law in general, which is to limit freedom in order to prevent harm, maintain order, and administer justice.

For example, as a general rule one should not hesitate to appeal to the courts when minor children are involved. The physicians treating the Christian Science child with meningitis should attempt to obtain a court order compelling treatment on the child. Courts generally grant such orders when minor children are at risk, even when the parents' wishes for nontreatment are grounded in their religious views. More complicated cases involve drug and HIV testing for pregnant women, as well as forced C-sections. For example, in the early 1990s the Medical University of South Carolina cooperated with local officials in a pilot program that forced drug testing and treatment on the pregnant women who came to the university's prenatal clinic.[20] Those who tested positive and refused the treatment program were sent to the police, and some went to jail. The program was later discontinued due to the controversy it generated. Since drug addiction by definition takes away much of a woman's autonomy, it could be argued that the treatment program was actually restoring her autonomy that was lost through the use of drugs. But the scenario in which pregnant women lose rights to privacy and bodily integrity simply because of their pregnancy seems problematic. To be sure, any pregnant woman has the moral responsibility to insure that her unborn child gets the best start in life possible. But the degree to which the law should coerce such behavior is difficult to determine. Should the law prohibit pregnant women from smoking and drinking, which are legal activities, since these cause harm to unborn children? Most people are very uncomfortable with such legislation, and justifiably so. At the least, drug-addicted women should be offered a treatment program, and rigorous counseling should be employed to persuade them to undergo the program. Perhaps a softer approach, without the threat of turning their records over to the police, would be less controversial and more effective in keeping vulnerable women coming to the university's clinic.

Even more controversial is the issue of forced C-sections, since a C-

20. Gaylin and Jennings, pp. 196-98.

section is such an invasive procedure. Clearly it is morally wrong for a pregnant woman to engage in any behavior that endangers her unborn child, and particularly to refuse medical care that is in her unborn child's best interests. But the degree to which the law should enforce that moral notion is a different question. It would be difficult to fault the hospital or physician for attempting to obtain a court order for a forced C-section. But there are some cases in which women deliver healthy children naturally despite warnings from the physician that the unborn child was in danger.[21]

Some cases in which autonomy is clearly abused have less of a gray area, though they are still the subjects of heated debate in the culture at large. For example, a woman's legal right to an abortion would seem to be an example of autonomy in excess. If one assumes that the unborn child is indeed a person,[22] then the law permitting pregnant women to take the lives of their unborn children is allowing them to exercise their autonomy at the expense of their unborn children. It allows them to place a higher priority on freedom than on life, which is virtually unprecedented in Western culture and has even less precedent in the non-Western world. Generally, when the exercise of freedom costs a person his or her life, the law clearly protects life at the expense of freedom. But not so with abortion law. Though the law assumes that the unborn are not persons at least until viability,[23] abortions are still allowed after viability, many of which are done out of respect for a woman's autonomous choice. If the unborn are indeed persons, then the law permitting abortion is an example of women having the autonomy to end the lives of their offspring simply based on their free choice to do it. There is no precedent for giving autonomy that high a priority, particularly when it costs a person in the womb his or her life. From a biblical perspective, with the unborn possessing personhood from conception onward, this is an egregious abuse of autonomy. Even if society expressed reservations about the personhood of the unborn and merely allowed the possibility that they might be persons, surely we

21. This was what happened in the case of the Pentecostal woman in Chicago in 1993 (see n. 18 above). She insisted on natural delivery, the hospital went to court to obtain an order to override her decision, and the court ruled for the woman. She delivered a healthy baby naturally the next morning.

22. See the argument for this controversial notion made in chapters 4 and 5. This is increasingly being recognized by some outspoken pro-choice advocates. See, for example, Naomi Wolf, "Our Bodies, Our Souls," *New Republic,* 16 October 1995.

23. Some would suggest that abortion is actually legal from conception right up until birth. See Francis J. Beckwith, *Politically Correct Death: Answering the Arguments for Abortion Rights* (Grand Rapids: Baker, 1993), who argues that *Roe v. Wade* and *Doe v. Bolton,* both 1973 Supreme Court decisions, actually allow women to procure abortions up until the point of birth.

ought to err on the side of caution and limit the autonomy of the pregnant woman, both morally and by the law, since the basic civil rights of the unborn are being violated each time a pregnant woman exercises her autonomy to end her pregnancy.

A second and similarly controversial abuse of autonomy is in the area of physician-assisted suicide.[24] It is an example of what Hastings Center founder Daniel Callahan called "autonomy run amok."[25] Autonomy is central to the argument in favor of physician-assisted suicide, and was one of the foundational elements of the Ninth and Second Circuit Court of Appeals justification of physician-assisted suicide as a constitutionally protected right. The justices of the Ninth Circuit Court of Appeals stated that "We first conclude that there is a constitutionally protected liberty interest in determining the time and manner of one's death . . . , we hold that insofar as the Washington statute prohibits physicians from prescribing life-ending medication for use by terminally ill, competent adults who wish to hasten their own deaths, it violates the Due Process Clause of the Fourteenth Amendment."[26] They argued that the precedent had been set by the abortion decisions, and that they were simply extending to physician-assisted suicide the notion of autonomy at the heart of the legal right to an abortion. They stated: "In deciding right to die cases, we are guided by the Court's [the U.S. Supreme Court] approach to the abortion cases. . . . These matters, involving the most intimate and personal choices a person may make in a lifetime, choices central to personal dignity and autonomy, are central to the liberty protected by the Fourteenth Amendment."[27] Thus autonomy, recognized as central to the abortion decisions, was now, in the justices' view, logically extended to decisions at the end of life. The Second Circuit Court of Appeals agreed: "What concern prompts the state to interfere with a mentally competent patient's 'right to define his own concept of existence, of meaning, of the universe, and of the mystery of human life,' when the patient seeks to have drugs prescribed to end life during the final stages of a terminal illness? The greatly reduced answer of the state in preserving life compels the answer to these questions: 'None.'"[28] Both these decisions underscore the critical place autonomy has in the justification of physician-assisted suicide.

24. See the more extended discussion of physician-assisted suicide in chapter 7.
25. See n. 6 above.
26. *Compassion in Dying v Washington*, No. 94-35534 (6 March 1996): 3109-3263, at 3117.
27. *Compassion in Dying v Washington*, p. 3133, citing *Casey v Planned Parenthood of Pennsylvania* (112 S. Ct. at 2807).
28. Quill v Vacco, No. 95-7028 (2 April 1996): 2095-2966, at 2935.

But upon appeal, the U.S. Supreme Court disagreed and held that physician-assisted suicide is indeed a case of autonomy run amok. The Court stated: "That many of the rights and liberties protected by the Due Process Clause sound in personal autonomy does not warrant the sweeping conclusion that any and all important, intimate and personal decisions are so protected. . . . Our discussions lead us to conclude that the asserted 'right' to assistance in committing suicide is not a fundamental liberty interest protected by the Due Process Clause."[29] The Supreme Court rightly suggested that the right to assistance in suicide did not follow from the legal right to an abortion, since there was no hint of a tradition sanctioning suicide in the United States — in fact, far from it.[30] Every state has had laws making suicide and assistance in suicide illegal, and there is no precedent for recognizing another right to privacy. This is reinforced by the harm that comes to others through the exercise of the right to assistance in suicide, as the evidence from the Netherlands makes clear.[31] Further, the Court rightly recognized that the state has legitimate interests in prohibiting assistance in suicide, such as preservation of human life, protecting the integrity and ethics of the medical profession, protecting the most vulnerable groups, such as the poor and elderly, and the state rightly fears that legalizing assisted suicide will "start it down the path to involuntary euthanasia."[32]

One final example of autonomy run amok has to do with the way in which HIV/AIDS has been reported to public health authorities. Though the interest in privacy and preventing discrimination was understandable, the public debate over HIV reporting focused almost entirely on this aspect and scant attention was paid to the public health consequences, that is, to the harm to the broader society that resulted from the failure to prevent the spread of the disease. With other sexually transmitted diseases public health takes precedence over many privacy concerns, and cases are reported to public health authorities and contact tracing is routine. But no such measures were taken until recently, when the law changed, with HIV. Some have argued that more restrictive public health measures such as closing many of the bathhouses, as well as more rigorous testing and contact tracing, would have contributed substantially to controlling the spread of HIV in the 1980s.[33] But they were not widely instituted out of deference to autonomy, which took precedence over public health and a concern for the common good.

29. *Washington v Glucksburg,* No. 96-110 (26 June 1997): 23.
30. *Washington v Glucksburg,* p. 18.
31. See the discussion of physician-assisted suicide in the Netherlands in chapter 7.
32. Washington v Glucksburg, pp. 27-28. See further the discussion of this in chapter 7.
33. See Gaylin and Jennings, pp. 242-43.

Conclusion

Restoring the tradition of beneficence to health care involves balancing respect for the patient's autonomy with a commitment to the patient's good. Patients routinely place themselves in the care of their physicians and expect that physicians will look out for their best interests and treat them in accordance with their values. They enter a covenant of trust with their physicians. When there is a conflict in the patient's values and the physician's judgment of the best interests of the patient, the physician should use all of his or her persuasive efforts on the patient and his or her family to consent to treatment that is in the patient's best medical interests. When dealing with minor children, physicians and hospitals should not hesitate to seek court orders to compel treatment that is in the child's best interests. Patients should aggressively protect their rights as patients, but should recognize that even when they are patients, they still have responsibilities to their families and the community that may involve placing the common good ahead of their own autonomy.

Protecting autonomy and restoring the tradition of beneficence are more challenging in today's managed care environment, where patients' choices are more limited by their health plans and physicians' decision making and resources in caring for their patients are more limited than in the past. Physicians lament the fact that more medical decisions are being taken out of their hands and put in the hands of health plan administrators. They further must make their resources stretch to take care of an entire patient population for which they are financially and medically responsible. There are new conflicts for physicians that could undermine both autonomy and beneficence, as they are being forced to balance the needs of individual patients against the needs of the entire patient population for which they have responsibility under the terms of their managed care contract. Patients may find that their wishes for treatment not covered by their plan will not be honored, undermining both their autonomy and the physician's beneficence. Physicians may find that they lack the resources to do everything medically appropriate for all their patients. They may find that there is a conflict between the patient's best medical interest and their financial self-interest, as structured by the managed care contract. As the managed care environment continues to mature, one hopes that the health care system can adequately manage these conflicts. Whether it can do so with managed care as its foundation is still an open question. Patients should be prepared for limits on their autonomy, and should consider the interests of others and the community as well as their own interests as patients.[34] Physicians should commit themselves to beneficence toward their patients, however complex that commitment becomes in today's managed care environment. The physician's covenant with the patient is "to place the good of the patient at the center of my professional practice and, when the gravity of the situation demands, above my own self-interest."[35]

---

34. See, for example, the provocative article by John Hardwig, "Is There a Duty to Die?" *Hastings Center Report* 27, no. 2 (1997): 34-42, in which he argues that people may have a moral duty to refuse some life-sustaining treatment if the costs to their family and others important to them would outweigh the benefits.

35. Edmund D. Pellegrino and David C. Thomasma, *For the Patient's Good: The Restoration of Beneficence in Health Care* (New York: Oxford University Press, 1988), p. 205.

CHAPTER 7

Death as a Conquered Enemy

Introduction: "Doctor, Please Do Everything!"

In a well-publicized case in the early 1990s, Helga Wanglie, an eighty-six-year-old woman, fell and broke her hip in her home.[1] After treatment she was placed in a nursing home, where she experienced respiratory failure only a few weeks later. As part of her treatment she was placed on a respirator to enable breathing with mechanical assistance. Physicians in the hospital where she was being treated tried unsuccessfully to wean her off the respirator for the next five months. As a result of these repeated failures, she was transferred to a ventilator-dependent unit, a unit that specializes in patients who are on respirators. During one of the many attempts to wean her off the respirator, she suffered a heart attack. She was administered CPR and successfully resuscitated, but only after enough time had elapsed for her to suffer severe and irreversible brain damage. This is not uncommon in the use of CPR with elderly patients, since it often takes a few minutes to resuscitate them, and the longer it takes the longer the brain is without oxygen, resulting in brain damage. This was the case with Mrs. Wanglie.

Prior to her heart attack, she was aware of her environment and could relate to her loved ones and caregivers. After her heart attack, when she had been readmitted to the acute care hospital, she was diagnosed to be in a permanent vegetative state with permanent respirator dependency. She was unaware of herself and her environment and unable to relate in any way to

---

1. This account of the *Wanglie* case is summarized from the account in the *Hastings Center Report* 21 (July-August 1991): 23-24.

anyone who visited her, and in the judgment of her physicians would not regain consciousness or improve. She had been treated aggressively for a variety of complications such as pneumonia and was being fed by artificial means.

With her extremely poor prognosis, her physicians suggested to her husband that any further treatment would not be beneficial to her. They suggested discontinuing treatment, giving her comfort care and allowing her various diseases to take their natural course. But the family (her husband and children) resolutely insisted that all forms of treatment be continued. They held out hope for a healing miracle from God and held that since only God can take life, it was not their place to make a decision to withdraw treatment as the physicians were suggesting.[2] Her husband claimed that his wife had made it clear to him that if she could no longer make decisions for herself and take care of herself because of illness, she did not want anything done that might shorten her life. In other words, she wanted everything done for her up until the very end of her life, and her family was faithfully representing her wishes.

During the next few months, the hospital agreed to follow the family's wishes temporarily while continuing efforts to resolve the conflict. There was no change in Mrs. Wanglie's condition, and as time went on the feeling of the hospital staff became more clear that further treatment should be discontinued. By the time the case went to court, she had been in the hospital and/or on a respirator for roughly one year. By the end of her stay, her hospital charges were in the hundreds of thousands of dollars.

Mrs. Wanglie's case involves a new and recurring conflict, between physicians and hospitals who judge further treatment of seriously ill patients to be futile and family members who insist on everything being done for their loved one.[3] Both the legal focus and ethical focus have shifted in recent years, resolving some situations but creating other dilemmas. The classic cases in end-of-life

2. This is a common rationale for continuing treatment in the face of a very poor prognosis. An alternative Christian vision for death and dying that focuses on resurrection and the afterlife will be proposed later in this chapter. See Russell B. Connors, Jr., and Martin L. Smith, "Religious Insistence on Medical Treatment: Christian Theology and Re-Imagination," *Hastings Center Report* 26 (July-August 1996): 23-30.

3. Two other cases in addition to *Wanglie* have contributed to courts sending a mixed message to physicians and hospitals about withdrawing or withholding futile treatment. In the case of Baby K in Virginia, the courts ruled for the family that they had the right to continued treatment even though the baby's physicians deemed it futile. In the *Gilgunn* case, decided in 1995, the court ruled that the medical center was not responsible for a patient's death should it elect to discontinue treatment that the patient's physicians were sure was futile.

ethics such as those of Karen Ann Quinlan (1976)[4] and Nancy Cruzan (1990)[5] set a precedent for competent adult patients to make their own decisions regarding their treatment, or let qualified surrogate decision-makers make them using what is called substituted judgment. That is, the surrogate decision-maker is responsible for making a decision based on what he or she thought the patient would have wanted under the present circumstances. The surrogate's judgment substitutes for the patient's. In those cases the conflict was between physicians and/or hospitals who wanted to continue treatment and patients or their surrogate decision-makers who wanted to discontinue it. Today the cases involve dying patients or their surrogates who request care at the end of life that their doctors consider futile. Case managers and administrators followed these cases closely because they have great impact on the financial management of the hospital. The care being requested is almost always very expensive, and can run into the hundreds of thousands of dollars. Though most hospitals have some sort of budget line item for uncompensated care (for the poor who cannot pay or who pay partially through Medicaid, and for the elderly, who pay partially through Medicare), it only takes a few cases like *Wanglie* to consume the entire budget in this area. This precludes the hospital from using those funds for other types of more beneficial care such as providing prenatal care for pregnant women or immunizing children.

Futile care at the end of life is just one of the many complex issues in bioethics at the ending edge of life. How to properly care for the dying has become a prominent subject in the medical and bioethics literature in the past few years, as studies are showing that the care of the dying in many hospitals is a serious problem.[6] The poor care for the dying has understandably fueled

---

4. In the *Quinlan* case (Karen Ann Quinlan, 355 A. 2d. 665, 1976), she had suffered a head injury that left her dependent on a ventilator for breathing, or so her physicians thought. Her family wanted the ventilator turned off, insisting that Karen would not want this treatment to keep her alive. The court ruled for the family, the ventilator was turned off, and to everyone's surprise, she kept breathing on her own. She lived for approximately another ten years.

5. The *Cruzan* case (*Cruzan v Missouri Dept. of Health,* 497 US 261, 1990) differed slightly from *Quinlan.* Nancy Cruzan had a serious head injury as a result of an automobile accident that left her in a persistent vegetative state. Her family wanted her feeding tubes removed. The hospital refused, and the Supreme Court ruled that with "clear and convincing evidence" that the patient did not want such life-sustaining treatment, the hospital would have to abide by the patient's wishes. However, at the time of trial in Cruzan's case, the Supreme Court ruled that there was not such evidence. The case was heard in a lower court following this, in which evidence that met the Supreme Court's standard was presented. The feeding tubes were then removed and Nancy died within a few days.

6. See, for example, the recent symposium, "Caring for Patients at the End of Life,"

interest in physician-assisted suicide, which has made its way all the way to the United States Supreme Court, where the justices decided that there is no constitutionally protected right to physician assistance in suicide.[7] End-of-life care has raised the important issue of proper pain management, particularly for patients with various end-stage cancers. The discussion of advance directives and DNR (do not resuscitate) orders also comes out of a growing concern about properly managing dying persons' last days, free from unnecessary pain and suffering and consistent with their wishes about how they want to be treated toward the end of their lives. Health care organizations are becoming more interested in what dying patients and their families really want from their health care providers, and that data is being made public. These issues need to be addressed from a theological perspective on death and dying. This perspective will set people free from an excessive dependence on medical technology to prolong life at any costs (known as vitalism), and yet it will also provide caution and skepticism about more extreme responses to the poor care for the dying such as physician-assisted suicide.

Background: Care for the Dying

Care for the dying is more difficult today than in past times because medical technology has given caregivers the ability to prolong life in increasingly poor quality-of-life circumstances. Decisions about withdrawing life-sustaining treatments ordinarily did not have to be made in the past, since that technology was not available and patients died more suddenly as a result. In the past, chronic disease was not nearly as common as it is today. People generally did not linger with a life-threatening disease; more often than not, they died suddenly and without much warning. They also generally died in the presence of the community, being cared for by the people in the community who were closest to them. Death was more of a public event than it is today. Death was viewed as a normal part of life, something over which mere mortals had little control. Medicine was limited in what it could provide for a cure, so it was more focused on providing dying patients with what comfort it could.

With the advent of sophisticated medical technology in the past thirty years, medical professionals have developed a remarkable ability to stave off

---

special issue of *Western Journal of Medicine* 163 (1995): 231-305. Since the SUPPORT study was published, the discussion in the bioethics literature on this issue has increased significantly.

7. *Washington v Glucksburg* and *Vacco v Quill* (117 S. Ct. 2258, 1997).

death. One result is that many people die in a hospital, surrounded by technology that they may not want and cared for predominantly by strangers. It is a very private affair, particularly since the physician relationship today is more technical and less trust related.[8] Death became an enemy to be conquered, and to be fought with all the available resources. Care for the dying involved aggressive treatment. There was less emphasis on helping people die comfortably.

Recent empirical data suggests that the quality of care at the end of life is less than desirable. For example, the widely publicized SUPPORT study, a five-year study (1989-94) with multimillion-dollar funding from the Robert Wood Johnson Foundation, was designed to track the experience of dying in the hospital setting.[9] It included roughly 9,100 patients who had one or more clearly identifiable life-threatening diseases. Patients were not admitted into the study unless they were in advanced stages of these diseases. In other words, admission to the study did not indicate a good prognosis for the patient. The study was conducted at five hospitals in the United States: Beth Israel Hospital, Boston; Duke University Medical Center; MetroHealth Medical Center, Cleveland; Marshfield Medical Research Foundation/St. Joseph's Hospital, Marshfield, Wisconsin; UCLA Medical Center. Included in this list are both teaching and community hospitals, located in both major metropolitan areas and smaller communities.

The study measured five critical components of the experience of dying in the hospital that reflected the assumptions of the investigators as to what constituted a "good death."[10]

1. If and when *DNR (do not resuscitate) orders* were written. The investigators involved with the study assumed that a timely DNR order was indicative of a more peaceful death, without expensive technology and repeated attempts at resuscitation.

2. Patient-physician agreement on *CPR preference.* The investigators assumed that patients had had meaningful communication with their physi-

---

8. For more on how the phenomenon of death has been changed by the introduction of sophisticated medical technology, see Daniel Callahan, *The Troubled Dream of Life* (New York: Simon and Schuster, 1993), pp. 23-56.

9. The SUPPORT Principal Investigators, "A Controlled Trial to Improve Care for Seriously Ill Hospitalized Patients," *Journal of the American Medical Association* 274, no. 20 (22/29 November 1995): 1591-98. Its findings were considered so important that the Robert Wood Johnson Foundation also funded a study by the Hastings Center to address the ethical implications of the study ("Dying Well in the Hospital: The Lessons of SUPPORT," special supplement of the *Hastings Center Report* [November-December 1995]: S1-S36).

10. The marks of a "good death" will be discussed later in this chapter.

cians about their preferences for CPR at the end of life. Such communication about patient preferences was considered essential for managing someone's dying process well.

3. Days spent in *ICU* or *on mechanical ventilation.* The investigators assumed that fewer days spent on a ventilator or in the ICU indicated a peaceful death without expensive and oftentimes burdensome technology to prolong the dying process.

4. Frequency and severity of *pain.* The investigators of the study assumed that adequate pain management was critical to a good death in the hospital.

5. Hospital *resource use.* The investigators assumed that the more resources a dying patient used while in the hospital, the more it indicated that the patient's physicians were employing expensive technology that only delayed an inevitable death.

One key element of the study was an intervention performed halfway through by specially trained nurses with multiple contacts with families, patients, physicians, and hospital staff. This was done to alert the hospital staff and physicians to some of the problems that the investigators had uncovered in the first two years of the study and to see if, by increased discussion of these issues with physicians and nurses, they could be corrected.

The *findings* of the study included some startling discoveries that surprised the general public and much of the professional health care community but were not a surprise to those who specialized in treating dying patients. The investigators discovered that:

1. Almost half of DNR orders were written within two days of death. That is, dying patients were considered a "full code" and were given all attempts at resuscitation, however futile, until roughly two days prior to their death. Though there are clearly occasions in which such a late DNR order can be justified, this finding indicates that most dying patients in the study were subjected to expensive and often painful and harmful resuscitation efforts when it was clear that their death was near. In some cases, however, a full code was ordered and recorded but not necessarily carried out.

2. Roughly half of the physicians did not know of patients' CPR preferences. This finding indicates a significant lack of communication between patients/families and their physicians. Though the pace at which physicians must work today makes good communication with patients and their families more difficult and costly, this was considered by the investigators to be basic communication that should have taken place with a dying patient or the family. The fact that in many cases CPR preferences were not even discussed suggests that the physicians in the study were operating with a presumption

for aggressive care, even though the patient was dying from a life-threatening disease. It further suggests that training in clinical care for the dying has not kept up with the changes in technology.[11]

3. Over one-third of irreversibly dying patients spent at least ten days of their hospital stay in the ICU. This finding suggests that dying patients were subjected to expensive and aggressive treatment as their prognosis became increasingly poor. The ICU is associated with the most expensive and aggressive care available in any hospital and is reserved for the most seriously ill patients. However, the place for the irreversibly dying patient with death near is not the ICU but a hospice, which specializes in providing comfort care for patients for whom aggressive care is no longer desired or effectual. This finding correlates with another well-known trend in the care of the dying, that most hospice consultations are not conducted in a timely manner, and patients are transferred to a hospice far too late in their dying process.[12]

4. Fifty percent of patients and/or families reported that the patient had been in moderate to severe pain during the last three days of life. This is the most troubling finding of the study, and contributed a great deal of impetus for the advocates of physician-assisted suicide. If patients are faced with the options of either dying in moderate to severe pain or having a physician assist them in committing suicide, the choice for assisted suicide seems obvious. The investigators rightly considered proper pain management a moral obligation, and this finding points out the shortcomings in medical education not only in caring for the dying generally but also specifically in controlling their pain adequately.

5. Median hospital charges were roughly $30,000.

Researchers estimate that there are approximately 400,000 hospital admissions of patients annually across the United States that meet criteria for admission into the SUPPORT study. The main investigators conclude that "we are left with a troubling situation. The picture we describe of the care of seriously ill or dying persons is not attractive."[13] Boston University health care law professor George Annas put his conclusion more pointedly: "if dying patients want to retain some control over their dying process, they must get

11. It should be noted that most of the facilities SUPPORT cites were tertiary-care hospitals, clearly committed to aggressive treatment for the dying. Many community hospitals do not share this commitment and operate without this presumption for aggressive care.

12. The reason for hospice transfer being so late is sometimes due to a patient's unwillingness to be considered a "dying" patient earlier in the process, thereby depriving themselves of helpful hospice care.

13. The SUPPORT Principal Investigators, p. 1591.

out of the hospital they are in, and stay out of the hospital if they are out."[14] These findings should encourage us to take seriously the appropriate desires of dying patients and, in upholding their dignity, give attention to appropriate levels of care, proper pain management, and good communication between patients/families and their caregivers. They further indicate a need for ongoing education aimed at dying patients and their caregivers. Otherwise the demand for measures like physician-assisted suicide will continue to grow. These findings raise important questions such as, what constitutes a good death? what does it mean to properly care for the dying? and, how should a Christian view the dying process?

Biblical Perspectives on Death and Dying

Much of the discussion of care of the dying has gone on without a great deal of theological reflection. The exception is the extensive network of Catholic hospitals and medical centers, which is striving to integrate general theological perspectives such as respect for human beings made in God's image, compassion to the vulnerable, and the obligation to serve the poor into health care. One good example is the Supportive Care of the Dying Project, sponsored by the Sisters of Providence Health System in conjunction with the Catholic Health Association and other Catholic health care organizations around the United States. But most of the discussion of care of the dying in the bioethics literature takes place without any explicit interest in theological or philosophical views of death and dying, except for discussion on how to deal with patients who have strong religious views. Good care of the dying raises important questions about our theological view of death and dying. For example, is death an enemy to be resisted at every turn? Is doing everything to delay death a necessary part of being consistently "pro-life"? Or is death a normal part of life, and should such a view suggest limits on how hard it should be fought? Is "death with dignity" an oxymoron or a goal to be pursued?

Throughout the Scripture human life is treated as a sacred gift from God. Human beings are made in the image of God, which gives them a status above the animals and a bit lower than the angels (Heb. 2:6-8). The sanctions against taking innocent life are grounded in the fact that human beings are the image of God (Gen. 9:5-6).[15] Innocent human life is to be protected

14. George J. Annas, "How We Lie," in "Dying Well in the Hospital," p. S13.
15. This is developed further in chapter 4 and will only be summarized here.

(Exod. 20:13; Deut. 5:17), with capital punishment prescribed for murder functioning as the strongest possible deterrent for taking innocent life. This has become a fundamental moral and political principle in most every culture in the ancient and modern worlds, suggesting that respect for the sanctity of human life may actually be grounded in natural law, or God's revelation of moral values outside of Scripture. Many of these cultures that have similar prohibitions for taking innocent life and similar sanctions when that principle is violated actually preceded the revelation of God in the Ten Commandments. Respect for human life is thus embedded into creation by God and has been discovered by human beings irrespective of their faith commitment. To be sure, it is clarified by God's revelation in Scripture and given authority as the written word of God. It is hardly accidental that virtually every civilization has had respect for the sanctity of life as one of its foundation principles underlying its political philosophy.

This respect for human life is applied differently in different cultural contexts and in different age groups. For example, it is well known that certain tribes of Eskimos practice and actually encourage euthanasia among their people. The reason for this is a religious belief about the afterlife, that people enter the afterlife in the same physical condition in which they die. There is no doctrine of the resurrection of the body as in Christianity. Thus to respect a person's dignity is to encourage that person to enter the afterlife before his or her body has had the chance to seriously deteriorate through old age and disease. Many Eskimos would look at the way people die in hospitals across the United States and suggest that by prolonging life we are actually doing a terrible injustice to them. The moral principle is the same — respect for human dignity — but the way it is carried out is very different. Thus this would not be an example of a value difference due to a difference in culture. There is actually agreement on the principle, but a difference in the way the principle is practiced.

The Mosaic Law expands this notion of the protection of innocent life by emphasizing the obligation to protect the most vulnerable in the society. With increased vulnerability comes a heightened obligation to protect people's lives and opportunities to care for themselves. The Law is replete with admonitions to care for the most vulnerable in the society. The poor, the immigrant (called the alien), and the powerless are given a safety net that protects their lives by providing their sustenance needs and their chance to support themselves. For example, the Law mandated a primitive form of workfare for the poor in the form of the chance to glean in fields of those who owned farmland and grew crops. Landowners were required by the Law to set aside the edges of their fields for the poor to harvest. In addition, the owners could not go back through the field a second time in order to harvest more thoroughly. What was left behind was for the poor and the immigrant, to allow them to avoid starvation (Lev. 19:9-10; Deut. 24:19-22; Ruth 2:1-3). The Law further mandated that the poor and immigrants not be taken advantage of in the courts in day-to-day business dealings (Deut. 24:10-18). They were to be paid their wages at the end of the day, and basic necessities taken as collateral for a loan were not to be kept overnight. Laws concerning the redemption of the land and the year of Jubilee suggest that the economically vulnerable are to be given regular opportunities to enter the workforce and support themselves (Lev. 25:8-31). The prophets repeatedly point out that among Israel's numerous failings as a nation, their neglect of the most vulnerable among them was considered a grievous sin (Isa. 58:6-7; Amos 2:6-7). There seems to be special emphasis in the Law and Prophets on taking care of the most vulnerable, focused on the poor and immigrant. This is closely related to the sacredness of human life and the respect due to human beings made in God's image. Human beings are not to be taken advantage of, treated like property, or oppressed as if they had no value. This is particularly the case since periodically such oppression actually resulted in the death of the vulnerable person. Though not specifically mentioned in the Law, it would seem to be a short step by way of application to include the elderly, the unborn, and the seriously ill in the group of the most vulnerable in the society. The greater the vulnerability of the individual or the group, the greater was the obligation to care for them and protect their lives and interests. Thus with the dying, whether the elderly or seriously ill newborns, their physical and, at times, mental vulnerability brings upon society the obligation to protect them and care for their needs. The biblical teaching on the sacredness of innocent human life and the obligation to protect the most vulnerable is one of the primary reasons for insuring proper care for the dying and why euthanasia as an alternative is problematic.[16]

Death became a reality with the entrance of sin into the world with the sin of Adam and Eve. One of the consequences of Adam's disobedience was the introduction of death into the realm of reality that he and Eve would experience from that point on. The Genesis account introduces the reality of death in poetic terms when God reminds Adam that

> "you [will] return to the ground,
>   since from it you were taken;

---

16. Euthanasia and physician-assisted suicide will be discussed in further detail later in this chapter.

for dust you are
    and to dust you will return." (3:19 NIV)

The apostle Paul makes it clear that death entered the world through the sin of Adam (Rom. 5:12; I Cor. 15:21-22). Thus death is not part of God's original design, but after the entrance of sin into the world death became a normal part of everyday life. In that sense death is a "natural" part of life, nature having experienced the curse of sin.

Death is thus a universal part of the experience of human beings on the earth. Death is seen in the Scripture as the great equalizer, that regardless of a person's position, wealth, influence, power, status, or wisdom, death is the common experience of all human beings (Eccles. 2:15-16; 3:19-21; 5:15-16; 9:1-6). For example, in the wisdom literature, when Solomon suggests that there is a time for everything, namely, a time to be born and a time to die, he is reminding his readers that life "under the sun," that is, this side of eternity, is a life in which there is an appointed time for death. It is a normal part of life in a fallen world (Eccles. 3:1-2).

Though the doctrine of resurrection and the afterlife is not thoroughly developed in the Old Testament, it does give some indication that there is hope beyond the grave for the person who trusts and knows God. Some of the texts that are used to indicate a hope in the afterlife could just as legitimately be interpreted to refer to people being delivered from the threat of death by the intervention of God (Pss. 17:15; 16:10).[17] However, other texts hint more clearly that there is hope beyond death, that death is not the final destination of every human being. For example, in Job 19:25-27 Job is envisioning what he thinks is his forthcoming death and states his hope as follows:

"I know that my Redeemer lives. . . .
And after my skin has been destroyed,
    yet in my flesh I will see God;
I myself will see him
    with my own eyes — I, and not another." (NIV)

The phrase "after my skin has been destroyed" is taken to suggest a figure of speech for death, and Job is indicating that after his death he will see God, or

---

17. Ps. 16:10 is a very controversial passage that is used in Acts 2:25-28 to indicate fulfillment of prophecy concerning the resurrection of Christ. There is debate about the original intent of the psalmist in Ps. 16, whether that refers to literal resurrection or deliverance from an earthly threat of death. For further information on this text, see Darrell L. Bock, *Proclamation from Prophecy and Pattern* (Sheffield: JSNT Press, 1985).

experience resurrection and afterlife. It is possible to take this text to indicate that Job believes that God will deliver him from the various earthly threats to his life which have put him in the grip of death. This view points to the phrase "yet in my flesh I will see God" to suggest that Job will again experience God on earth after God has delivered him from his present troubles. That is, God will not allow him to be conquered by his present troubles and will rescue him from imminent death. It is possible that this passage gives a hint of the afterlife, but it is likely not clear enough to make a definitive suggestion. Perhaps the clearest indication of eternal life in the Old Testament is found in the prophetic puzzles of Daniel 12, in which Daniel predicts resurrection and afterlife as part of the prophetic culmination of the end times (Dan. 12:2).[18]

However, the New Testament is abundantly clear that the afterlife is a reality and that the grave is not a person's final destination. Jesus refers repeatedly to the hope of resurrection and life after death. He refers to himself as "the resurrection and the life" (John 11:25-26) and teaches about the reality of eternal hope on numerous occasions (John 5:24; Luke 14:14; Matt. 22:31). The Epistles continue this development as a promise that every believer in Christ will experience eternity with God (Phil. 3:10-11, 20; Col. 3:1-4; I Tim. 1:16). Perhaps the most often quoted and powerful indication of the hope of the afterlife comes from I Corinthians 15:29-57, which climaxes with the notion of death as a conquered enemy. Paul writes in reference to Christ's victory over death with his death and resurrection:

"Death has been swallowed up in victory.

"Where, O death, is your victory?
   Where, O death, is your sting?"

The sting of death is sin, and the power of sin is the law. But thanks be to God! He gives us the victory [over death] through our Lord Jesus Christ. (15:54-57 NIV)

Death is an enemy which has been vanquished by the death and resurrection of Christ. Death is a result of the entrance of sin into the world, the culmination of the consequences of sin and diametrically opposed to God's original design for creation. Because it has been conquered by Christ, his victory over

---

18. A final Old Testament text that may suggest the afterlife is found in Isa. 26:19, in the context of Israel's restoration. But this may be a figure of speech for Israel's return from exile or, depending on one's eschatological views, for Israel's restoration prior to the return of Christ. It is probably not clear enough to make a definitive conclusion about the afterlife in the Old Testament.

death has brought the reality of life beyond death. Thus death is seen in Christian perspective as the doorstep to eternal life, the means by which individuals are ushered into eternity in God's presence. For the believer, death is not something to be feared. To be sure, there are inevitable losses involved with a person's death, and these are not to be minimized. Premature death, especially for children, is a terrible tragedy because it cuts off a person's contributions before he or she has a chance to live a full life. For the person's bereaved loved ones, premature death is very difficult and painful. But for the Christian who has lived a full life and is physically deteriorating, death is not something to be feared, since it provides the passageway into an eternity with God. Death is at the same time an enemy, though conquered, and a normal part of life.[19]

The notion of death as a conquered enemy has many ramifications for a Christian perspective on death, dying, and caring for the dying at the end of life. It is true that death is an enemy in that it was not a part of God's original design for human beings, and that in some sense the notion of death with dignity is an oxymoron. In light of the cause of the reality of death, the notion of a dignified death seems difficult to maintain since the death and the deterioration that accompanies it involve the temporary victory of sin. The late Protestant theologian and ethicist Paul Ramsey suggested that we ought not speak of death and dignity in the same sentence. He put it this way: "Good death, like 'good grief' is ultimately a contradiction in terms."[20] However, Ramsey's view seems to understate the fact that death has been conquered and the sting removed from it by the death and resurrection of Christ. If death has been conquered and is ultimately not to be feared (though death is an unknown and it is not wrong to be afraid of the unknown), then death need not be resisted at every turn. Caregivers need not provide every aggressive treatment to forestall death, and patients and their families need not request all available aggressive treatments to delay an inevitable death. Of course, when there is a good prognosis and hope for a restoration to function and health, then aggressive care should generally be pursued. But when the prognosis is poor and further treatment is futile to turn around the overall deterioration of the patient's condition, then one should realize that death is

19. For further discussion of the theological background to death and dying, see Dennis P. Hollinger, "Theological Foundations for Death and Dying Issues," *Ethics and Medicine* 12, no. 3 (1996): 60-65.

20. Paul Ramsey, "The Indignity of Death with Dignity," *Hastings Center Report* 2 (May 1972): 47-62, cited in Allen Verhey and Stephen Lammers, eds., *On Moral Medicine: Theological Perspectives in Medical Ethics,* 1st ed. (Grand Rapids: Wm. B. Eerdmans Publishing Co., 1987), pp. 185-96, at 186.

not the ultimate enemy that must be fought at every turn. It has been conquered, and doing everything necessary to delay death is not required, nor is
it a necessary part of being consistently pro-life. Of course, there is not always
a clear line that separates futile and beneficial treatment, though that line can
become clearer when the patient and the physician have a relationship built
on trust and openness, in which the physician has cared for or knows the patient. Viewing death as a conquered enemy should preclude vitalism, or the
view that keeping someone alive regardless of the medical circumstances has
value. One wonders about the reality of a patient's or his or her family's eternal hope when they tenaciously continue to request that all aggressive treatment be provided when the prognosis is extremely poor. Though it is true
that the desire for self-preservation is part of the human constitution, there
are times when it is appropriate to let go of the desire to live and accept death
as the doorstep into eternal life. When this happens, caregivers are obligated
to preserve as much of the patient's dignity as possible, which is normally
what is meant by proponents of a "death with dignity." This is surely a worthy
goal to be pursued in the care of the dying.

Seeing death as a normal part of life and the universal experience of all
human beings suggests that there are limits on how hard death should be
fought. This is particularly true since death has been vanquished and the
sting of death has been removed by Christ. Since it is a universal experience,
death should be seen as the ultimate end point of all medical treatment. Even
the deterioration of life and the aging of human beings is a part of the dying
process, even though it may begin decades prior to one's death. It is important to see all of life as a continuum in this way, thereby minimizing the fran-
tic avoidance of "facing death" at the end of life. Ethicist Daniel Callahan suggests that

> Death is that to which medical care should be oriented from the outset in
> the case of all serious, potentially life threatening illnesses or of a serious
> decline of mental and physical capacities as a result of age or disease. Of
> each serious illness, especially with the elderly, a question should be asked
> and a possibility entertained: could it be that this illness is the one that ei-
> ther will be fatal, or since some disease must be fatal, should soon be al-
> lowed to be fatal? If so, then a different strategy toward it should come into
> play, an effort to work toward a peaceful death rather than fight for a
> cure.[21]

21. Daniel Callahan, "Toward a Peaceful Death," *Hastings Center Report* 23 (July-
August 1993): 33-38, at 34.

Callahan is rightly suggesting that the culture needs to reexamine its view of death and move away from the death-denying trends that are so prevalent today. Medical training today overwhelmingly reflects a legacy of aggressive treatment for disease, with little emphasis on how to care for people who will eventually succumb to a particular disease. Yet if death is a conquered enemy, then a perspective like Callahan's makes sense. Since death is a normal part of each person's experience, and all of life should be seen as part of the dying process and a preparation for death, then medical care should be oriented toward caring for the dying when aggressive treatment to cure disease is no longer feasible or desirable. Likewise, since death has been conquered, it is not necessary that it be treated like an enemy to be subjugated with the full focus of human medical efforts. That is not to say that medicine should not continue its aggressive research into cures for various diseases. But death cannot be conquered by human ingenuity. Just because medicine finds cures for various diseases, that has put us no closer to conquering death, since new fatal diseases have arisen to take the place of the ones for which medicine has found a cure. In reality, though medicine's cures for many previously fatal diseases have had an undeniable net benefit, one result of medicine's success is that many people are now living long enough to suffer from dementia-producing conditions such as Alzheimer's disease. In addition, many people are living longer but with chronic diseases that seriously affect their quality of life. Many elderly people are living in almost total isolation, both physically and socially, in nursing homes with Alzheimer's and other dementia-producing conditions which leave them virtually incapable of human relationships.

Caring for the Dying in Christian Perspective

Undergirded by Christian moral values such as the sacredness of life, respect for the dignity of persons made in God's image, compassion for the vulnerable, and a view of death as a conquered enemy, caring well for the dying is a moral obligation for professional caregivers and loved ones who take care of dying family members. Far too often the dying are essentially abandoned, and they feel alone, isolated, and powerless, unable in many cases to speak for themselves, and frequently when they can, having their wishes ignored. When they are also unable to care for themselves, it is not difficult to see how they can feel stripped of their dignity. Good care for the dying helps compassionately restore the dignity at which physical and sometimes mental deterioration chips away. Good care for the dying does what is possible to create the possibility of a "good death" for the patient and his or her family. How one understands good care for the dying patient will reflect the definition of a "good death." Good care for the dying must have as its basis an openness to the understanding of the meaning of death for the patient. It is clear that some patients are very resistant to any discussion of the meaning of death, but many dying patients will participate eagerly in the discussion of the meaning of their life and death, where they expect to be after death, and what their hopes are for life after death. Leaving these aspects of the patient-physician relationship undiscussed, as frequently happens with competent medical technicians, may rob a dying patient of participation in some very important discussion, which benefits both the patient and the physician. Just as the SUPPORT investigators assumed certain elements of a good death and crafted their investigation and recommendations as such, any description of proper care for the dying will assume the central aspects of a good death.

Proper Pain Management

Virtually everyone in health care agrees that a fundamental part of a good death is adequate relief of pain and suffering. Roughly half the patients in the SUPPORT study died in moderate to severe pain, an alarming conclusion.[22] Inadequate pain management is unethical because of the way it assaults the dignity of the patient and subjects him or her to unnecessary suffering. It is further a tragedy because the medical profession has at its disposal the means to manage virtually all pain successfully. That does not mean that medicine can relieve all pain successfully, but that it can be managed so that no patient needs to be subjected to prolonged, intractable pain. The failure of medicine to adequately treat pain is one of the driving forces behind the demand for physician-assisted suicide, because, if left with the choices of dying in pain or assisted suicide, most people would understandably choose assisted suicide. As Dr. Mitchell Max of the Pain Research Clinic at the National Institute of Dental Research put it, "pain is the reason Jack Kevorkian has been so successful."[23]

But arguing that assisted suicide is needed to relieve pain is to present a

22. See also Charles S. Cleeland et al., "Pain and Its Treatment in Outpatients with Metastatic Cancer," *New England Journal of Medicine* (3 March 1994): 592-96.

23. Cited in Shannon Brownlee and Joannie M. Schrof, "The Quality of Mercy," *U.S. News and World Report*, 17 March 1997, pp. 54-67, at 56. It should be noted that many of Kevorkian's "patients" are suffering from chronic mental and physical deterioration, and he assists them in suicide in order to preclude more suffering even though they may not be in pain.

false dichotomy. There is an alternative that makes assisted suicide practically unnecessary. If pain is properly managed, most people would not choose assisted suicide. Medicine has at present the tools to adequately manage almost all pain that a patient will endure in the dying process. Palliative care is becoming a well-developed specialty within medicine, particularly within oncology. It is true that some pain management scenarios are more challenging than others, and that at times it does take a pain specialist to meet the challenge. It is further true that medical training has traditionally emphasized palliative care, similar to care of the dying in general. But that is changing, and there are more specialists in this area than ever before. It is also true that not all patients have access to advanced pain management techniques, but if society is given the choice between putting resources into making these techniques more accessible and putting them into the structures that will be necessary to insure that assisted suicide, should it become legal, will not be abused, society should choose to invest in more widely accessible pain management.

If all the tools to manage pain are at medicine's disposal, why then do studies such as the SUPPORT investigation show that so many patients die in pain? A number of factors help explain this, including lack of education on pain; inadequate assessment of pain, including caregivers' frequent skepticism of patients' reports of pain; fear of addiction; fear of hastening a patient's death due to slowing down his or her respiratory system from pain medication; reluctance by physicians to prescribe opioids (opium-derived painkillers such as morphine, recognized as the most effective treatments for pain), due to fear of investigation for overprescribing them; and some patients' reluctance to take morphine because of the side effects on their mental alertness.

In response to these barriers to good pain management, education on pain management is improving, but is still far from optimal in most medical training. Assessment tools are improving as well, and the skepticism of caregivers can be addressed by simply believing patients' reports of pain when they give them. When patients say they are in pain, they should be believed, unless there are compelling reasons not to. The burden of proof should be on caregivers to show that the skepticism is warranted, not on patients to show that they are in the kind of pain they say they are.

Fear of hastening a patient's death is understandable, but if the intent of administering the medication is to relieve pain and not to kill the patient, most pain management groups and the AMA have supported what is called the principle of double effect. This is invoked when a morally legitimate action (such as pain relief) has anticipated but unintended consequences that would normally be avoided (hastening the patient's death). The negative consequences do not render the original act that caused them immoral.[24] There is some debate over how frequently this principle needs to be invoked, since the respiratory system develops a tolerance for pain medication, as does the nervous system.[25] Fear of investigation for overprescribing opioids is changing, and more physicians are prescribing the level of pain medication that is necessary to manage the patient's pain irrespective of the oversight threat, which many physicians suggest is overstated. Reluctance to take morphine due to its impact on mental alertness is understandable, but caregivers should recognize that pain medication is not the only means available to manage pain. A variety of techniques can be used to supplement medication, such as psychosocial and spiritual means, alternative therapies, massage, and other types of techniques.

A final alternative to insure good pain management for dying patients is a timely referral to a hospice, or to hospice care that can be provided at the patient's home. Hospices are one of the most underutilized health care facilities and can be employed much sooner than they normally are. This requires early education of the patients and their families that hospices are not "places of death," but people and systems who help them finish living their lives to the fullest extent possible.

Respecting the Patient's Wishes

A second feature of good care for the dying upon which virtually everyone in health care agrees is the need to elicit and respect the treatment wishes of the patient and/or family. With the emphasis on patient autonomy in recent years, most medical practice has moved away from the kind of paternalism that often characterized the patient-physician relationship. However, with end-of-life care, patient wishes are often ignored, even when stated clearly,

24. The literature on the principle of double effect, particularly in Catholic bioethics circles, is voluminous. See, for example, Task Force on Pain Management, "Pain Management: Theological and Ethical Principles Governing the Use of Pain Relief for Dying Patients," *Health Progress* (January-February 1993): 30-40, at 36-38.

25. In correspondence from the Wisconsin Cancer Pain Initiative to the Council of Ethical and Judicial Affairs of the AMA, they stated, "Death from respiratory depression is exceedingly rare in patients with cancer who chronically receive opioid analgesics for pain. As a person nears death, there is deterioration in respiratory function. However, these respiratory changes should not be confused with the effects of opioids." Cited in Task Force on Pain Management, p. 37.

and in many cases the seriously ill are treated as though they were incompetent.

Since the early 1990s, with the introduction of the Patient Self-Determination Act (PSDA), patients at the end of life have had additional protection of their rights to make their own informed decisions about end-of-life treatment and care. The PSDA mandated that all hospitals offer all incoming patients an opportunity to complete an advance directive, a document that specified for physicians and nurses the kind of care patients did and did not want should their condition become terminal. There are two specific kinds of advance directives: the living will, which lays out the patient's instructions to caregivers about the types of treatment desired; and the durable power of attorney for health care (DPAHC), which designates someone (a surrogate or proxy decision-maker) to make treatment decisions for the patient in the event the patient cannot make them for himself or herself. Most advance directives contain both elements, and the surrogate, or proxy, decision-maker is responsible for interpreting and insuring that the desires of the loved one are carried out. Today relatively few people in the general public have completed advance directives, and many are not well written. As a result there is usually some element of interpretation involved, and often a question about whether it is appropriate to invoke the directive at any given point during the patient's illness.

Closely related to an advance directive is what is called a "do not resuscitate" order (DNR). These are generally issued with the consent of the patient or surrogate decision-maker, and usually with the agreement of the family as well. A DNR order indicates that if a patient who is seriously ill with very poor prognosis has a heart attack, cardiopulmonary resuscitation (CPR) will not be instituted and the person will be allowed to die a natural death. The reason for DNR orders is that CPR is often invasive and expensive and can leave the patient in a worse condition after it is applied than before. In other words, it can produce a greater burden than benefit for the patient. A DNR order is usually issued prior to removing life-supporting treatments and can be seen as the first step in allowing death to take its natural course. Patients or surrogate decision-makers can request DNR orders, physicians can suggest them, and in some cases physicians can issue them without the consent of the family.[26]

26. There is a significant amount of debate over unilateral issuance of DNR orders. Most agree that physicians at least are obligated to communicate to the family that a DNR order has been issued. It is somewhat rare for physicians to actually issue DNR orders without family consent, though there is more discussion that would empower physicians to do

Advance directives are an important part of insuring that a person's autonomy will be respected and his or her wishes followed at the end of life. When properly completed, they are legally binding and cannot be overridden without compelling reasons. However, in many hospital settings they are sometimes overridden, often because many families cannot "let go" of their loved one and keep insisting on aggressive treatment. The Wanglie example cited above is a good example of families, especially ones with a religious belief in miracles, having difficulty letting go. This also happens because it is difficult for physicians to "let go" as well; trained as they are to cure, they find it difficult to admit the implicit (and misguided) sense of failure involved when a patient fails to respond to treatment. Physicians also have an understandable fear of litigation that often drives them to provide aggressive treatment beyond the time when it is appropriate. A vivid example of a patient's wishes being ignored comes from this narrative of one family member's experience.

> The doctor said he wanted to continue to build him up. I said, "No, that was not his wishes," and I wouldn't do it. I said, "I don't know why you're asking these things; you've got this living will and you can follow that." I said, "He told you he wanted no machines and he wanted to die a natural death if he could, with the least amount of pain and to be made comfortable." The doctor said he had two hours to live. My husband made arrangements that he wouldn't have to live on machines. So when we followed him out in the hall, they said we had to leave because they were going to treat him. They put an oxygen mask on him with 100 percent oxygen to take the fluids out from around his heart. They broke his nose. He had a welt that went from one side of his chin to the other. His ears were blackened from the tight mask. He specifically wished that he would have no machines to prolong his life because he was in a lot of pain. A pressure mask that's trying to remove the fluids from around his heart was uncalled for. They asked me if they could call the doctor in to break his chest bone to go in and take the fluid around his heart. This man had cancer cells everywhere!! Why would you do something like that?[27]

Scenarios like this illustrate why it is important not only to put one's wishes in writing, but also to designate a surrogate decision-maker to in-

---

that. See Frank H. Marsh and Allen Staver, "Physician Authority for Unilateral DNR Orders," *Journal of Legal Medicine* 12 (1991): 115-65; Giles R. Scofield, "Is Consent Useful When Resuscitation Isn't?" *Hastings Center Report* 21 (November-December 1991): 28-36.

27. Alicia Super et al., *Living and Healing during Life-Threatening Illness* (Portland, Ore.: Supportive Care of the Dying, 1997), p. 8.

sure that those wishes are properly understood and followed. However, in light of the above narrative, taking those steps may not guarantee that a person's wishes will be followed. After putting these wishes in writing, one should discuss them with one's personal physician and the person who has been appointed the surrogate decision-maker. A copy of the advance directive should be kept in the patient's medical records so that it can be easily accessed, both by caregivers and family members, who may not be aware of their loved one's wishes. In order to avoid putting family members in the very uncomfortable position of having to make difficult decisions for a loved one without a clear understanding of what that person's wishes are, it is important to have an advance directive in writing and to discuss among family members what is meant by the directive's contents.[28] Even with advance directives, there is still a need for a long-term relationship of trust with a primary caregiver who understands the will of the patient and family and who can advocate for them within the health care system. In many cases patients are transferred to specialists who do not know them well, and who may not communicate at all with the patient's primary-care physician. Increasingly, with the separation of office- and hospital-based physicians in many HMO arrangements, maintaining a relationship of trust with a primary-care physician is more difficult. Advance directives are helpful, but they are no substitute for ongoing discussions with the physician and patient/family, since patients do change their minds about what they want during the course of treatment.

Both the law and bioethics recognize the rights of competent patients to refuse any life-sustaining treatments.[29] This right is the foundation for encouraging people to make their wishes known so that they can be protected. In general, it is morally legitimate to refuse a treatment if there is no hope for changing an irreversible course of disease. Rather than fighting off death as the ultimate enemy, when treatment is futile or more burdensome than beneficial it is appropriate and theologically consistent to let death take its natural course and anticipate the afterlife. To see death as a conquered enemy involves letting go of the fight when it cannot be won on

28. For more information on planning for end-of-life care, see Joan M. Teno, T. Patrick Hill, and Mary Ann O'Connor, "Advance Care Planning: Priorities for Ethical and Empirical Research," special supplement to the *Hastings Center Report* 24 (November-December 1994): S1-S36.

29. In most cases, it is probably better to refer to these treatments as death delaying or dying-process-prolonging rather than life sustaining. Though they are clearly sustaining life, that term is usually not helpful in encouraging family members to appropriately let go of dying loved ones.

earth. The victory over death has been won already by Christ, and in light of that it makes little sense to treat death as the enemy that must be vanquished by medicine. When the treatment is futile, or imposes a burden that is greater than the benefit, then the patient or family is under no obligation to request it. Health care providers are under no obligation to offer or provide treatment that is refused by a competent patient, is more burdensome than beneficial, or is futile. This includes feeding tubes that are used to provide nutrition and hydration by medical means.[30] There is little difference between medical means to provide nutrition and hydration and medical assistance in breathing, which a ventilator provides. Yet there is no debate about the morality of removing the treatment of ventilator assistance. There are also no legal obstacles to removing feeding tubes from patients with an advance directive indicating that they do not want such treatment, from patients for whom it is futile, or from patients for whom it is more burdensome than beneficial. Wishes to refuse treatment, including feeding tubes, are generally appropriate wishes that should be followed by health care professionals as part of respecting patient wishes.

However, there are limits to patient autonomy.[31] That is, there are some wishes that will not and should not be recognized. For example, autonomy does not include the right to assistance in suicide. As the Supreme Court recently ruled, there is no constitutionally recognized right to die.[32] Neither does autonomy include the right to treatment that one's physician judges to be futile.[33]

---

30. The issue of medically provided nutrition and hydration is still debated, though the consensus in bioethics circles is that it constitutes a form of medical treatment that can be refused. The Supreme Court in the *Cruzan* decision ruled that with "clear and convincing evidence" that a patient did not wish to be on a feeding tube, it can be withdrawn. For further discussion on this issue, see Scott B. Rae, "Views of Human Nature at the End of Life," in *Christian Perspectives on Being Human: A Multidisciplinary Approach,* ed. J. P. Moreland and David M. Ciocchi (Grand Rapids: Baker, 1993), pp. 252-55.

31. This is discussed in further detail in chapter 6.

32. This will be addressed further later in this chapter.

33. The literature on the futility debate is voluminous. Some of the most widely mentioned contributions include John J. Paris and Frank E. Reardon, "Physician Refusal of Requests for Futile or Ineffective Interventions," *Cambridge Quarterly of Healthcare Ethics* 2 (1992): 127-34; Daniel Callahan, "Medical Futility, Medical Necessity: The Problem without a Name," *Hastings Center Report* 21 (July-August 1991): 30-35; Tom Tomlinson and Howard Brody, "Futility and the Ethics of Resuscitation," *Journal of the American Medical Association* 264, no. 10 (12 September 1990): 1276-80; Lawrence J. Schneiderman, Nancy S. Jecker, and Albert R. Jonsen, "Medical Futility: Its Meaning and Ethical Implications," *Annals of Internal Medicine* 112, no. 12 (15 June 1990): 949-53; Tom Tomlinson and Diane Czlonka, "Futility and Hospital Policy," *Hasting Center Report* 25 (May-June 1995): 28-35.

The issue of futile treatment is a difficult one and involves a number of complicated issues.

The central issue is whether or not physicians and health care institutions have a moral obligation to provide expensive life-sustaining treatment that is judged futile if the family or surrogate decision-maker requests it. But before that issue can be resolved, what we mean by "futile" care must be established.

What exactly does it mean that a treatment is futile? Does it mean that it will not work, as antibiotics for a virus simply won't work? Or does it mean treatment that does not provide a benefit to the patient? There is long-standing consensus that treatment that will not work need not be provided. For example, if it is certain that CPR would not resuscitate the patient, then it is futile. But a distinction needs to be made between a benefit of treatment and an effect of treatment. Treatments that have a positive effect do what they are designed to do, but that effect may or may not be a benefit to the patient. For example, CPR may successfully resuscitate a terminally ill patient but leave him or her in such a deteriorated state that it may not have been a benefit to that patient. In addition, antibiotics for pneumonia in a terminal cancer patient with only a few weeks to live may kill the infection, but it may also prolong a painful dying process. Thus simply keeping someone alive, or even trying to keep him or her alive, may or may not benefit that person.

The definition of futility goes right to the heart of the goals of medical treatment. The goals of any treatment would seem to go beyond simply maintaining physiological functioning. Other definitions of futile treatment include the following:

1. Treatment that does not contribute to integrated functioning of the whole person is futile.
2. Treatment that only preserves permanent unconsciousness or a persistent vegetative state is futile.
3. Treatment that cannot end dependence on continued life support or other intensive care medicine is futile.
4. Treatment that only prolongs the dying process is futile.
5. Futile treatments are those that are not medically indicated, offer no long-term benefit, or are harmful to the patient.

Unless the treatment is clearly physiologically futile, that is, has no positive effect, there are still questions about the definition of futility. Some suggest that a policy on this be procedural, not substantive, since virtually any definition can be seen as flawed.[34] Most agree that treatment that offers no benefit to the patient is futile, but the definition of a benefit seems to involve a value judgment that is imposed upon the patient. In the best circumstances, a futility determination would be a value judgment that is determined with the patient. Most evaluations of a benefit of treatment involve quality-of-life assessments, which also involve value judgments about what quality of life is acceptable to a particular patient. A patient understandably may not want others deciding what is an acceptable quality of life for him or her. The conclusion that a treatment is futile is not always a matter of objective medical fact; it is also a value judgment that physicians should be careful about imposing on patients. On the other hand, they also need to educate patients about the wisdom of utilizing scarce medical resources when a patient's prognosis is poor. Physicians have no obligation to present physiologically futile options to patients, but they should be careful about making unilateral decisions of futility when quality-of-life judgments must be made.[35]

Some hospitals have developed futile care policies in order to provide institutional support to physicians who think it appropriate to withdraw futile end-of-life care. Some have even developed cooperative policies in order to prevent patients from hospital hopping, looking for one that will provide otherwise futile treatment. One well-publicized example occurred in Houston, with roughly fifteen hospitals joining efforts to develop a standard approach to handling requests for futile care.[36] Their perspective is not to provide any standard definition of futility but to set up a procedure for handling disputes between physicians, the medical center, and patients/surrogates. Any good approach to mediating these disputes should involve clear communication with the patient/surrogate, institutional review, and recognition of the patient's right to be transferred.

34. See the article by Tomlinson and Czlonka, "Futility and Hospital Policy," which makes this point explicitly.

35. Patients and families need to realize that physician decisions in these circumstances depend on the physician's age, experience, specialty, faith commitments. Optimally, the patient should expect the physician to be an expositor of the known treatment possibilities and the known probable effects and side effects, advocating for the patient to place his or her own values in the decision mix.

36. Houston City Wide Task Force on Medical Futility, "A Multi-Institutional Collaborative Policy on Medical Futility," *Journal of the American Medical Association* 276, no. 7 (21 August 1996): 571-74.

Clear and Timely Communication

Respecting the dignity of persons and offering compassionate care at the end of life involve clear and consistent communication with patients, surrogate decision-makers, and families. There is little doubt that the fast pace of medical practice today, particularly in a managed care context, has made it much more difficult for physicians to take the time to communicate well with patients and their families. In some instances nursing staff are empowered to communicate more fully the aspects of the patient's care that physicians may not have time to do. But the results of the SUPPORT study indicate that frequently patient/family–physician communication is less than desirable.

Communication that is timely and consistent is important so that dying patients do not feel abandoned, a common complaint. Part of the reason for this is that caregivers often feel inadequately trained in communicating with patients in general, and especially with the dying.[37] A further reason for this inadequacy in communication is the discomfort of both physicians and patients in facing their mortality, particularly physicians facing their "failures," namely, sick people who die under their care. Of course, this is not necessarily a failure, but a recognition of the inevitable. Because of this inadequacy, caregivers often emotionally withdraw from dying patients and their families, only adding to the sense of isolation and abandonment that the dying often feel. Another reason for this abandonment is the erroneous equation of DNR orders with permission to stop caring for the DNR patient. DNR is often referred to as a "no code" status, meaning that if the patient has a heart attack, no code is to be called, that is, no efforts at resuscitation are to be administered. A common misconception in many hospitals is that "no code = no care." This is a violation of patients' dignity and constitutes less than compassionate care for the dying. It is crucial for caregivers to carefully explain the illness; the best estimate of the prognosis, particularly since that may change on a regular basis; and the treatment options with their probabilities of success, including the option of comfort care only, instead of aggressive care.

Whether or not they ask directly, studies show that dying patients want to know the truth about their prognosis and what they can expect in the dying process.[38] They frequently become distressed when their questions go unanswered or are not answered to their satisfaction. Family mem-

37. Super et al., pp. 9-10.
38. Super et al., p. 5.

bers sometimes hide the truth from their dying loved ones, thinking that if they knew their disease and prognosis, they would give up on living, thereby hastening their death. Families from different cultures often value truth telling differently, thinking that not disclosing the truth to the patient will ease the burden of the patient's illness.[39] Families from these cultures view their responsibility as shouldering as much of the burden of the patient's illness themselves as possible. However, most patients generally want to know the truth and have a good intuitive sense that something is wrong. In addition, a patient entering the dying process without knowing that death is relatively imminent may not sense the urgency and seize the opportunity to take care of unfinished relational business prior to his or her death. Respecting patients' dignity involves telling them the truth, or at least giving them the opportunity to hear the truth for themselves. If a patient knowingly chooses to not hear the truth about his or her diagnosis and chooses to let the family bear the burden of his or her illness, that is that patient's right. But to withhold the truth from the patient without finding out if that is the patient's wish is problematic, irrespective of the patient's cultural background.

No Legalized Assistance in Suicide

Compassionate care for the dying should not be undermined by offering assistance in suicide.[40] Though widely seen as an option by the general public, assisted suicide is against the law in every state except Oregon, which passed the issue in a public referendum in the fall of 1997, after having passed it into law in 1995.

On 28 June 1997 the U.S. Supreme Court decided the first "right to die"

39. Leslie J. Blackhall et al., "Ethnicity and Attitudes toward Patient Autonomy," *Journal of the American Medical Association* 274, no. 10 (13 September 1995): 820-25.

40. The literature on assisted suicide and euthanasia is extensive. Some of the best works (both pro and con) include James Rachels, *The End of Life* (New York: Oxford University Press, 1986); M. Scott Peck, *Denial of the Soul: Spiritual and Medical Perspectives on Euthanasia and Mortality* (New York: Harmony Books, 1997); Carlos Gomez, *Regulating Death: Euthanasia and the Case of the Netherlands* (New York: Free Press, 1991); Robert N. Wennberg, *Terminal Choices: Euthanasia, Suicide, and the Right to Die* (Grand Rapids: Wm. B. Eerdmans Publishing Co., 1989); David C. Thomasma and Glenn C. Graber, *Euthanasia: Toward an Ethical Social Policy* (New York: Continuum, 1990); Bonnie Steinbock and Alastair Norcross, eds., *Killing and Letting Die* (New York: Fordham University Press, 1994). There have been numerous articles and symposia in the bioethics journals such as the *Hastings Center Report*.

case.[41] It overturned two appeals court decisions: a Washington case *(Washington v. Glucksburg)* heard by the Ninth Circuit Court of Appeals, which covers the seven Western states, Alaska, and Hawaii; and a New York case *(Vacco v. Quill)* heard by the Second Circuit Court of Appeals, which covers New York, Connecticut, and New Jersey. Both courts of appeals had affirmed a constitutional right to physician-assisted suicide.[42]

The Court ruled that there is a significant difference between refusing life support and assisted suicide. The justices said, "we think the distinction between assisting suicide and withdrawing life-sustaining treatment, a distinction widely recognized and endorsed in the medical profession and in our legal tradition, is both important and logical; it is certainly rational." They pointed out that there is a different cause of death, and that the intent is different, and recounted physician testimony that "patients who refuse life-sustaining treatment may not harbor a specific intent to die, and may instead fervently wish to live but to do so free of unwanted medical technology, surgery or drugs."

They reminded us that the legal precedent in cases concerning life-sustaining treatment, such as the 1990 case of Nancy Cruzan, established that a competent patient has the right to refuse unwanted medical treatment, grounded in the right of bodily integrity and freedom from unwanted touch-

41. The concept of the right to die has been the subject of much discussion. See, in particular, Yale Kamisar, "Are Laws against Assisted Suicide Unconstitutional?" *Hastings Center Report* 23 (May-June 1993): 32-41; Leon R. Kass, "Is There a Right to Die?" *Hastings Center Report* 23 (January-February 1993): 34-43.

42. The Ninth Circuit Court of Appeals stated it this way in its decision: "Today we are required to decide whether a person who is terminally ill has a constitutionally protected liberty interest in hastening what might otherwise be a protracted, undignified and extremely painful death. If such an interest exists, we must next decide whether or not the state of Washington may constitutionally restrict its exercise by banning a form of medical assistance that is frequently requested by terminally ill people who wish to die. *We first conclude that there is a constitutionally protected liberty interest in determining the time and manner of one's own death*, an interest that must be weighed against the state's legitimate and countervailing interests, especially those that relate to the preservation of human life. After balancing the competing interests, we conclude by answering the narrow question before us: We hold that *insofar as the Washington statute prohibits physicians from prescribing life-ending medication for use by terminally ill, competent adults who wish to hasten their own deaths, it violates the Due Process Clause of the Fourteenth Amendment.*"

The court based its decision on arguments from personal autonomy, the logical extension of the *Cruzan* decision, that there is no significant difference between refusing treatment and requesting assistance in suicide, there is no threat to the integrity of the medical profession, there is no reason to believe that abuses would occur, and that concern about preventing suicide is not an issue with the terminally ill. They are in a different category altogether.

ing.[43] But that is not the same thing as a right to assisted suicide. The Court held that denying assisted suicide does not treat classes of the seriously ill differently. The law grants the right to refuse unwanted treatment to everyone, and the right of assistance in suicide to no one.

The Court further ruled that the rights of personal autonomy do not extend to the right to assistance in suicide. The *Cruzan* case was based on the right to refuse unwanted medical treatment, rooted in the right of bodily integrity. The Court ruled that "(in Cruzan) we certainly gave no intimation that the right to refuse unwanted medical treatment could be somehow transmuted into a right to assistance in committing suicide."

The Court also rejected the parallel with the Casey abortion decision in 1992.[44] The petitioners in that case argued that the precedent for liberty in the Constitution and other Supreme Court rulings, especially on abortion, made it clear that the right to die should also be protected. The Court rejected that parallel, saying the fact that "many of the rights and liberties protected by the Due Process Clause sound in personal autonomy does not warrant the sweeping conclusion that any and all important, intimate and personal decisions are so protected."

The Court recognized that there are legitimate state interests in prohibiting assistance in suicide. It recognized that states have valid concerns about legalizing assisted suicide. Some of the valid state interests include:

a. *Preservation of human life.*
b. *Prevention of suicide,* especially among vulnerable groups such as the poor, the disabled, and the elderly.
c. Many people who request assistance in suicide are suffering from *treatable depression and physical pain.* The Court cited "research that indicates that many people who request physician assisted suicide withdraw that request if their depression and pain are treated."[45]
d. Preservation of *the integrity of the medical profession.* Assisted suicide is incompatible with medicine's healing role and could undermine the patient-physician trust relationship.
e. Permitting assisted suicide may lead to *involuntary euthanasia.* "Thus, it turns out that what is couched as a limited right to physician assisted

---

43. *Cruzan v Missouri Department of Health,* 110 S. Ct. 2481 (1990).

44. *Planned Parenthood v Casey,* 112 S. Ct. 2791 (1992).

45. See H. Hendin, *Seduced by Death: Doctors, Patients, and the Dutch Cure* (1997), and New York Task Force on Life and the Law, *When Death Is Sought: Assisted Suicide and Euthanasia in the Medical Context* (1994).

suicide is likely, in effect, a much broader license, which could prove extremely difficult to police and contain."

States are now free to pass their own laws in regard to assisted suicide. Most have laws on the books prohibiting it. These are not unconstitutional. Neither does it appear that laws allowing it would be unconstitutional. The Court's decision did not end the debate. It only allowed it to continue and encouraged it to do so.

In the debate over euthanasia and physician-assisted suicide, one must be careful to distinguish between different types of hastening one's death. Refusal of treatment, once called passive euthanasia, is generally morally acceptable under one of three conditions: if a competent patient requests it, if treatment is futile, and if the burden of the treatment outweighs the benefit. Physician-assisted suicide is when a physician assists the patient in taking his or her own life. In this the patient actually initiates the suicide with the assistance of the physician, usually in the form of prescribing sufficient medication for the patient to take in order to kill himself or herself. But in some cases the patient is too seriously ill to take his or her life. The physician must do it for the patient. This is commonly called active euthanasia. In this the physician introduces an overdose of medication into the patient's IV line, and death occurs usually within twenty minutes to a half hour.

The Case for Assisted Suicide Analyzed

The most common arguments in favor of physician-assisted suicide have been articulated by Dr. Jack Kevorkian, who has kept the issue in the headlines. Other participants include organizations like the Hemlock Society (and its founder Derek Humphry) and Compassion in Dying. Many of these groups articulate similar arguments for the morality of assisted suicide. There is, first, an argument from mercy, that assisting a terminally ill person in suicide is a compassionate thing to do, in some ways parallel to human beings putting animals "out of their misery" by killing them. Some have even suggested that assisted suicide fulfills the Golden Rule, since it is assumed that no one would want to suffer interminably at the end of life.[46]

However, this argument is misdirected and, in effect, is an example of "burning down the barn to roast the pig." It is undoubtedly true that far too many people spend their last dying days in pain. The SUPPORT study is clear

---

46. See Rachels, chap. 2, for further discussion of this point.

proof of this unfortunate reality. But the solution to the problem of pain at the end of life is better pain management, not legalizing assistance in suicide. Physicians have at their disposal today the means to adequately control the pain of virtually every patient who is terminally ill.

Why people still die in pain is a good question, and the reasons include physicians' reluctance to adequately medicate patients in pain due to fear of addiction (though with the terminally ill this seems to be a moot point) and fear of investigation for overprescribing pain medication, and their failure to believe patients when they complain of pain. There is little doubt that poor pain management in hospitals is one of the driving forces behind the euthanasia movement, but the solution should stop far short of legalizing assisted suicide. It should include more timely referrals to hospices, one of the most underutilized health care institutions. Hospices specialize in the art of pain control particularly for the terminally ill. Far too many people die in hospitals, pursuing aggressive care, when they could be spending their last days with their pain under control, their depression (from being terminally ill) being treated, and not subject to expensive and burdensome aggressive medical technology.

A second argument in favor of assisted suicide is from personal autonomy. That is, individuals have the right to make life's most private and personal decisions on their own, apart from government interference. The law recognizes the right of people to make decisions about their beliefs, marriage, procreation, child rearing, and many other areas in the protected zone of privacy. Proponents of assisted suicide argue that surely the time and manner of one's death should be included in these protected and private decisions. Yet autonomy is clearly not an absolute. There are some things that persons cannot do to their own body, such as put illegal drugs into it and engage in prostitution. Traditionally, liberty has been trumped when the exercise of that liberty produces tangible harm to others. One can make a good case that in places where assisted suicide is legal, such as the Netherlands, voluntary euthanasia is giving rise to nonvoluntary euthanasia. People who are being put to death without their consent are clearly being harmed.[47]

A third argument is that there is no morally relevant difference between killing a person and allowing a person to die.[48] Since refusing life-sustaining

---

47. Data on the Dutch practice of euthanasia will be addressed later in the chapter.

48. Philosopher James Rachels makes this point with his well-known analogy of the nephew in the bathtub. Suppose your ten-year-old nephew is the sole heir to a sizable fortune. Should he die, you would inherit the fortune. You walk into the bathroom and, at the precise moment you enter, witness your nephew as he hits his head against the faucet and falls unconscious under the water. You elect to do nothing; that is, you al-

treatment means that someone will allow the patient to die, which is generally acceptable, so too must be assistance in suicide. However, there are some very important differences. The cause of death is different. When treatment is refused, the cause of death is the underlying disease or condition of the patient. But when euthanasia is performed, the cause of death is the direct action of the physician or the patient to end life. In addition, the intent is different. With refusal of treatment, the intent is to let the patient's disease take its natural course and allow the patient to live out his or her last days free from burdensome medical technology. It is true that sometimes when treatment is refused, death does result in a relatively short time period. But the intent is not to end the patient's life in most cases. With euthanasia the intent is always to end the patient's life. Intent does make a moral difference, though it can be difficult to ascertain. But intent has traditionally been an important component of a moral action, and is sometimes the only difference between two otherwise identical acts.[49]

A fourth argument for assisted suicide is that it is consistent with the Hippocratic oath and thus does not undermine the integrity of the medical profession. In fact, in the time of Hippocrates, there was no sophisticated medical technology and little chronic disease like there is today. Generally, when people got sick, they either got well soon or they got worse and died in a relatively short time period. Proponents of assisted suicide argue that had Hippocrates been around today, he would have likely seen the suffering of the terminally ill and might not have said in his oath that physicians should not kill their patients. However, the oath is clear that physicians must not be active agents in the death of their patients. Given the appropriate distinction between killing and allowing to die, what Hippocrates prohibited in the oath is precisely what some physicians want the freedom to perform under the legalization of assisted suicide. Further, given that most pain for the dying patient can be adequately managed, thus making the argument from mercy much less valid, there would seem to be very few occasions in which physicians would have to violate the oath by assisting in suicide in order to best care for their patients.

---

low him to die. Rachels argues that there is no moral difference between that act and holding your nephew's head under the water and drowning him. For more on Rachels's position and a critique, see Rae, pp. 244-47.

49. In the case of a gift and a bribe, the intent is the only difference between two otherwise identical actions.

Assisted Suicide in the Netherlands

For roughly the past two decades, assisted suicide has been loosely legalized in the Netherlands, making it an appropriate venue in which to observe the practice and see how well or how poorly it has worked. Euthanasia is technically still against the law there, but physicians are exempt from prosecution if they follow guidelines prescribed by the Royal Dutch Medical Association,[50] which is responsible for prosecuting physicians who might abuse the freedom to assist patients in suicide. The guidelines are as follows:

1. Assistance in suicide must be entirely voluntary. No coercion of patients to sign a euthanasia consent is acceptable.
2. Euthanasia must be employed as a last resort in order to deal with unacceptable (to the patient) levels of pain and suffering.
3. The request for euthanasia must be well considered and from a stable desire to have euthanasia performed. That is, the request must be well thought out and must have been repeated over a period of time. The patient cannot make the request one day and have euthanasia performed on the next. Further, the request must come from a competent patient who is not overly influenced by pain and things like depression, which often afflict the terminally ill.
4. Euthanasia must be performed in consultation with another health care professional. There are to be no "lone rangers" assisting patients in suicide, working apart from professional consultation and discussion.

For some time it was difficult to ascertain many things about the Dutch practice of euthanasia. For example, even determining the number of cases in which euthanasia was performed was complicated, and estimates varied from 200 to 400, the number of cases actually reported to the Justice Ministry, to 20,000, the estimate of the opponents of euthanasia.[51] One reason for this difficulty is that Dutch physicians would sometimes state the cause of death on the person's death certificate as "respiratory failure" or some other "natural" cause, rather than clearly identifying that euthanasia had been performed. A further difficulty is that at times cases would not be reported at all, thus the disparity between the number of cases reported and the actual occurrences,

---

50. These were drafted by the Dutch Royal Medical Association in 1984 and were approved a year later by a government-appointed commission on euthanasia.

51. In the years 1987-90, there were 122, 181, 336, and 454 cases reported, respectively. Cited in John Keown, "On Regulating Death," *Hastings Center Report* 22 (March-April 1992): 39-43, at 41.

which most agree is far more than the roughly 200 to 400 cases reported annually.

Of more interest to the public and the groups responsible for overseeing euthanasia is the degree to which physicians were following the guidelines for exemption from prosecution. Were they insuring that patients were giving full consent for euthanasia? Were the patients' requests well considered and from a stable desire? Were patients requesting euthanasia as a last resort, only in cases of intractable pain and suffering? And did physicians consult with other health care professionals prior to administering euthanasia? The answers to these questions were important and provided some indication whether or not the Dutch were heading down a "slippery slope."

In the early 1990s the Dutch government published two studies of physicians' practice of euthanasia in order to determine how they were following the guidelines. In 1991 the medical examiner Gerrit van der Waal surveyed general practitioners and found that physicians varied widely in both their interpretation and application of the guidelines. For example, take the guideline that mandates that the request for euthanasia be well considered and from a stable desire. The survey by van der Waal found the time span between the first request for euthanasia and its performance ranged from a day (13 percent of cases) to no more than a week (35 percent of cases) to no more than two weeks (17 percent of cases). For roughly two-thirds of the cases, the time between the first request for euthanasia and its administration was two weeks or less. In approximately two-thirds of the cases the request was oral only, with no written document that the patient had signed with a proper witness.[52]

The survey found similar concerns about the requirement for consultation with another health care professional. More than 25 percent of general practitioners admitted that they had no consultation before performing euthanasia, and more than 12 percent did not have any form of discussion with any other caregivers. The consultation was infrequently put in writing, and when consultation did occur it was done informally and usually by a colleague, not an independent physician. Fewer than half of the general practitioners consulted the patient's nurse about the patient's request for euthanasia. As a result of these findings, van der Waal concluded, "a substantial proportion of general practitioners is not (yet)

---

52. G. van der Waal et al., "Euthanasie en heup bij zelf doding" (Euthanasia and medically assisted suicide), *Medisch Contact* 46, no. 7 (1991): 212-14. This is cited in Keown, "On Regulating Death," p. 43.

operating in accordance with current procedural precautional require-ments."[53]

The most extensive data has been correlated by the government-appointed Remmelink Committee, which issued its findings in 1990 and up-dated them in 1995.[54] Physicians who participated were guaranteed immu-nity from prosecution for whatever they revealed. The committee reported that, in 1990, physicians administered euthanasia without the consent of the patient in roughly 1,000 cases, about 20 percent of the estimated total deaths from euthanasia.[55] Physicians further revealed that in 8,750 cases in which they intended to hasten death by withdrawing treatment and in a further 5,000 cases in which they intended to hasten death by administering opioids (pain medication), the patient had not requested such hastening of death. British law professor John Keown summarizes the data this way: "In short, doctors stated that in 1990 they sought to accelerate death in some 20,000 cases, in almost three-quarters of which there had been no request by the pa-tient."[56] Based on this data, Keown points out that even some of the support-ers of euthanasia admit that there is a lack of control on the administration of euthanasia and that, in the current context there, adequate control of the practice may be very difficult if not impossible.[57] The reason for this is the private nature of the discussions between the patient, his or her physician, and the patient's family members and loved ones. Without intolerable inva-sions of privacy, there is virtually no way of knowing whether or not a termi-nally ill patient has been coerced into requesting euthanasia, either by loved ones or the physician. Enforcing the guideline that euthanasia must be fully voluntary and consensual would seem to be almost impossible.[58]

The 1995 data from the Remmelink Committee has been variously in-

---

53. G. van der Waal, "Toetsing in geval van euthanasie of hulp bij zelfdoding" (De-termining cases of euthanasia or assisted suicide), *Medisch Contact* 46, no. 8 (1991): 239-41, cited in Keown, "On Regulating Death," p. 43.

54. P. J. van der Maas, J. J. M. Van Delden, and L. Pijnonborg, *Euthanasia and Other Medical Decisions concerning the End of Life* (New York: Elsevier Science Inc., 1992). Also published in the journal *Lancet* 338 (1991): 669-74.

55. Herbert Hendin, Chris Rutenfrans, and Zbigniew Zylicz, "Physician Assisted Suicide and Euthanasia in the Netherlands: Lessons from the Dutch," *Journal of the Ameri-can Medical Association* 277, no. 21 (4 June 1997): 1720-22, at 1720.

56. Keown, "On Regulating Death," p. 42. See also the work of Keown in "The Law and Practice of Euthanasia in the Netherlands," *Law Quarterly Review* (January 1992), and Gomez, *Regulating Death*.

57. Keown, "On Regulating Death," p. 42.

58. Daniel Callahan, "Self Determination Run Amok," *Hastings Center Report* 22 (March/April 1992).

terpreted as either an encouraging sign that euthanasia can be successfully administered or as a danger sign that voluntary euthanasia is leading to nonvoluntary euthanasia.[59] The new data can be encouraging when one looks at the category of "ending life without request," which declined slightly from 1990 but still constitutes roughly 15 percent, down from approximately 20 percent reported in 1990.[60] However, when the figures include the category of death resulting from administration of opioids, or pain medication, and when they are examined using an estimate from the researchers that roughly 80 percent of deaths in these categories occurred without the patients' explicit consent, then the results are more alarming.[61] There has actually been an increase in the incidence of euthanasia without consent since 1990, though as a percentage of total deaths from euthanasia it has declined slightly.[62] Though the 1995 figures indicate a decrease in the percentage of deaths without consent, it is still an alarming figure (38 percent, down from 44 percent) and hardly a model for effective oversight.

The risks of legalizing assisted suicide and euthanasia are significant, particularly for those at the margins of life such as the poor, the elderly, and the disabled. With the resources available for effective pain management and

---

59 For the interpretation that suggested that euthanasia is being adequately regulated, see Paul J. van der Maas et al., "Euthanasia, Physician-Assisted Suicide and Other Medical Practices Involving the End of Life in the Netherlands, 1990-1995," *New England Journal of Medicine* 335, no. 22 (28 November 1996): 1699-1705; Gerrit van der Waal et al., "Evaluation of the Notification Procedure for Physician Assisted Death in the Netherlands," *New England Journal of Medicine* 335, no. 22 (28 November 1996): 1706-11; Marcia Angell, "Euthanasia in the Netherlands: Good News or Bad?" *New England Journal of Medicine* 335, no. 22 (28 November 1996): 1676-78. For a different interpretation see Hendin, Rutenfrans, and Zylicz, "Physician Assisted Suicide and Euthanasia in the Netherlands."

60. In 1990 the committee reported 1,030 deaths from euthanasia without consent. This constitutes less than 1 percent of the total deaths in the Netherlands, but roughly 20 percent of all deaths by euthanasia. The committee estimated that there are close to 5,000 deaths from euthanasia annually. In 1995 those figures had been reduced to 948 deaths without consent, out of an approximate estimate of 6,300 deaths from euthanasia. See Hendin, Rutenfrans, and Zylicz, p. 1720, for a table summarizing these figures.

61. However, there is a medically and morally fine line between hastening death as a side effect of proper use of pain medication and active euthanasia with the intent to kill with opioids. The former may be morally justifiable under the notion of double effect.

62. Assuming the 80 percent estimate of the Dutch researchers, the number of cases of euthanasia without consent increases in the 1990 figures to 2,110 out of an estimate of 4,813 total deaths from euthanasia, or close to 44 percent. In the 1995 figures, it increased to 2,464 deaths without consent, out of an estimated 6,368 total deaths from euthanasia, or 38 percent. This is calculated using the data from the summary table in Hendin, Rutenfrans, and Zylicz, p. 1720.

with hospices underutilized, physician-assisted suicide and euthanasia are draconian responses to a very real problem of people dying in unacceptable circumstances. The Christian call to care for the dying is aptly illustrated by the following narrative of a "good death."[63]

> As I sit writing this, my father-in-law is 3 feet away, lying in a bed in a coma, in his last hours of life. He is 81 years old, and has widespread cancer. He is now passing on right in front of my eyes. His spirit and self are in the process of leaving the house that is his earthly body, soon to inherit a heavenly body unencumbered by poor lungs, oxygen tubes, morphine frop pump, and Foley catheter. I am honored to be part of his passing and delivery into eternal life. Rarely do family members get to experience death with their loved ones these days. Many are afraid; many cannot let go; many do not know they can, or how rich and good and deep an experience it can be. The example of my father in law is in peaceful contrast to the tyranny of life's urgencies. His death in our house, while not acknowledged beyond a small circle, was a celebration of relationship. He was aided by a few friends, family members, medical professionals, and Hospice personnel. With pain, struggle, and success, it all fit together. When the hour of his death came, we were rewarded rather than shattered.
>
> Jacob's ladder seemed to descend from the Heavens as the veil between the material and spiritual worlds parted in our presence. We were in a holy place and we all knew it. My father in law's eyes gradually closed and his breathing slowed to a stop as he "walked home" into eternal life. He was gone from here; the shell of his body clearly no longer housed *him*. We all sobbed gently in sadness, in relief for him and in celebration of his life. One of our close friends looked over at me and through bright sparkling wet eyes and tear-washed cheeks, whispered, "Look what Kevorkian is stealing from people." We had all experienced something more than we could have ever planned for, yet we knew it was not unique. His death, awfully wonderful, was a foreshadowing that all humans could experience. The elements that helped make this death such a deeply fulfilling human experience are available to everyone: faith, forgiveness, family, friends, and the help of professionals, especially hospice. These things didn't take away the real, daily details of pain, fear, loneliness, blocked bowels, sleepless nights, yelling out, bedpans, crying fits, fighting kids, medication, side effects or exhaustion. But they did help make them manageable and meaningful, and they have the potential to make death a blessing rather than a curse. We had all experienced the blessing. This is the way it was meant to be.

63. This is an excerpt from D. Andrew Macfarlan, M.D., "The Death of Roy Kuhn," *The Journal of Family Practice* 39, no. 1 (July 1994): 81-82. Used with permission.

CHAPTER 8

Distributive Justice and Health Care Delivery

Introduction

Dr. A. is finding that the way he practices medicine has changed dramatically in the past few years. When he started his private practice years ago after finishing his residency, he was a sole practitioner with a loyal group of patients with whom he anticipated a lifetime of caring for their medical needs. He had time to talk with them in his office, and they paid for his expertise and procedures either personally or through their insurance company. The insurance company rarely questioned whether or not a particular test or procedure was necessary. It paid what he indicated was the cost for the care. When patients had to be hospitalized, he treated them in the hospital and provided all the follow-up care for them in his office. He felt well qualified to provide medical care for his patients and their families because he knew them well and had built a relationship of trust with them. In fact, he considered his patients more than paying customers for his services. He knew he was responsible for their long-term health, as much as was in his power, and considered his relationship to them a covenant to care for them. Over the years his practice grew and he gradually took on other physicians to help him share the load. He treasured his close connections to his patients. He encouraged the other physicians who practiced with him to adopt a similar approach to medicine, and since he hired some of his associates right out of their residencies, he was able to successfully pass on these values to them. He wanted to be a role model for younger physicians about how to practice medicine correctly. As a Christian, he considered this the Christian way to practice medicine as well.

But today he realizes that he is being nostalgic for a form of medical practice that no longer exists, or at least is much more difficult. Today he is part of an enormous multidisciplinary group of physicians. He can count on one hand the number of colleagues who are in sole practice. He has contracts with numerous health maintenance organizations (HMOs) and operates under a dizzying array of payment schedules that include deep discounts on his services that he is forced to accept as payment in full in order to qualify as a preferred provider.

Other contracts include what is known as capitation, or accepting a fixed payment each month to cover all the medical needs of the patient. If the patient does not need any care that month, the practice keeps the payment, but if the patient's needs exceed the capitation amount, the practice must pay the difference. He now has far more patients than he can adequately care for, yet his income has decreased by roughly 30 percent in the past few years. If he were a specialist, he would have taken a greater decrease in pay. He finds it ironic that the pay of his colleagues is also dropping, yet he reads in the paper about the bonuses given out to the executives of the area's most profitable HMOs. To even speak of profitable HMOs is puzzling to him, since for most of his career, hospitals and health care organizations have been nonprofit organizations.

He finds that he has little time for important conversation with his patients, since he must see so many per day to meet the demands of the HMOs for whom he works. In fact, some HMOs have guidelines as to how much time he can spend with certain classes of patients. The average time allotted for a routine office visit is now roughly five minutes. For some of his patients he is only the office physician, and another physician cares for them when they are hospitalized, disrupting the patient-physician relationship. He feels like he is practicing assembly line medicine, and he longs for the days when his practice was not so frenetic in its pace. In years past he could order tests, hospitalize patients, and perform procedures as he saw fit, with only the patient's best interests to guide him. Today he finds that patients cannot get access to some kinds of tests and prescription drugs. He finds that he must get preapproval from the HMO or insurance company to hospitalize certain patients or run certain tests, and he wonders at times if the corporate administrators are really the ones practicing medicine.

He finds that he does have quite a bit of power since he is the "gatekeeper," or the general practitioner who must be seen prior to the patient going to a specialist. He often makes the call as to whether or not a patient can see a specialist. He feels like the HMO, not to mention the hospital's case managers and utilization review office, is looking over his shoulder as he practices, and is not sure that he wants to continue practicing medicine in this way. He is discouraged to read that the Medicare program, the funding source for many of his older patients, is increasingly turning to the managed care model for those patients covered by Medicare. He wonders what Hippocrates would think if he saw the way physicians practiced medicine today.

The Changing Health Care Delivery System

The way health care is delivered has changed dramatically in the past decade. The rise of managed care medicine has virtually replaced the traditional fee-for-service medicine. HMOs and large insurance companies control the financing of health care and, with the federal and state governments, fund almost all health care today. Many of these private health care organizations are for-profit, and the market share of not-for-profit health care organizations has been steadily diminishing. Some fear that medicine might become entirely for-profit in the next decade. Physicians are faced with new conflicts of interest under managed care, chiefly those incentives which encourage them to limit costs and "unnecessary" care. In 1993 President Clinton proposed a wide-ranging set of changes in the health care delivery system, for which the public was not ready. But his initiative kept the issue before the public and underscored how important the issue was. Most agree that the costs of health care must be controlled, but there are numerous debates about the best way to accomplish that.

Three primary factors contributed to the changes in health care delivery, particularly the rise of managed care medicine in the United States. First, the American skepticism of a government-run, central-payer health care system, as exists in Canada and much of Europe, has put the burden for health care reform on the back of the private sector, thus opening the door to market solutions to the current health care crisis. The second factor is the spiraling costs of health care, due in part to the overuse and overavailability of expensive technology, which has increased longevity in increasingly poor quality-of-life circumstances, and in another part to the growing number of Medicare and Medicaid patients, a problem which will become more acute in the next twenty-five years as the baby boomer generation hits retirement age. Third, as a result of spiraling costs, a growing number of persons are without any health care access or coverage. Premiums became out of reach for many people, and the managed care industry filled a market niche profitably.[1]

The changes in health care delivery in the past few years have created a new vocabulary for health care. *Managed care* stands in contrast to traditional *fee-for-service* medicine, in which medical care was treated like any other service or commodity. One paid the physician/provider and received the care one needed. The provider was rewarded for overtreating patients. As insurance assumed the role of payer to the physicians and hospitals, the patient became more removed from direct responsibility for paying for his or her health costs, paying a premium to the insurance company instead. This arrangement, coupled with the increase in more expensive technology, has contributed significantly to the spiraling increase in health care costs. Managed care organizations offer essentially two different types of services, a *PPO* arrangement, which is a discounted fee for service, and an *HMO*, in which you pay a premium each month for a specific array of medical services. Most HMO arrangements depend on what is called *capitation*, in which a physician or physician group is paid a flat fee each month to cover the costs of treating a group of patients. Some, such as Kaiser, directly employ physicians rather than contract with them, paying them a salary instead of through capitation. With capitation there is financial incentive to undertreat patients.

The debate over health care delivery has focused on both the specific physician practice and the broader questions of what type of delivery system is best. Three primary delivery systems are at the forefront of the debate. For some, the pure market system is the best because the market most efficiently distributes all goods and services. Medicine is simply another commodity that should be distributed through the market. The rise of managed care medicine is an example of the market generating creative solutions to distribution problems. There is little doubt that managed care has delivered on its central promise, to control health care costs, but many wonder if the price for such cost containment has been the quality of medical care.

The notion of health care as a commodity is somewhat problematic since health care is quite unlike most other commodities or services. For example, there is an enormous disparity in the level of knowledge about the product between the consumer and the provider. One cannot acquire the expertise to intelligently shop around, since that would require attending medi-

1. For a discussion and ethical analysis of these and other changes in health care, see John F. Kilner et al., eds., *The Changing Face of Health Care: A Christian Appraisal of Managed Care, Resource Allocation, and Patient-Caregiver Relationships* (Grand Rapids: Wm. B. Eerdmans Publishing Co., 1998); and Kenman L. Wong, *Patients and Profits: An Ethic for Managed Care* (Notre Dame, Ind.: University of Notre Dame Press, 1999).

cal school. In addition, that expertise is precisely what the patient is paying the physician for. Therefore it is very difficult for the patient to be a truly informed consumer given his or her relative ignorance of medicine. A further problem with the notion of health care as a commodity is that when people need the product, they are very vulnerable because they need the physician's services at that time. When people become ill, they do not have the luxury of shopping around for the best price for the procedure or medical services which they urgently need.

At the other end of the spectrum is what is known as a single-payer system. Some refer to this as socialized medicine. This is the system which exists in Canada and much of western Europe, though some of those countries are moving toward more of a market system. In this system all physicians are employed by the government. The people pay into the system in the form of either premiums and/or taxes, and their health care needs are provided for. This system guarantees universal coverage for all citizens, but has been widely criticized for its inefficiency, long waiting periods for many treatments, and debatable quality of care, especially when it comes to specialist care.

In many single-payer systems people who have the money to pay for health care on their own and who want better quality or fewer delays in obtaining care usually end up going outside the system into the market. The American system is characterized by a two-tiered system such as this. There is a single payer for people who cannot afford to pay for medical care or insurance premiums. The government pays for the care of the uninsured, mainly the poor, through Medicaid, and for the elderly through Medicare. Public health facilities such as county hospitals and clinics provide the care for the poor, and Medicare routinely pays for quality care at the country's best hospitals. But people who want more control over their care and better quality can obtain it through the market, which constitutes the majority of health care in the United States. This is done either through private payment or some sort of insurance/HMO arrangement, the latter being known as a third-party payer arrangement. This system seems to assume that a minimum level of health care is a right that society should provide for all who cannot afford it. But above the minimum level, health care is seen as a commodity, to be purchased through market means. This is a third alternative between the market and single-payer systems.

The Relationship between Business and Medicine

The rise of managed care medicine, particularly with for-profit managed care organizations (MCOs), has raised a growing concern about the blend of business and medicine. There is widespread public skepticism about the ability of MCOs to choose the health interests of their customers when those interests conflict with the interests of their shareholders in maximizing their return on investment. Indeed, numerous bits of anecdotal evidence are now available that have not been encouraging and have added to the public skepticism about this new intersection of business and medicine. In a growing number of disturbing stories, patients either have been denied care or given substandard care apparently for cost reasons, and have suffered or even died as a consequence.[2] There is further a growing call for an ethic that can effectively govern the managed care industry.

It is widely assumed in this discussion that there are two different sets of ethical standards that are in fundamental conflict. The traditional medical ethic emphasizes patient well-being and the physician's obligation to the patient. This stands in apparent conflict with the way business ethics is largely perceived, with its emphasis on profit maximization. Many assume that these cannot be brought together and that managed care is an attempt, largely succeeding, to subvert the traditional medical ethic with a business ethic that is only concerned with the bottom line. Numerous observers have stated that, at some level, obligations to the bottom line will directly conflict with duties to serve the needs of patients.[3] A representation of this assumed conflict between medical and business ethics can be seen in the proceedings of a symposium on managed care that appeared in 1995 in the well-respected *Journal of Law, Medicine and Ethics*. Wendy K. Mariner puts it like this:

> The ethical principles that promote free and fair competition are quite different from the ethical principles that preserve the integrity of the physician-patient relationship and specifically those that protect patient welfare, and these principles can lead to quite different outcomes. MCO's were created to achieve economic objectives that may be fundamentally incompatible with traditional principles of medical ethics. Even if it is possible to agree that certain principles ought to apply to managed care, the market may make it impossible to live fully by those principles.

2. See, for example, David R. Olmos, "Cutting Health Costs — or Corners?" *Los Angeles Times,* 5 May 1995, pp. A1, 22-23.

3. See Arnold Relman, "What Market Values Are Doing to Medicine," *Atlantic Monthly,* March 1992, p. 106; Bettijane Levine, "He Might Have the Cure for All Ills" (interview with AMA president Lonnie Bristow), *Los Angeles Times,* 18 July 1995, p. E1; and Cardinal Joseph Bernardin, "The Case for Non-Profit Health Care" (speech delivered at the Harvard Business School Club of Chicago, 12 January 1995). Relman makes the pointed statement that "Medical care is in many ways uniquely unsuited to private enterprise. It cannot meet its responsibilities to society if it is dominated by business interests."

She further argues that in the normal course of business, MCOs can act as "ordinary business organizations with no moral obligations, or, at least, obligations that have little to do with traditional medical ethics."[4] She adds that when "an MCO's financial goals conflict with its service methods, little in the field of business ethics argues for giving subscribers priority."[5] Or, as William Healey, M.D., put it, more bluntly and in biblical imagery, in the journal *Business Ethics*, "No doctor can serve two masters — patients and HMO's."[6] Many people in health care believe that asking a business ethic and medical ethic to co-exist together is like putting Albert Schweitzer and Ivan Boesky together at the top of the same organization.[7]

Much of the objection to the participation of shareholder-owned business organizations in managed care stems from concerns over the ethical challenges raised by the profit motive. Simply put, it is believed that there will be inevitable and irreconcilable conflicts in mixing business with medicine because the traditional "good" for medicine, dating back to the Hippocratic oath, has been the health of the patient, while the "good" for business has been and continues to be profit.[8]

We want to first call into question the assumption underlying this dichotomy between business and medicine, that medicine is patient centered and business is profit centered. For most of this century health care has been big business. To say that only now there are conflicts of interest for physicians and hospitals is naive and ignorant of medical history. For example, there are now, and have been for some time, financial incentives for physician referrals in addition to physician investment/ownership in treatment and diagnostic facilities to which physicians refer patients. These are conflicts of interest that could undermine the fiduciary duty of physicians to their patients and would not have been acceptable in business settings where there are fiduciary relationships. They are not new and do not come from the current mixture of medicine and business. There is a significant correlation between the posi-

4. Wendy Mariner, "Business Ethics vs. Medical Ethics: Conflicting Standards for Managed Care," *Journal of Law, Medicine and Ethics* 23 (1995): 236-46, at 236.

5. Mariner, p. 238.

6. William V. Healey, M.D., "The Ethics of Managed Care," *Business Ethics* (November/December 1994): 8-9, at 8.

7. This dichotomy was coined by Andrew C. Wicks in "Albert Schweitzer or Ivan Boesky? Why We Should Reject the Dichotomy between Business and Medicine," *Journal of Business Ethics* 14 (1995): 339-51, at 339.

8. We are indebted to William W. May for stating this in such a poignant and insightful fashion. See William W. May, "Managed Care: Insurers, Values, and the Bottom Line on Care" (paper presented at the American Academy of Religion panel, New Orleans, 25 November 1996).

tions of the AMA on health care reform, managed care, Medicare, and Medicaid, and the financial interests of the physician members. The patient-centered model surely overestimates the charitable and altruistic nature of the health care professions.[9] We say this not to cast aspersions on the integrity of the profession — we are around numerous physicians who are exemplary in their commitment to their patients, at times to the detriment of their self-interest — but clearly, in a fee-for-service arrangement, physicians' financial incentives work to lead them to overtest and overtreat (to be sure, the litigious environment contributes a great deal to this also). As the CEO of a hospital with which one of us consults put it, in response to the incomes of HMO executives, "doctors and hospitals have had their day at the trough too." He was highlighting the fact that financial self-interest has always been a motivating factor in provider behavior.

The typical *response* to this is to somewhat grudgingly acknowledge the business element of medicine but to argue strenuously that overtreatment (from fee-for-service incentives) is far better for patients than undertreatment (from managed care incentives). In fact, most patients would rather be overtreated and overtested than undertreated and undertested. However, the rejoinder to this response is twofold: *First,* overtreatment is not always benign, but can be harmful. Iatrogenic harm is well documented in the medical literature, and it is clear that unnecessary surgery, X rays, and other types of invasive procedures can produce harm to patients. For example, it is widely accepted now that many cesarean sections have been performed unnecessarily, and though most of the women recover, they have been placed at increased risk.[10] *Second,* the response incorrectly assumes that the only harm that counts is harm that comes to individual patients. Even if no patient were ever harmed from overtreatment, harm still occurs. It occurs when the costs of care rise to a point where millions are cut off from access to the health care system, and when indemnity insurance premiums go out of the reach of the average working person. In a world of scarce medical resources, the costs of overtreatment incur to society and to other sick persons who need care and cannot get it. Harm may have occurred on a broader scale, but it is harm nonetheless.

Not only has there always been a marriage between business and medicine, but scarcity of resources is increasingly forcing a closer relationship that is changing the way bioethics is done. In a managed care context, in which capitation is the payment mechanism for physicians, they must balance their

9. Wicks, pp. 341-42.
10. George J. Annas, "Protecting the Liberty of Pregnant Women," *New England Journal of Medicine* 316, no. 19 (1988): 1213-14.

commitment to their individual patients with their responsibility, under the terms of the managed care contract, to the entire population of lives to whom they have been entrusted.[11] In other words, physicians cannot simply look out for the isolated interests in the individual patient. They are also stewards of the resources that are earmarked for care of their entire population. This is an enormous paradigm shift for physicians and puts them in very difficult positions. The conventional wisdom on conflicts of interest in managed care is that the physician's self-interest is pitted against the patient's best medical interest, and in some cases that is true. But the more difficult balancing act is between the patient's best interests and the interests of the entire patient population for which the physician is responsible. It is an ethic of stewardship, not autonomy. Bioethics is just beginning to give helpful guidance to physicians on how to properly balance these conflicts.[12]

Not only can we critique the "medical ethic" in this dichotomy, but we can also critique the "business ethic" as represented by those who are concerned about the business ethic dominating the medical ethic. To suggest that a business ethic is only concerned with profit maximization is to misunderstand what business ethics is about (we suspect that those who fear the encroachment of business into medicine are also assuming that there is a dichotomy between business and ethics). However, we admit that the conduct of some HMOs around the country does reinforce the notion that all they are interested in is profit, and at any price. But we would argue that a business ethic of profit maximization as the sole goal of business is an oxymoron, and that some HMOs have been acting unethically in their pursuit of profit.

It is a standard maxim in most business schools in the United States that the sole goal of a corporation is to maximize shareholder wealth. The classic statement of this is from Milton Friedman, who holds that corporations exercise all the social responsibility they need to simply by making a profit. In doing so they provide the public with a useful product or service and provide jobs for people in the community. He further argues that for corporations to act in socially responsible ways that do not contribute to their profit is actually stealing from shareholders.[13] Friedman's paradigm has been

---

11. We prefer the term "entrusted lives" to the customary term "covered lives."

12. For some general guidelines see Susan Wolf, "Health Care Reform and the Future of Physician Ethics," *Hastings Center Report* (March-April 1994): 28-41.

13. Milton Friedman, "The Social Responsibility of Business Is to Increase Its Profits," *New York Times Magazine,* 13 September 1970, pp. 33, 122-26. This article has been reprinted in numerous anthologies on business ethics. See, for example, Scott B. Rae and Kenman L. Wong, *Beyond Integrity: A Judeo-Christian Approach to Business Ethics* (Grand Rapids: Zondervan, 1996), pp. 241-45.

challenged by stakeholder theory, which suggests that the interests of stake-holders, such as employees, the community, the environment, etc., should be taken into account along with those of shareholders in the decisions a company makes.[14] Others favor a conception in which moral duties are "nonfiduciary" in nature, but are also significant and are owed to other stake-holders, thus preserving the special status of shareholders.[15] We would argue that most investors would not consider it theft for the firms in which they invest to be socially responsible, even at the expense of profit. For example, most mission statements contain elements like excellence in the service/product, service to the community, and a fair rate of return for the company's investors. No mission statement of which we are aware promises investors that the company will do everything within the law in order to maximize their return. Of course, the degree to which a mission statement is actually followed varies widely, but it is the one piece of information available to the investing public that informs them of the philosophy of the company into which they are investing. In addition, a growing body of empirical evidence suggests that investors would be willing to take less return in exchange for the company acting in a socially responsible way. The work of Georgetown finance professor Pietra Rivoli suggests that investors who consider social and ethical concerns and act on those concerns constitute a significant portion of equity investment in the United States. As she puts it, "wealth maximization is a constrained objective, and the constraints are social and ethical values."[16]

Real-life examples of corporate self-restraint are not difficult to find. The well-publicized actions of then seventy-three-year-old Aaron Feuerstein are a good case in point. Citing his commitment to the community, Feuerstein rebuilt his burned-down manufacturing plant that was a vital economic lifeline to the town of Muthen, Massachusetts, despite the fact that he could have simply retired on the insurance money. Other corporations which are shareholder owned, such as Merck, Starbucks, Johnson and Johnson, and many others, function according to a stakeholder model that views their social commitments as being perfectly consistent with their financial success.[17]

A good example of this kind of socially responsible mixture of business and medicine is the pharmaceutical giant Merck. A scientist at Merck

14. Kenneth Goodpaster, "Business Ethics and Stakeholder Analysis," *Business Ethics Quarterly* 1, no. 1 (January 1991): 53-73.

15. Goodpaster, p. 69.

16. Pietra Rivoli, "Ethical Aspects of Investor Behavior," *Journal of Business Ethics* 14 (1995): 265-77.

17. Wicks, p. 346.

discovered that a drug the company was selling to fight parasites in farm animals could be adapted to cure the Third World disease of river blindness. It too came from a parasite that, upon entering the body, grew to up to two feet in length and caused such suffering that victims frequently opted for suicide instead of enduring the agony. It eventually reached the eyes, causing blindness. The drug becoming available was great news to the victims, but the problem for Merck was that none of its potential "customers" could afford to pay for the drug. Merck was faced with a difficult decision, whether or not to invest the money necessary to develop the drug with no anticipation of any return on its investment. Merck had hoped to raise funding from a variety of public and private sources, but to date the company has not been successful in so doing. It essentially faced the decision of whether or not to give the drug away. It would cost the company roughly $20 million annually to produce and deliver the drug, which it decided to do, forever. The reason was not necessarily because the firm was doing charity, though it was. This was *mission driven*. Merck's corporate philosophy puts it this way: "We try never to forget that medicine is for the people. It is not for the profits. The profits follow, and if we have remembered that, they have never failed to appear. The better we have remembered it, the larger they have been."[18] The company's mission was not profit maximization at all costs; it was service for which the company could expect a reasonable return on investment.

This is precisely the spirit of the moral philosopher and ideological founder of free-market capitalism, Adam Smith.[19] Smith considered business a profession in which service to the community through one's product/service was the mission, and profit was an anticipated by-product of excellence in that service. The service, not the profit, was the end. The bottom line was not the bottom line. His legacy for modern capitalism is not the one widely attributed to him, that the sole goal of a corporation is to maximize shareholder wealth. In addition, for Smith, enlightened self-interest was the engine of capitalism. He never suggested, in the words of mergers and acquisitions specialist Gordon Gekko in the film *Wall Street*, that "greed is good." He distinguished between greed and self-interest, as does the Bible (Phil. 2:4, "look out not only for your own interests, but also for

18. The Merck case is cited in Wicks, p. 345.

19. For further discussion on the contribution of Smith to business ethics, see Patricia Werhane, *Adam Smith and His Legacy for Modern Capitalism* (New York: Oxford University Press, 1991). For a specific application of Smith to the business of medicine in managed care, see "The Ethics of Health Care as a Business," *Business and Professional Ethics Journal* 9, nos. 3-4 (fall-winter 1990): 15.

the interests of others"). But more importantly, he assumed that individuals possessed the internal resources necessary to show restraint in their pursuit of self-interest. That is, ethics and self-restraint play critical roles in the proper functioning of the market and everyday market transactions. He was very sensitive to this, out of his profession as a moral philosopher, and he assumed that the Judeo-Christian moral consensus that existed in his time would function as the source of this restraint. Of course, that consensus is not what it used to be. But restraint of self-interest is still necessary for a properly functioning economic system. As Catholic theologian Michael Novak argues, "A firm committed to greed unleashes social forces that will sooner or later destroy it. Spasms of greed will corrupt its executives, anger its patrons, injure the morale of its workers, antagonize its suppliers and purchasers, embolden its competitors and attract public retribution."[20] There is such a thing as virtuous self-interest — that is not an oxymoron. We would suggest that it takes a reservoir of virtues in order for an economic system to properly function. Without values like trustworthiness, keeping of promises (contracts), truth telling, and so on, an economic system would look like the system that now exists in the former Soviet Union.[21] Though it is true that some firms operate on the "greed is good" corporate philosophy, to characterize a "business ethic" as such is both inaccurate descriptively and an internal contradiction. The kind of enlightened business model that Adam Smith proposed provides an alternative to the predominant ethos of business today.[22] This is an improvement over the traditional medical ethic and the profit maximization practice of business. Patients and profits can coexist. They always have.

Distributive Justice and Health Care Delivery

Nearly everyone agrees that health care, however it is delivered, must be deliv-

---

20. Michael Novak, *The Spirit of Democratic Capitalism* (Lanham, Md.: University Press of America, 1991), p. 92.

21. Philip Boyle, "Business Ethics in Ethics Committees?" *Hastings Center Report* (September-October 1990): 37. For a detailed discussion of the trust necessary for an efficient economy, see Francis Fukuyama, *Trust: The Social Virtues and the Creation of Prosperity* (New York: Free Press, 1995).

22. William Evan and R. Edward Freeman, "A Stakeholder Theory of the Modern Corporation: Kantian Capitalism," in *Ethical Theory and Business*, ed. Thomas Beauchamp and Norman Bowie, 4th ed. (Englewood Cliffs, N.J.: Prentice-Hall, 1993), pp. 75-84.

ered fairly, in accordance with commonly held norms of justice. Of course, since we do not live in an ideal world, a rough justice is likely the best for which society can hope, but its ideals should be high nevertheless. Health care delivery debates are actually discussions about what philosophers call distributive justice, or the just distribution of the goods of society, health care being one of the principal goods that society has to offer. The basis on which society distributes its goods is the crux of distributive justice.[23] The criteria on which health care is distributed are the point of debate in the discussion over a just health care delivery system.

In the early 1960s, when dialysis machines were first introduced into health care, the demand overwhelmed the available supply. The administrators of the first dialysis centers faced some difficult distribution questions when they had to decide who got access to the machines and on what basis. This is similar to the issues that arose around the first heart transplants as well as other organ transplants, in which the demand for the available organs was and still is far ahead of the available supply. Other types of health care distributive dilemmas include triage in emergencies when the available medical personnel is limited and the number of casualties is overwhelming. Physicians are making allocation-of-resource decisions more routinely at the bedside, when faced with patients whose families are requesting care that is costly and futile.[24] The way our health care system works involves care being limited or unavailable for those who are uninsured or cannot otherwise pay for it. Because so many people have limited access to health care, and because proper health care is so critical to a person's flourishing in life, the question of the justice of the health care delivery system becomes very important. The way Medicare and Medicaid are distributed is a critical distributive justice question, since those tax dollars are limited and the number of elderly who will be eligible for Medicare is growing substantially as the baby boom generation moves toward retirement. On what basis should those limited resources for health care of the poor and elderly be distributed?

We will explore this issue with an hypothetical scenario. Imagine the di-

23. The literature on distributive justice theory is extensive. For a survey of this material, see Karen Lebacqz, *Six Theories of Justice* (Minneapolis: Augsburg, 1986). For one of the landmark theoretical works in this field, see John Rawls, *A Theory of Justice* (Cambridge: Harvard University Press, 1972).

24. See, for example, the discussion of bedside rationing in E. Haavi Morreim, *Balancing Act: The New Medical Ethics of Medicine's New Economics* (Washington, D.C.: Georgetown University Press, 1995). See also Peter A. Ubel, M.D., and Robert M. Arnold, M.D., "The Unbearable Rightness of Bedside Rationing: Physician Duties in a Climate of Cost Containment," *Archives of Internal Medicine* 155 (25 September 1995): 1837-42.

lemmas faced by the administrator of the first dialysis units made available in the early 1960s. His facility possessed only three machines, and as soon as he made it known that they were available for use, he was overwhelmed with requests. Among the first people who came to him were the following (in no particular order):

1. A sixty-two-year-old company president, with a wife, three grown children, and six grandchildren.
2. A twenty-eight-year-old single woman, employed by a local university as a researcher in biochemistry.
3. A ten-year-old boy in the fourth grade at school.
4. A thirty-four-year-old single mother, with three children, ages eight, five, and two.
5. A forty-one-year-old single man, a priest at a Catholic church in the community.
6. A thirty-six-year-old man, currently unemployed, having recently been released on parole from prison, where he had been doing time for armed robbery.
7. A fifty-five-year-old woman, widowed and working as an administrative assistant for a local company, with three grown children.
8. A fifty-seven-year-old married man with two grown children, who is the governor of the state.

Since the administrator has only three machines, clearly not everyone on the list will be able to begin dialysis immediately. Let's assume that all these people need to begin treatment as soon as possible, so that no one is more medically needy than another. The administrator must make the decision about who gets access to the machines. His board of directors has asked him to think carefully about the criteria he will use for making his decision. The board wants his decision to be the most just and fair decision possible, since it does not want the medical center to be portrayed in the press as being unfair. Who gets the treatment, and on what basis does the administrator make his decision? Welcome to the world of distributive justice.

Think about the different criteria the administrator could use to make this decision. He could base it on *need,* that those who have the greatest need for the treatment have the greatest claim on the resources. That criterion probably won't help in this decision, and though it is a good baseline principle, need alone will not be sufficient to enable one to make many distributive justice decisions, since those with need for the resource will often exceed the available resource. Where it is helpful is in triage situations, in which emergency medical resources are often distributed based on who has the most pressing need for treatment. Triage has to with the division of the wounded into three groups: one with superficial wounds, whose treatment can wait — they have need but it is not urgent; one is comprised of those too injured for any treatment to be helpful — they have less need; and a third group in the middle, the members of which have significant needs which could be helped by immediate treatment. Based on the principle of need, one would justly give the majority of the treatment to the middle group, because their need and potential benefit are maximized. In the dialysis scenario, need could be relevant if the administrator considers one's socioeconomic as well as medical need. That is, which family would be most adversely affected if access to treatment for the patient were denied? Using this criterion, the single mother (person 4) could be considered the most needy, since if she were denied treatment, she would die leaving three children as orphans.

Secondly, the administrator could base his decision on *merit* — those most deserving of the resource would be entitled to it. Of course, how one measures merit is open to debate. Related to merit is the *ability to pay*, which is merit measured in financial terms. The people likely to obtain the treatment on this basis would be the executive (person 1) and the governor (person 8). Only those who can pay for the treatment would merit it.

A further criterion that is related to merit is *social worth*, where a person is considered more deserving of the resource because of his or her worth to society, either demonstrated in the past or potentially in the future. On this basis the researcher (person 2), because of her potential for social contribution; the priest (person 5), because of his past and future contribution to people's lives; and the governor (person 8) would be at the top of the list and would receive first access to the treatment. The difficulty in measuring social worth is considered one of the principal problems with this criterion. A second difficulty is illustrated by the early 1990s case of then governor of Pennsylvania, Robert Casey, who received a dual heart and liver transplant only days after being diagnosed with life-threatening heart and liver disease. It appeared to the public that because of his position as governor, he jumped ahead of many people who had been waiting for some time for a heart and liver. This led many in the public to conclude that social worth criteria were used to justify his access to a new heart and liver. These same people expressed unease that judgments of social worth would be used in this way.

A third criterion for distributing the dialysis machines would be based on *desert*, the opposite of social worth. One's lack of merit for the resource in question would disqualify him or her for access to it. To put it another way, when one's life choices are causally related to one's declining health and need for treatment, this would make access for him or her a lower priority than for others who have not made such poor life choices. One of the clearest examples of this criterion being invoked in health care occurred when baseball Hall of Famer Mickey Mantle received a liver transplant. It was well known that Mantle had abused alcohol for decades — clearly the main reason he needed a new liver. Though he died within a year after receiving a new liver, his case raises the question of whether he deserved a new liver after destroying his own due to alcoholism. The same question comes up when people who smoked for a lifetime end up with severe health problems, requiring expensive treatment that society often pays for in the form of Medicare. Not only are medical considerations relevant to the principle of desert, but, as was the case with social worth, socioeconomic factors are to be considered. No one on the dialysis list should be medically disqualified on the principle of desert, except perhaps the drug-abusing single mother (person 4). But one can raise questions of desert about the man recently released from prison (person 6). The case against him on the basis of desert would be stronger if he were currently in prison, say, for a murder charge. Then one could argue that by virtue of his crime, he has lost the right to flourish in life and thus lost the right to access to lifesaving medicine. Desert as a criterion suffers from the same shortcoming that social worth does, being difficult to measure and to rank, thus making it very difficult to be fair in such an assignment. In addition, though one should reap what one sows, society tends to have great compassion on those who have life-threatening disease, regardless of how they came to be in that position. Many people are uncomfortable with desert as a criterion for the same reasons that social worth makes them uneasy. Both criteria beg an important question of who decides the merit, or demerit, of a person for lifesaving medical treatment.

A further criterion for the dialysis machines that has been used in Europe for health care distribution overall is the criterion of *age*. In some countries in Europe, after age sixty-five, certain expensive treatments such as types of transplants are no longer available under the government-financed health care system. Of course, patients desiring such treatment can obtain it if they have the ability to pay. This criterion has strong intuitive appeal in the dialysis case, since the ten-year-old boy would be at the top of the list (person 3). However, employing that criterion at the other end of the age spectrum is more difficult. The appeal of the age criterion is, of course, that younger people, particularly children, have their lives ahead of them, and thus have more of a claim on the health care resources than people who have already lived full lives. Using this criterion in the dialysis case, the executive (person 1), the governor (person 8), and the administrative assistant (person 7) would be the last to obtain access to the treatment. Of course, the problem with age-based criteria is that they are arbitrary, and if used alone, lead to distribution decisions that are likewise arbitrary.

Though not useful in the dialysis case, a criterion that is used in some areas to distribute public health resources is *type of disease*. That is, the state will allocate health care resources for only certain treatments and not for others. For example, the state of Oregon, in its landmark reform of the state public health system, used a disease-based system to allocate state tax dollars designated for health care. One of the first test cases involved a young boy who needed a liver transplant, a condition that the state had decided it would not pay for because of its high cost and relatively rare occurrence. The state deemed that the money spent on these rare and expensive treatments could be better spent treating more common and less costly conditions. Though the boy was not well qualified medically to receive the transplant, the parents appealed to the community to raise the money needed to pay for it. They failed to raise the money, and the state refused to allocate tax dollars for the treatment. Tragically the boy died of liver failure. This case illustrates the arbitrary nature of such a disease-based criterion, and raises questions about the fairness of such an arbitrary measure.

One final, commonly used criterion for distributive justice is *equality*. That is, equal persons are to be treated equally, and in health care, persons with similar conditions are to receive similar treatment. This is rooted in the principle of fairness and respect for human dignity, ultimately rooted in the image of God. To treat similarly situated persons unequally is the equivalent of immoral discrimination. This criterion has broad intuitive appeal, yet it is difficult to use in bedside rationing decisions. Many of the other criteria were formulated because the equality principle was not sufficient on its own to direct distribution decisions. It can be used in the dialysis case, however. Treating all eight of the potential patients equally would suggest a random approach to deciding who gets access to the machines. To be entirely fair under the equality principle, one would have to draw lots to see who receives first access. Then the random approach would mandate a first-come, first-served approach after the initial distribution. This is the approach in use today in most organ transplant procedures. When one is considered medically qualified to receive the transplant, one is placed on a list and stays there until one gets to the top and the needed organ becomes available. Tragically patients do die before they get to the top of the list, and it is not uncommon for them to become less medically qualified the longer they remain on the list. That is, their condition deteriorates as they wait on the transplant list, making them less suitable candidates for the transplant since it will be more difficult for them to survive the surgery and complete a full recovery.

Distributive Justice in Theological Perspective

The question remains concerning what the Scripture teaches about these criteria for distributing the goods of society, namely, health care. Though the Bible does not give any systematic view of distributive justice, general theological principles can be gleaned from biblical teaching that can be applied to health care distribution. Since Scripture does not address the question directly, there will be some degree of debate over the application of these theological principles. Nevertheless, we will attempt to draw out relevant theological themes and suggest a direction in which Scripture points for distributive justice.

The Old Testament civil law set up the formal parameters for the distribution of society's goods, and thus gives a few more clues toward distributive justice than the New Testament. Of particular interest is how the Old Testament mandates care for the poor, since that involves a sort of redistribution of society's goods from those who have them to those who do not. There is little doubt that there is a high place for the poor throughout the Scripture. God has a special concern for the poor that is captured in the Old Testament and was something for which Jesus became well known in his public ministry. For example, the Psalms speak repeatedly of God's concern to deliver the poor (Pss. 9:18; 34:6; 40:17; 72:12). God commands generosity toward the poor (Deut. 15:7-11) and links caring for the poor with honoring God (Prov. 14:31; Isa. 58:6-7). The prophets continually remind Israel of its covenant obligation to care for the poor and indict it for failure to do so (Amos 4:1; 8:4). Jesus continues this concern in his preaching and personal ministry by upholding the poor and caring for them himself (Luke 4:18; 6:20 ["Blessed are the poor"]; 14:12-14; Matt. 25:37-46). The apostles maintain this emphasis on care for the poor and the soft place in the heart of God for them (James 2:1-13).

The Law mandated that the community care for the poor, including the immigrant, in numerous statutes. For example, the immigrant was not to be oppressed or taken advantage of since the Israelites were once poor immigrants themselves in Egypt (Exod. 23:9; Lev. 19:33). The laws concerning the Jubilee (Lev. 25:8-17), right of redemption of property (Lev. 25:25-43), and gleaning as the privilege of the poor (Lev. 19:9-10; Exod. 23:10; Deut. 24:19-22) all provide for the poor another opportunity to make a living, by taking land from those who had accumulated it (i.e., bought it from them) and redistributing it to those who were in need (by making them sell it back to the person or a close relative), or by collecting food from the harvest of prosperous landowners.[25] The high place for the poor in God's economy suggests that *need* as a criterion for distribution counts for a great deal.

However, *merit* plays an important role in distributive justice as well. It is assumed in both Testaments that if people are able to work to earn their share of society's goods, they are obligated to do so. If they are able and unwilling to work, they do not merit a share of society's goods (I Thess. 5:12-14; II Thess. 3:6-10). The economic system was not to be tilted against those who could and did work for their living. The Law was clear that dishonest gain and taking advantage of the economically vulnerable were offensive to God (Exod. 23:7; Deut. 24:14-15). Poverty is seen as a misfortune at times, and at times the result of a lack of moral character. For example, Proverbs repeatedly links one's diligence with prosperity and laziness with poverty (Prov. 6:6-11; 10:4-5; 24:30-34), suggesting that one's merit or lack of it (desert) is key to the share of society's goods to which one is entitled.

Even the laws set up to care for the poor appear to assume a degree of merit in order to take advantage of such provisions, as opposed to merely a handout. For example, the laws that gave the poor permission to glean in the fields of the prosperous assumed that the poor would take the necessary initiative to go out into the fields where the crop was set aside for them to harvest for themselves. The laws of the Jubilee and redemption did not give property or goods to the poor as a handout, but rather gave them a fresh start to apply themselves in order to earn a living. If they failed to apply themselves and take advantage of this new opportunity, then they were returned to poverty, and the likelihood that relatives would tire of redeeming their property became very high. The place of merit is underscored by the New Testament concept of the poor as those who were in some way unable to work, not those who were able but unwilling to work.[26] The Old Testament wisdom literature suggests that those who were able but not willing to work are the sluggards

---

25. See chapter 6 for a more detailed description of the laws concerning the Jubilee, gleaning, and redemption of property. These laws are not analogous to a forced redistribution of property by the tax system or socialism, since the person giving up property received fair market value for it. He or she was simply forced by law to resell it to the original owner when that owner or a close relative was able to purchase it back.

26. The situation of the poor is a bit more complicated today than in biblical times, suggesting a bit more latitude for the poor today than is taken by some conservatives or libertarians. The poor face structural obstacles to earning a living in many cases. That is, they are willing and able to work but unable to find jobs due to factors in the economic system that are beyond their control.

and the lazy for whom there is little compassion and no deserved share of society's goods (Prov. 24:30-34).

The Scripture seems to suggest a blend of distribution based on *need* for those who cannot provide for themselves and *merit* for those who can. The responsibility for redistribution of resources from those who have to those who do not is in part mandated by the Law in the Old Testament, and in both Testaments it is dependent upon the generosity of the prosperous toward the poor. With the end of the Old Testament era and the corresponding close of the Old Testament theocracy, the poor in the New Testament era were increasingly dependent on the generosity of their fellow believers. The churches took it upon themselves to provide out of their resources for their brothers and sisters in other churches who were less fortunate (Acts 2:44-45; 4:32-35; 11:27-30; II Cor. 8–9), and this pattern continued in much of the Western world until this century, when governments took over the responsibility for caring for the poor from the churches and forcibly redistributed society's goods from the prosperous to the poor.[27]

This blend of need- and merit-based criteria for distribution can also apply to the health care delivery system. Clearly there should be a high place for health care resources delivered on the basis of need. The public health facilities, though overburdened at present, are society's best efforts at meeting this need. In places with a single-payer system, need is balanced by other considerations such as age and disease. Thus people with genuine needs are denied access because the system cannot pay for everyone who has a medical need. Thus there is also a legitimate place for merit, as measured by the ability to pay. In single-payer systems merit comes into play when people choose to spend their own resources and opt out of the system in order to get care more to their specifications. In the American system, ability to pay plays a major role in distributing health care, through private payment and insurance premiums to third-party payers. For those who have genuine need and no ability to pay, our theological principles drawn from Scripture would suggest that society has an obligation to meet this need. For those who have need and the ability to pay, society has no obligation to pay for their health care resources. One direction for reform along this line might be for those over sixty-five who are receiving Medicare and who have considerable resources to pay for their own health care. Society would no longer have the obligation to provide Medicare for them; rather they would be dependent on their own resources or private insurance. The movement in recent years toward the medical savings account (MSA) reflects this notion that

---

27. For a chronicle of this transition, see Marvin Olasky, *The Tragedy of American Compassion* (Washington, D.C.: Regnery, 1992).

those who can pay for their health care resources should assume responsibility for those costs. The question that remains for the health care system is in efforts to reform it: Will reforms be crafted with greater emphasis on need, which would involve expanding the public sector for health care, or on merit, which would involve expanding the private sector through the market and increasingly through managed care medicine?

Ethical Issues in Managed Care Medicine

Managed care formats for medicine are increasingly the instruments of change in the health care delivery system and appear to be a part of the health care landscape for the foreseeable future. More frequently, managed care has forced allocation-of-resources decisions on physicians and hospitals to be made at the bedside, and has dramatically changed the practice of medicine. As our physician in the introduction to the chapter reflected, delivering health care today is quite different from in the past. Managed care has introduced a variety of ethical dilemmas for physicians that they did not face as frequently in years previous. As managed care continues to become more dominant in the health care marketplace, more physicians and hospitals will be faced with these ethical issues.

There is little doubt that managed care medicine has succeeded in one of its primary objectives, that of keeping costs of medical care under tighter control. But the question that critics of managed care frequently raise is, at what cost to the quality of care? To be sure, as the managed care industry matures, it is focusing more attention on quality. Though there are still anecdotal bits of evidence of lack of quality, managed care as a form of delivery is continuing to grow aggressively, and in some major metropolitan areas such as Los Angeles it dominates the health care market.

Some of the most common criticisms of managed care medicine include maternity units having to send newborns and new mothers home too soon, now rectified by federal law; generally inadequate mental health coverage in most plans; physicians being discouraged from using certain uncovered medications that they believe would benefit the patient; pressure from in-house colleagues to ration care, which may compromise the patient's best interest; unacceptable delays in getting patients to see specialists when necessary; plan and insurance administrators actually practicing medicine; insurers forcing prices of reimbursement down below what hospitals realistically treat due to employers' demands for lower premiums; and requirement of a gag rule in some contracts, preventing providers from disclosing to patients some important information.[28] However, these are not the foundational ethical issues created by managed care. At the root of the dilemmas created by managed care are the changes in the patient-physician relationship and the conflicts of interest created by managed care.

The changes in the patient-physician relationship are well documented, and include threats to this relationship such as less time for patient interaction, disruptions in continuity of patient-physician relationships (due to deselection, job changes, employer changing plans, dichotomy between office physicians and hospitalists), and less opportunity to be available to patients when they are making difficult decisions about treatment. Patients who have their health care in an HMO cannot be sure that they will see their physician in the office or when they enter the hospital. Since the relationship between patient and physician is a long-standing part of good medical practice and important for good quality of care, managed care has put pressures on this relationship that create conflicts for physicians. If they spend the time they think is necessary with a particular patient, they may not meet their productivity requirements and it may cost them financially.[29]

A second area of issues in managed care concerns the conflicts of interest it creates. It was noted earlier in this chapter that conflicts of interest for physicians are not new, but they are more acute in today's climate because managed care, in its attempts to contain costs, provides a temptation for physicians to limit care based on financial incentives to the physician. In systems such as capitation, it is not difficult to see how this could be a conflict of interest. Insurers, HMOs, and physician practice groups have tried to insulate physicians and hospitals from direct and immediate conflicts of interest by paying physicians straight salaries, or having the group rather than the individual physician be responsible for the cost of treating a patient. Nonetheless, this is a potential conflict of interest that bears watching.[30]

The more difficult conflict that physicians must increasingly face is the

28. In speaking on this subject to various hospital ethics committees and physicians, we have found these to be the most common criticisms of managed care.

29. For more on the patient-physician aspect of managed care, see Ezekiel J. Emanuel and Nancy Neveloff Dubler, "Preserving the Physician-Patient Relationship in an Era of Managed Care," *Journal of the American Medical Association* 273, no. 4 (25 January 1995): 323-29.

30. For more discussion of this issue, see Marc A. Rodwin, *Medicine, Money, and Morals: Physicians' Conflicts of Interest* (New York: Oxford University Press, 1993); E. Haavi Morreim, "The Ethics of Incentives in Managed Care," *Trends in Health Care, Law and Ethics* 10, no. 1/2 (winter/spring 1995): 56-62; Dan Brock and Allan Buchanan, "The Profit Motive in Medicine," *Journal of Medicine and Philosophy* 12 (1987): 1-34; Marc A. Rodwin, "Conflicts in Managed Care," *New England Journal of Medicine* 332 (1995): 604-7.

one between the needs of the individual patient and the needs of the group of patients for which the physician has responsibility. This was cited earlier in this chapter as an example of the way bioethics is changing. Managed care has pressed upon physicians and hospitals the reality that health care resources are limited, and in a context of scarce resources, difficult decisions must be made about balancing the needs of all of the patients for whom the physician must provide care. In many cases the physician or group has a limited amount of money available to care for a specific group of patients. Increasingly a physician must be willing to make decisions about allocation of resources in order to protect the interests of all his or her patients. Physicians are increasingly calling on clinical ethics committees to help them make these resource allocation decisions. The physician ethic is changing due to heightened recognition of scarcity of resources. Helping providers to make these kinds of decisions or to know when to advocate for their patients will be a primary role for ethics committees in the future.[31]

The physician may find himself or herself in one of two different situations in regard to making these difficult decisions.[32] In the first, the physician is faced with a decision whether or not to advocate for his or her patient within a particular health plan for a potentially beneficial treatment. The plan either clearly excludes the treatment or may be ambiguous about its exclusion, or may not have been tested. The greater the likelihood that the proposed treatment will prevent harm (and the greater the harm prevented), the more aggressively the physician should advocate for the patient. For all proposed treatments in which the plan is ambiguous about inclusion or exclusion, the physician should advocate for the patient for any treatment he or she believes would prevent harm or confer a benefit. In a second scenario, the physician has discretion within a health plan to provide treatment, which may be costly to him or her financially. Here again, the greater the likelihood that the proposed treatment will prevent harm (and the greater the harm prevented, the greater the obligation), the stronger the duty to provide the treatment. Though this is only a beginning, much more work is needed to help physicians and hospitals manage these conflicts.

31. See, for example, the article by Wolf, "Health Care Reform and the Future of Physician Ethics."

32. These scenarios and the principles are taken from Wolf, pp. 35-36.

Conclusion

The moral issues in health care delivery will continue to be pressing for the foreseeable future, since the delivery system affects so much of medical practice at the bedside. There is no reason to be skeptical in principle of the blend of business and medicine, since they have always mixed. The mixture of profits and patients has made for acute ethical dilemmas, with which physicians, ethicists, nurses, and administrators will continue to grapple. At this point it is unclear what the overall shape of the health care delivery system will look like when attempts to reform it are complete. The Scripture places emphasis upon criteria of need and merit for a just distribution system, the benchmarks by which the fairness of the system should be measured.

PART III

EMPLOYING A CHRISTIAN APPROACH

CHAPTER 9

Christian Bioethics in a Secular Culture

Introduction

Imagine a Christian physician in the state of Oregon, where in the fall of 1997 physician-assisted suicide was approved by a voter referendum and became legal, subject of course to guidelines to prevent abuse. This physician has been asked by his state medical association on more than one occasion in the past few years to testify before the state legislature on this issue, because of his prominence in the medical community. As a Christian he opposes assisted suicide on theological grounds. But he realizes that not everyone in the state shares his biblical view of the world. It is not enough to simply suggest that assisted suicide should be prohibited because the Bible says, "Thou shalt not murder." He realizes that for public policy, in a pluralistic society in which biblical authority is increasingly discounted or ignored, his reasons for opposing physician-assisted suicide must have more in common with people who do not accept his theological worldview. He finds this experience to be similar to the one he had trying to persuade the ethics committee at the hospital where he is affiliated that it should not participate in physician-assisted suicide.

To take the above scenario further, the physician is now seeing one of many elderly patients who are considering requesting his assistance in suicide should their condition result in an unacceptable quality of life. Of course, the physician could tell that patient gently but firmly that he is a Christian and opposes assisting anyone in suicide, and thus will not be able to participate in aiding the patient in taking her life. But chances are that the patient will find someone else to assist her, and thus the only thing the physician has accomplished is enabling himself to sleep better at night, knowing that he did not violate his conscience and perhaps has created some doubt about assistance in suicide for his patient.

But he wants to do more than simply opt out of procedures with which he is morally uncomfortable. He wants to be able to tell his patients why he thinks physician-assisted suicide is a bad idea, not only for society, but also for them individually. His patients come from a wide variety of cultural and religious backgrounds, many of which have little in common with his faith. How does he explain to them that requesting assistance in suicide is a poor option, not to mention unethical for any physician, without depending on the Bible or his theology to persuade them? Though he acknowledges that communicating God's Word has power to transform people's thinking,[1] he realizes that most of his patients do not accept biblical authority and will not find such reasoning persuasive. What reasons does he use to explain to them that physician-assisted suicide is not a moral option?

There is another group with whom he will have to discuss this issue very soon. The handful of HMOs with whom he contracts are subtly and quietly suggesting that all physicians who contract with them participate in physician-assisted suicide with their patients who request it. They argue that assistance in suicide is legal, that it avoids the high costs of end-of-life treatments and care, and thus should be honored if it is requested. Though these HMOs never come out and explicitly state it, our physician senses from his dealings with these organizations that they will put more pressure on him as time goes on. It would not surprise him if he were threatened with deselection, that is, removed from consideration as a preferred provider by these HMOs, if he chooses not to participate in assisted suicide. This would likely cost him many of his patients and could have a very detrimental effect on his practice. His peers in his physician group are getting the same sense from the HMOs, but they are willing to participate, and after discussing it with our physician, they cannot see why he thinks it is immoral. Like his patients, they embrace a variety of worldviews, and they reflect the secular nature of the culture at large. They too find our physician's biblical and theological defense unpersuasive. How does he talk about his views on assisted suicide to the HMO executives with whom he arranges contracts? How does he reason with his colleagues in practice about his views on this issue?[2]

---

1. Isa. 55:11.

2. We cite this issue as an example of the need for publicly accessible reasons for one's theologically grounded views. We have outlined some of the reasons for our opposi-

Or imagine a Christian OB-GYN in private practice in a large group setting. As is the standard of practice, this physician offers a variety of prenatal tests to the pregnant women she sees in her office. Though she is a bit uneasy about the risks of amniocentesis, she has no problem making it available for women over the age of thirty-five, who statistically are at higher risk for some birth defects such as Down syndrome. However, she is growing more disturbed at the number of couples who are opting to end their pregnancies when they find out that their unborn child is suffering from a genetic anomaly. Though she makes it clear that she does not do abortions for any reason except in the rare emergency cases in which the mother's life is endangered, she wants to do more. She wants to do what she can, and what is appropriate, to encourage these couples not to end their pregnancies. She has firm convictions from Scripture about the personhood of the unborn, but she realizes that not everyone will find those reasons convincing. How does she talk to these patients about the fact that these unborn children are persons, and no less persons because of the genetic defect from which they are suffering? She realizes that she must have these discussions without dependence on Scripture. Rather she must use reasons that are compelling to these couples. Of course, she is aware that for some couples, no amount of persuasion will change their minds, no matter what the reasons. But she feels the obligation to these unborn children to undertake the discussion.

Or imagine a Christian serving in the state legislature. This man represents a broad spectrum of cultures and ethnic backgrounds in his district and realizes there are numerous religious and philosophical views of the world to which he must be sensitive. He is an attorney by profession, specializing in family law, and ran for the legislature because he saw the need to change many of the laws dealing with families and children. He grew weary of "picking up the pieces" from what he considers ill-advised laws, and wants to make more substantive, institutional changes in the law.

One issue that has troubled him from the beginning of his legal practice is the growing phenomenon of surrogate motherhood. Couples have asked him in the past if he would broker surrogacy arrangements, and he has refused, sensitively but firmly citing his opposition to assisting couples in procreating in that way. This issue is currently before his subcommittee in the legislature, and he has the chance to influence the way in which surrogacy law in his state will be crafted. As a Christian, he opposes surrogacy because it violates the biblical notion of the family and procreation. But he

tion to assisted suicide in chapter 7. Our approach there, though brief, reflects the perspective we will develop in this chapter.

realizes that not everyone shares this concept of the family. In his district single women and lesbian couples are having children using donor sperm, insisting that they are a family even though they do not fit the traditional or biblical model of a family. He has heard public testimony from gay couples who want to use a surrogate mother so that they can have a child and be a family too. On his committee are libertarians who insist that as long as there is no clear, tangible harm to others, people have the right to make a family in any way they choose and with whomever they choose. But he is very uncomfortable with surrogacy as a reproductive option for virtually anyone. How does he persuade these various constituencies that surrogacy is morally problematic, without depending on his theology of the family?

Christian Public Policy in a Secular Culture

Any discussion of bioethics, particularly as it relates to public policy issues, from a Christian perspective must begin from the biblical and theological roots in the issue at hand.[3] For the Christian in public policy, theological considerations must provide the parameters for all policy alternatives. No specific policy option that ends up outside those boundaries can be seriously considered by the Christian in the public arena. However, articulating the implications of our theology for public policy and with others who do not share our view of the world is another matter entirely. Here appeals to Scripture and theology alone are likely not adequate, since an increasingly secular public policy sector dismisses if not distrusts views with a religious origin.[4] Theological views must be communicated in a way that is persuasive to this public policy sector without excessive reliance on a worldview that it does not accept. This is not to say that appeals to Scripture and theology are not important, but since many public policy makers do not accept the Christian view of the world and thus do not frame the issues in this way, it is important not only to help them see the issues from within a Christian framework but also to make

---

3. In chapters 3 through 8 we attempted to formulate our argument in this way: we laid out the theological foundations first, then applied the principles to areas of medical practice and bioethical social policy where they have a bearing.

4. See, for example, the recent work by Yale law professor Stephen L. Carter, *The Culture of Disbelief* (New York: Basic Books, 1993), in which he documents the bias against religiously grounded public policy views. That this is detrimental to civil society is argued by Richard John Neuhaus in *The Naked Public Square* (Grand Rapids: Wm. B. Eerdmans Publishing Co., 1983).

sense of a Christian perspective on the issue without dependence solely on Scripture and theology.

In the earlier parts of this century, there was a well-defined Judeo-Christian moral consensus in the United States and many parts of the West. There was a commitment to pluralism as well, and other views of the world were tolerated with varying degrees of civility. But pluralism involved toleration of views with which the general public disagreed, and could say publicly that they considered ideas or practices immoral. Pluralism today seems to involve not only toleration but also acceptance of other worldviews as equally valid. Part of this shift in the notion of pluralism comes from the privatization of one's view of the world, especially if it is derived from religious views. Those are considered private, subjective, and not subject to scrutiny, and therefore must be accepted as valid starting points. One does not normally make a moral or philosophical judgment in the public arena on the worldview of another. This notion of pluralism is, of course, contrary to the admonitions of Scripture, which urge the church to critique other worldviews from the perspective of the gospel and to present the truth of Christianity as a philosophically viable and consistent alternative (see, e.g., I Pet. 3:15; II Cor. 10:5; Acts 17:22-34; Col. 2:8). Today, as the culture moves toward the next millennium, the Judeo-Christian moral consensus which characterized much of the history of the West no longer holds persuasive influence in an increasingly secularized culture.[5] Public debate on most important issues is framed in terms that exclude religious ideas, since they are widely considered private and thus relevant only to the adherents of those beliefs.

The type of approach in which one uses publicly accessible reasons for one's position is not only necessary in the current cultural context for bioethics. It also has precedent in the Scripture. For example, the wisdom literature is widely considered to be addressed to an international audience, intended for readers outside the boundaries of the nation of Israel. This is one reason why, for instance, Solomon's wisdom was well known around the world (I Kings 10:1-13). The parts of the Old Testament that were primarily addressed to God's covenant people Israel, that is, the Law and the Historical

5. Though it is true that the numbers of Christian believers specifically and religious believers in general continue at high levels in the United States, much higher than in other parts of the West (the Third World is still overwhelmingly religious and much of it Christian), in terms of influence in the culture, Western culture is increasingly secularized. This means that religious ideas, symbols, and institutions no longer have the influence over the culture that they once did. For insightful critique of the secularization thesis in general, see Richard John Neuhaus, *Unsecular America* (Grand Rapids: Wm. B. Eerdmans Publishing Co., 1988).

Books, contain a good deal of material that is conspicuous by its absence in the wisdom literature. To be sure, the overarching themes of obedience to God and the importance of a relationship with him are continued, but the Wisdom Books are framed without mention of many themes that dominated the Law and Historical Books. Motifs such as the Law of Moses; God's covenant with the people, including the blessings/cursings for obedience/disobedience; the Promised Land; the sacrificial system; the myriad of religious festivals; and the ceremonial laws of diet and purification are scarcely if ever referred to. The reason for these omissions seems to be that these themes were neither relevant nor persuasive for non-Israelites. The writers of the Wisdom Books, particularly Proverbs, used more publicly accessible reasons to persuade their audience to adopt their wisdom propositions. Proverbs is replete with appeals to the observable track record of consequences of certain types of unwise and immoral behavior. It contains virtually no references, apart from Proverbs 1, which suggests that the fear of the Lord is the beginning of wisdom, to its authority coming from the fact that the proverbs enumerated therein are the inspired Word of God. The writers of the Wisdom Books do not doubt that this is true, but they use other means of persuasion that will more likely be accepted by their worldview-diverse audience. The parts of the Old Testament addressed to Israel use motifs that would be persuasive to Israelites, such as the themes just mentioned.

This pattern is continued in the New Testament as well. Though the apostles and early church clearly proclaimed the gospel message, they used the most appropriate and likely to be effective means of persuasion at their disposal. For example, when reasoning with the Jews, both common people and religious leadership, they used the language of the Old Testament and showed how Jesus fulfilled Old Testament prophecy and patterns (Acts 17:1-2). With others, they used the clear and indisputable fact of Jesus' resurrection.[6] One of the clearest examples of the apostles' making the message persuasive in terms conducive to their audience occurs when Paul debates the Greek philosophers on Mars Hill in Acts 17:22-34. His message is clearly the gospel, with the coming judgment and Jesus' resurrection at the heart of his presentation. But he reaches his audience by interacting with their objects of worship, their writers and poets, and the fact of the resurrection of Jesus. He frames his argument in terms that they would find persuasive, and in fact, some of them do. His central message does not deviate from the gospel message, but his means of communicating the message are

---

6. Of course, the apostles preached the resurrection to the Jews too, but they explained its meaning explicitly from the Old Testament.

dependent on what will best convince his audience of the truth of that message.

Not only does Scripture open the door for using the most persuasive method to communicate God's truth, most public policy organizations, particularly government panels, which develop policy guidelines on bioethical issues insist on publicly accessible reasons for one's public policy conclusions. In addition, most health care institutions serve very diverse communities with a variety of worldviews to which they must be sensitive. When formulating policies on different bioethical issues, they must appeal to reasons that are persuasive to the community they are serving.[7] Furthermore, patients who do not share their physician's specifically Christian view of the world need other reasons to persuade them to accept what the physician considers the most morally appropriate thing to do. Of course, the physician is not obligated to provide care that violates his or her conscience or religious views, but is obligated to attempt to explain the reasons for such views in terms that the patient or family who does not share the physician's view of the world might find persuasive.

Take, for example, the National Bioethics Advisory Commission (NBAC) report on human cloning. Though the commission made a laudable attempt to solicit the views of religious leaders on cloning, its report made clear that it does not consider religiously grounded reasons alone sufficient for discourse in a pluralistic, democratic society. Public policy discussion requires reasons that are not restricted to a religious perspective. The report acknowledges the importance of publicly accessible reasons for moral discussion appropriate to a pluralistic culture. The commission report puts it this way in the introduction to the chapter entitled "Religious Perspectives":

> For purposes of recommending public policy in a democratic society, the Commission was also interested in the extent to which moral arguments in various religious traditions rest on premises accessible to others outside those traditions. Sometimes religious thinkers appeal to categories such as "nature," "reason," "basic human values," and "family values" that may speak to citizens outside their traditions because these categories do not necessarily

---

7. Even Catholic health care institutions, which operate explicitly according to the church's ethical and religious directives for health care, attempt to persuade their communities of patients and physicians that the directives make good sense for health care. Of course, Catholic hospitals maintain their directives even if the patients and physicians disagree with them. Physicians who do not care to work under these guidelines can seek affiliation elsewhere. Patients who are seeking procedures that the directives prohibit, such as elective abortion and nonmedically indicated sterilization, are free to obtain the care they need at non-Catholic hospitals.

depend solely on particular faith commitments, scripture, revelation, or religious authority. Such categories therefore contribute to a broader societal discussion of the ethical arguments for and against cloning humans.[8]

In the most direct statement in the entire report, in which the panel addresses the place of morality in public policy formation, it insists that in formulating public policy in a widely diverse culture, consensus and persuasive argument are critical to developing a policy that will find acceptance in the public. Theological arguments that it holds are restricted to one religion or sect cannot be the basis for such a consensus. The panel states that "Americans share some but not all of their ethical and cultural traditions, and no single set of approaches that balances conflicting values in particular ways enjoys universal acceptance. Some theological analyses provide answers to their adherents, but these are incapable of serving as the sole basis for policy making in a religiously diverse nation committed to separation of church and state."[9]

Whether or not this is the way it should be, of course, is a matter for vigorous debate.[10] The Christian should not idly stand by while his or her theological convictions are marginalized in public policy debate. The Christian can point out that the First Amendment did not prohibit theological convictions from informing public policy. In fact, the Founding Fathers were insistent on the importance of religion and morality for the success of democracy. The First Amendment simply guaranteed religious freedom by prohibiting the establishment of a state church and government sanction of any particular religion or sect. It did not demand neutrality toward religion in general, nor did it prevent theological views from being relevant to public policy.[11] Of course, there is con-

---

8. National Bioethics Advisory Commission (NBAC), *Cloning Human Beings: Report and Recommendations of the National Bioethics Advisory Commission* (Rockville, Md.: NBAC, 1997), p. 39.

9. NBAC, p. 93. The panel cites the Supreme Court in the *Planned Parenthood of Southeastern Pennsylvania v. Casey* decision, in which the Court held that "In order to be legitimate, the State's interest must be secular; consistent with the First Amendment, the State may not promote a theological or sectarian interest," 112 S. Ct. 2791 (1992). To say the least, it is open to debate whether the intent of the First Amendment prohibited the state from advancing a theological interest. One can argue that for most of U.S. history, the Judeo-Christian theology was promoted, with no suggestion that it violated the separation of church and state. For more on the background to the church-state separation issue, see Neuhaus, *The Naked Public Square*.

10. One example of this debate is found in Robert Audi and Nicholas Wolterstorff, *Religion in the Public Square: The Place of Religious Convictions in Political Debate* (Lanham, Md.: Rowman & Littlefield, 1997). Our position more closely resembles that taken by Audi.

11. For more discussion on this, see A. James Reichley, *Religion in American Public Life* (Washington, D.C.: Brookings Institution, 1985), pp. 89-106. His argument is summa-

siderably more religious diversity today than in the times of the Founding Fathers. But part of the Christian role in being salt and light in the world is expanding the influence of Christian ideas, symbols, and institutions in the culture. Nothing in the First Amendment prevents the church from fulfilling its public and prophetic role in heralding the truth to issues of public policy.

The NBAC report does represent accurately the way things are when it comes to religious views in public policy. Appeal to religious or theological views alone is not very persuasive in a secular and diverse culture. Thus the Christian attempting to advance his or her issue with colleagues or public policy institutions should be clear on the position being advanced and the theological underpinning for it. Christian positions in bioethics must be thought through at the theological level, since theology provides the parameters outside of which no position can be seriously entertained. No position that is contrary to orthodox theology should be advanced. But the foundations for a position and the means used to persuade others who do not share an evangelical view of the world can be very different. In this effort at persuasion it is essential that the position taken be identifiably Christian, but the means of persuasion need not and should not be limited to theological and biblical notions.

Application to Current Bioethical Issues

The Unborn

One example of how the theological foundations and the means of persuasion to a secular culture can be different comes in the notion of the personhood of the unborn. In chapter 4 we cited a variety of theological arguments, particularly the image of God and the incarnation, that indicate that the image of God is present in the unborn child from the earliest points of pregnancy. Further, we cited several examples, notably from Psalms 51 and 139, that show a continuity of personal identity from in utero to mature adulthood. We then applied these concepts to important aspects of medical practice such as informed consent and confidentiality. These doctrines touch on other important issues, which have social policy implications, such as abortion, reproductive technologies, and embryo and fetal tissue research. When it comes to establishing public policy in a widely diverse culture on these controversial issues, however, more than our theological foundations is required to make our views persuasive. If the

---

rized in Scott B. Rae, *Moral Choices: An Introduction to Ethics* (Grand Rapids: Zondervan, 1995), pp. 235-37.

only means of persuasion we have at our disposal is our biblical and theological arguments, then the person who does not accept biblical authority is not likely to find that these arguments carry much weight. The person or organizations we are attempting to persuade will likely dismiss these arguments as sectarian, religious, and not relevant to public discussion.

For example, the 1994 National Institutes of Health panel on embryo research which was convened following the announcement of successful embryo cloning[12] suggested that religious views of the personhood of the unborn be viewed in the context of a pluralistic approach to public policy. This pluralistic approach appears to be at the heart of the panel's desire to approach the public policy aspects of embryo research independent of any particular worldview. In justifying its pluralistic view, it stated that "Public policy employs reasoning that is understandable in terms that are independent of a particular religious, theological or philosophical perspective, and it requires weighing of arguments in light of the best available information and scientific evidence."[13] Interestingly, the panel appeared to place philosophical traditions in the same category as religious convictions, both under the umbrella of private perspectives and thus not suitable for public policy. This would seem to leave the panel with at least an implicit commitment to empiricism (the worldview that holds that the only things that are knowable are empirically verifiable facts) as its starting place, given its emphasis on the available scientific evidence on the moral status of the embryo.

However, personhood is not a scientific concept, but a philosophical one that is by definition worldview-dependent. The panel's deliberate omission of philosophical considerations seems particularly problematic here. In addition, it actually was not followed by the panel itself. Ethicist Daniel Callahan suggests that "the report has in fact adopted a particular philosophical viewpoint on the purpose of law, on the imperative of scientific research and on the moral status of the fetus. If the Panel did not notice that, just about everyone else will."[14] The panel's view that religious and philosophical perspectives are private and not relevant to public policy should, of course, be vigorously challenged. Simply because one holds to religiously grounded views should not disqualify one from participation in public debate. But the panel's views of what counts as valid reasons for a particular public policy po-

12. See the discussion of both embryo and somatic cell cloning in chapter 3.

13. National Institutes of Health Embryo Research Panel, *Report of the Human Embryo Research Panel* (Washington, D.C.: National Institutes of Health, 27 September 1994), pp. 50-51.

14. Daniel Callahan, "The Puzzle of Profound Respect," *Hastings Center Report* 25 (January-February 1995): 40.

sition suggest that more than theologically grounded reasons need to be offered in order to be persuasive in the public debate on these issues.

This is why we offered a defense of the personhood of the unborn in chapter 5 from the perspective of a substance. This view does not require any religious convictions prior to accepting it as valid, but is consistent with the theological analysis of the unborn. We would offer the material in chapter 5 as a means of persuasion that is independent of one's religious views on the unborn and could appeal to a broad spectrum in the culture. Of course, whether or not such a means of persuasion would be effective is another question. Perhaps it would not be, particularly with the Embryo Research Panel's prior commitment to empiricism, which could be challenged as well. But it seems incumbent on the Christian attempting to communicate his or her religious views on the unborn in an arena broader than simply the church to appeal to arguments other than those which would be persuasive to fellow believers.

Physician-Assisted Suicide

A second example of how extrabiblical means of persuasion might be used in public debate is in the issue of physician-assisted suicide.[15] The biblical notion of "Thou shalt not murder" is the foundation for opposition to assisted suicide, because all human beings are made in the image of God and are entitled to this inalienable right. The image of God is present in a person up until the point of death, as the biblical notion of the continuity of personal identity suggests. The substance view of a human person is also relevant in that no elderly, terminally ill, or permanently vegetative person can be said not to be a person. Many advocates of assisted suicide insist that at the end of life those who would desire assistance in suicide are no longer persons, but both the theological view of the continuity of personal identity and the philosophical notion of a person as a substance suggest otherwise. Other reasons that should be advanced in opposition to assisted suicide include the idea that proper pain management makes assisted suicide unnecessary to relieve pain and suffering, the limits on personal autonomy entailed in the practice, and the dangerous potential to move from voluntary to involuntary assistance in suicide, as is the case in places such as the Netherlands, where physician-assisted suicide is not prosecuted.

---

15. For more detailed discussion of this issue, see chapter 7.

Surrogate Motherhood

A third example is the controversial reproductive arrangement of surrogate motherhood. In all cases of surrogacy, the couple who contracts the surrogate expects her to give up the child when it is born. To do this the surrogate must sign a waiver of parental rights, similar to what is done in adoption proceedings. As explained in chapter 3, the great majority of surrogacy cases are both commercial and genetic. The surrogate is paid to conceive, gestate, give birth to, and waive parental rights to a child to whom she is genetically related. If she changes her mind and wants to keep the child, she is normally sued for breach of contract. Generally when this happens, the surrogate shares custody of the child with the natural father, similar to what might happen in a divorce. There is considerable debate over the rights of a gestational surrogate to the child she bears. Some hold that genetics gives a woman maternal rights, and thus the surrogate would have no rights to the child she bears since it would not be her child.[16] Others hold that the traditional view of motherhood should decide these cases, that the woman who gives birth to the child should be the mother with maternal rights.[17] In these cases the surrogate is the mother and has maternal rights to the child she bears. If she chooses to give up the child to the contracting couple, she does so knowing that it is hers to give or keep. If one holds the traditional view, then there is no difference in maternal rights between genetic and gestational surrogacy.

Surrogacy is theologically problematic because it violates the creation norm for marriage, family, and procreation by introducing a third-party contributor, either in the form of a womb donor or a womb and egg donor. As such, surrogacy should not normally be used by the Christian since it is contrary to the biblical notion of the family. But when it comes to making public policy and the law on surrogacy, the biblical notion of the family is not likely to be considered persuasive for the substantial part of the population that does not share a biblical concept of the family and a biblical view of the world. How might Christian legislators address their colleagues in the legislature and constituents back home about the issue? To what could they appeal to make their biblical position persuasive to people who do not share their view of the world?

16. This is the view of the California Supreme Court in *Johnson v. Calvert,* the most widely discussed case of gestational surrogacy to date. 851 P. 2d 776 (Cal.).

17. For a summary of these views, see Scott B. Rae, "Parental Rights and the Definition of Motherhood in Surrogate Motherhood," *Southern California Review of Law and Women's Studies* 3, no. 2 (spring 1994): 219-77, and Rae, *The Ethics of Commercial Surrogate Motherhood* (Westport, Conn.: Praeger, 1994).

Since the majority of surrogacy cases are both commercial and genetic, in which there is little debate that the surrogate is the legal mother,[18] what makes surrogacy problematic is that it constitutes the sale of children.[19] As such, it violates the Thirteenth Amendment to the Constitution, which prohibited slavery, because the purchase and sale of human beings was considered immoral and a fundamental violation of their dignity and rights to life, liberty, and the pursuit of happiness. Undergirding this perspective is the notion that human beings possess inherent dignity that makes them what legal scholar Margaret Radin calls "market inalienable."[20] That is, they should not be subject to barter in the marketplace. Virtually everyone agrees that human beings possess fundamental dignity and should not be treated as objects of commerce. For the Christian, the view of human beings created in God's image and for whom Christ died gives them inestimable value and mandates that they should not be exchanged for money or other consideration.[21] This

18. Legal precedent for this was established in the well-publicized Baby M surrogacy case, which reached the New Jersey Supreme Court before it was resolved. The court ruled that when the surrogate contributes the egg and gives birth to the child, she is the legal mother (see *In the Matter of Baby M*, 537 A. 2d, 1227 [1988]). The only debate about assigning maternal rights in this way comes from those who favor a strict contract view of surrogacy in which the preconception intent to parent is weighted more heavily than either gestation or genetics. Advocates of this view include Andrea Stumpf, "Redefining Motherhood: A Legal Matrix for the New Reproductive Technologies," *Yale Law Review* 96 (1986): 197-208, and Majorie Maguire Schultz, "Reproductive Technology and Intent-Based Parenthood: An Opportunity for Gender Neutrality," *Wisconsin Law Review*, no. 2 (1990): 297-398. For a critique of these views, see Rae, *Ethics of Commercial Surrogate Motherhood*, pp. 94-105.

19. For an extended discussion of surrogacy as baby selling, see Rae, *Ethics of Commercial Surrogate Motherhood*, pp. 29-75.

20. Margaret J. Radin, "Market-Inalienability," *Harvard Law Review* 100 (June 1987): 1849-1937.

21. One might wonder how the Old Testament institution of slavery is consistent with the notion of human beings made in God's image. Slavery in the Old Testament was fundamentally different by design than slavery in other parts of the ancient world. Slaves in Israel were to be treated as the virtual equivalents of family members, and when time came for them to be released, they were to be sent away with enough provisions to enable them to adequately support themselves. For others, slavery functioned as the equivalent of the welfare system, in which destitute people could align themselves with a family as slaves in exchange for their service. If the system of slavery had been abolished, many destitute people would have had no means of survival. Even when slaves were "purchased," they were subject to the right of redemption in which they could be released if a family member reimbursed the family who took them in. They were further subject to the provisions of the Jubilee, or automatic release in the fiftieth year. As with other issues such as divorce — about which Jesus explains that God temporarily allowed the practice in Old Testament

shared value of respect for human dignity is the foundation for appeal to a broader audience. The primary task for Christian legislators is to persuade their colleagues that surrogacy is indeed the equivalent of baby selling, and should not be allowed. If the parties in a surrogacy scenario were involved in an adoption, they would clearly be in violation of the law and public policy. The term normally used for the sale of a child to an adoptive couple is "black market adoptions," since it is illegal to sell human beings.

The way a surrogacy arrangement is set up strongly suggests that the surrogate is paid for the production of a child and delivery of that child over to the contracting couple. To suggest that the surrogate is only paid for gestational services rendered misses the obvious point, that under this scenario if she wants to keep the child, the couple who contracts her cannot accuse her of breaching her contract, since her obligation to the couple was fulfilled the moment the child was born. The reaction of the contracting couple in cases in which the surrogate elects to keep the child indicates that they are expecting, in return for their payment to the surrogate, that she deliver a child to them, not that she simply gestate and give birth. Those are obviously necessary elements, but they are not sufficient for the terms of the agreement to be fulfilled. The couple expects a product, not a process. They normally keep up to half of the surrogate's fee in an escrow account until she signs a waiver of parental rights and turns over custody of the child to them. She is clearly paid for giving up her rights to her child, something that is illegal in adoption set-tings. The only difference is that the arrangement is made prior to conception in surrogacy, rather than during the pregnancy as in most adoption settings.[22]

One can appeal to widely shared values such as respect for human dignity to undergird the argument against surrogacy. If surrogacy is baby selling, then it violates dignity by making the most vulnerable of the human community, newborn children, the objects of commerce, and is thus unethical. It further violates the Constitution, and thus one can make a good case that it should also be illegal. Roughly one-third of the states have passed laws concerning surrogacy, and the majority of states have agreed that when done commercially it is baby selling and should be pro-

---

times as better than the alternative of no divorce (Matt. 19:3-9) — the New Testament clarifies that the norm God intends is stricter: in this case, no slavery. For example, Paul advises slaves to leave slavery where possible (I Cor. 7:21) and the slaveholder Philemon to release his slave Onesimus (Philem. 16).

22. Others have argued that surrogacy is very different from black market adoptions. For discussion and critique of this position, see Rae, *Ethics of Commercial Surrogate Motherhood*, pp. 38-46.

hibited.[23] Thus legislators can articulate their theological position on surrogacy, grounded in their theology of the family and procreation, in terms that appeal to a broader, more pluralistic audience. They do this by appealing to values that are widely shared in that audience and using a means of persuasion that is not dependent solely on theological notions that would likely not be accepted as compelling. Articulating the issues in this way is more comfortable for those who accept the notion of natural law in ethics, the view that God has revealed moral values outside of Scripture as well as in his biblical commands and principles.[24]

Conclusion

Doing Christian bioethics in a secular society involves thorough grounding in the theological notions underlying bioethics, but articulating those positions in ways that are not solely dependent on one's theology. Scripture itself opens the door to such an approach, and the public policy institutions generally demand that religiously grounded views be presented with publicly accessible reasons. Some are skeptical that such an approach can actually be effective, and they suggest more of a countercultural approach. Ethicist Mike McKenzie puts it this way:

> If the prevailing attitudes continue, this suggests that the public square will continue to exclude Christian values and norms, no matter how explicitly expressed. This development in turn will result in Christians turning to their own institutions, both ecclesiastical and social, for relief. For example, Christians may opt for more reliance on private hospitals in which the bioethical square still has room for Christian values and norms. It was here where the concept of hospitals began, and perhaps it is here where the future of values can continue.[25]

23. For a survey of state laws in surrogacy, see Rae, *Ethics of Commercial Surrogate Motherhood,* pp. 146-60.

24. For more discussion of the controversial issue of natural law in ethics, see Rae, *Moral Choices,* pp. 35-41; J. Budziszewski, *Written on the Heart: The Case for Natural Law* (Downers Grove, Ill.: InterVarsity, 1997); and Michael Cromartie, ed., *A Preserving Grace: Catholics, Protestants, and Natural Law* (Grand Rapids: Wm. B. Eerdmans Publishing Co., 1997).

25. Michael McKenzie, "Christian Norms in the Ethical Square: An Impossible Dream?" *Journal of the Evangelical Theological Society* 38, no. 3 (September 1995): 413-27, at 426.

This may indeed be true, and to rely on institutions that are more friendly to one's values is not to abandon the public square. The Catholic Church, with its extensive network of hospitals and medical centers, has done precisely this. But Catholics have also engaged the public debate on bioethical issues directly, and have been successful in some cases, most recently with their campaigns in various states against assisted suicide and at the federal level against human cloning. Though it may be necessary to have counterinstitutions, that should not mean that Christians are removed from the public debate on bioethical issues. Christians are called to be faithful to Jesus' command to be the salt of the earth and the light of the world, which among other things mandates involvement in the culture, contending for righteousness and persuading the culture of the truth of the Word of God.

CHAPTER 10

A Model for Bioethical Decision Making

Case 1 — "Attempted Suicide"?

One afternoon a nonambulatory, morbidly obese, arthritic, and chronically depressed woman in her late sixties who was in chronic pain and addicted to drugs was brought to the emergency room (ER). She had been injured by an apparent self-inflicted gunshot wound. Her husband had called the paramedics and she was brought to the ER. He said that had he known at the time he called the paramedics that she had shot herself in the head, he would not have called. She was taken to surgery and found to have sustained considerable damage to her head but not much damage to the brain except to the frontal lobes. The surgeons indicated that though the patient was intubated because of the mechanical damage and edema in her neck, they felt she would be extubated shortly. Because her brain damage was minimal and involved only the frontal lobes, she was not expected to have neurologic motor or sensory deficit.

Shortly after her arrival at the ER, her husband brought a durable power of attorney for health care (DPAHC) signed by the patient and dated approximately three months earlier. The patient had designated the husband as her DPAHC agent to make all necessary medical decisions for her should she become unable to make them herself. He told the hospital doctors and staff that he and his family were aware of the emotional and physical pain and suffering the patient had had over the years and understood that she was depressed, but she wanted to end the suffering and he wanted them to stop the emergency treatment and let her die. Some specific requests by the patient in the DPAHC seemed to contradict the agent's expression of her wishes, however. For example, "If the extension of my life results in mere biologic existence, devoid of cognitive function, I do not desire any form of life-maintaining procedures. My agent should ask the question, 'Is the proposed treatment an aid to recovery or merely a prolongation of inevitable death?' I desire that my agent act after a reasonable time for observation and diagnosis." Clearly, if the proposed treatment were an aid to recovery, she desired such treatment.

The medical center's lawyer presented the staff with the current law, which essentially says that if a patient enters a hospital as an attempted suicide, the suicide attempt should not influence the interpretation of the wishes expressed in the DPAHC. On this basis emergency treatment was continued despite the emotional and persistent protests of the husband and the family, who wanted to let the patient die. Even after a two-to-three-hour conversation with members of the ethics committee, the husband was still insistent on having the treatment removed.

The committee suggested that the above-quoted section of her recently signed DPAHC did not seem consistent with the wishes of someone who wanted to die. The husband responded by pointing out that her DPAHC was a standard form known to the patient for at least two years, written by an attorney friend, but not signed until recently. He and the family emphasized to the committee that this document did not represent her current desires and may not have been fully read by her at the time of signing, and that she didn't want to live and suffer from her infirmities any longer. As her agent, he stated he was expressing to the committee her real desires regardless of what was stated on the form. The committee expressed to the family its concern that it was obliged to follow the DPAHC because of ethical and legal considerations. Since the patient was apparently beginning to recover, all the treatments currently undertaken would be representing an "aid to recovery" and not a "prolongation of inevitable death." Further, there was concern that the family was requesting the medical center staff to "complete" the failed attempted suicide.

Should the medical center follow the agent's wishes and terminate all life-sustaining treatments and allow his wife to die? Or should it follow the expressed written terms of her directive and keep her on the ventilator until she could be weaned off of it?

Other critical issues raised by this case include the following:

1. What should the proper relationship be between the patient's written directive and the agent's role as a proxy decision-maker? Is the agent's role to carry out the written instructions, or can the agent modify or

"interpret" the directive in a way that he or she thinks is consistent with the patient's desires?

2. How should the ethics committee handle the dynamics involved in an ethics consultation like this one?

Perhaps as good a question as *what should we do* in this situation? is the question, *how should we decide what to do* in this situation? The process of making a moral decision can be as important as the decision itself, and many ethical decisions that people encounter are so complex that it is easy to exhaust oneself talking around the problem without actually making any progress toward resolving it. The response to many moral dilemmas is "where do I start?" and the person who is faced with these decisions often needs direction that will enable him or her to move constructively toward resolution and "see the forest for the trees."

The following is a model that can be used to address the ethical dilemmas that people encounter regularly and to insure that all the necessary bases are covered. This is not a formula that will automatically generate the "right" answer to an ethical problem. Rather it is a set of guidelines designed to make sure that all the right questions are being asked in the process of ethical deliberation.

Given the ethnic and religious diversity of our society, it is important that the model can be used comfortably by people with a variety of cultural, ethnic, and religious backgrounds. This is not a distinctively Christian model, though it is consistent with the Scripture and any Christian can use biblical principles in utilizing it. What makes many moral dilemmas so difficult is that the Scripture does not directly address many issues, and thus does not speak to them as clearly as one would prefer. More general principles can be brought to bear on the issue at hand. However, in these instances there is often disagreement about which biblical principles are applicable to the specific issue under discussion. For example, in a situation where disclosing information will harm one person and not disclosing it will harm another (as in case 2 below), the principle of compassion can be invoked as a reason both to disclose and not to disclose. It is not clear that appeal to principles alone will conclusively resolve this case. Thus to insist that all ethical dilemmas are resolved simply by appeal to biblical principles seems to be an oversimplification. Certainly many moral questions are resolved conclusively by appeal to Scripture. But there are other cases in which that does not happen. That is not to say that Scripture is not sufficient for the believer's spiritual life, but that the special revelation of Scripture is often supplemented by the general revelation of God outside Scripture. This model makes room for both general and special revelation, and gives each a place in helping to resolve the difficult moral dilemmas facing people today.

Here are the elements of a model for making moral decisions:[1]

1. Gather the Facts

Frequently ethical dilemmas can be resolved simply by clarifying the facts of the case in question. In those cases that prove to be more difficult, gathering the facts is the essential first step prior to any ethical analysis and reflection on the case. In analyzing a case, we want to know the available facts at hand as well as any facts currently not known but that need to be ascertained. Thus one is asking not only "what do we know?" but also "what do we need to know?" in order to make an intelligent ethical decision. This is not always an easy process because there are different sets of data and differing empirical judgments. Participants can perceive the facts differently, and that affects their reasoning in the steps that follow.

2. Determine the Ethical Issues

The ethical issue(s) are stated in terms of competing interests or goods. It's these conflicting interests that actually make for an ethical dilemma. The issues should be presented in a _____ versus _____ format in order to reflect the interests that are colliding in a particular ethical dilemma. One should keep in mind that there can be more than two competing interests in any given case. For example, many ethical decisions, especially at the end of a patient's life, can be stated in terms of patient autonomy (or the right of the individual to make his or her own decisions about medical care) versus the sanctity of life (or the duty to preserve life).

3. What Norms Have a Bearing on the Case?

In any ethical dilemma, certain moral values considerations, or norms, are central to the competing positions being taken. It is critical to identify these norms,

---

1. This model is adapted from the seven-step model of Dr. William W. May, School of Religion, University of Southern California, from his course "Normative Analysis of Issues."

and in some cases to determine whether some norms are to be weighted more heavily than others. Clearly, biblical principles will be weighted the most heavily, but other principles from other sources may also speak to the case. Constitutional principles or principles drawn from natural law may supplement the biblical principles that come into play here. Not only principles should be considered, but also character virtues and broader theological paradigms. The narrative of one's life and community may have a bearing on the case as well.

Although earlier in this book we critiqued the overreliance on principles in the methodology of Beauchamp and Childress, their insights regarding the principles of autonomy, beneficence, non-maleficence, and justice are helpful within the parameters of Scripture. For example, individuals do have rights to bodily integrity based on the notion of human dignity, rooted in the creation of every person in God's image.[2] Further, health care professionals have the obligation to act in the best interests of patients and to not bring harm to them. These obligations are grounded in the biblical notions of compassion, love, and service to others, which fundamentally involve seeking people's best interests, even, at times, when it involves personal sacrifice and placing one's own interests as a lower priority.

4. List the Alternatives

Part of the creative thinking required for resolving an ethical dilemma involves coming up with various alternative courses of action. Though some alternatives will be ruled out without much thought, in general the more alternatives that are listed, the better the chance that one's list will include some high-quality ones. In addition, one may come up with some very creative alternatives not previously considered.

5. Compare the Alternatives with the Norms

At this point, the task is one of eliminating alternatives according to the moral norms that have a bearing on the case. In many instances the case will be resolved at this point, since the norms will eliminate all alternatives except one. In fact, the purpose of this comparison is to see if there is a clear decision that can be made without further deliberation. If a clear decision is not forth-

2. See the detailed discussion of this in chapter 4.

coming, then the next part in the model must be considered. At the least, some of the alternatives may be eliminated by this step of comparison.

6. Assess the Consequences

If the principles do not yield a clear decision, then a consideration of the consequences of the remaining available alternatives is in order. Both positive and negative consequences are to be considered. They should be informally weighted, since some positive consequences are more beneficial than others and some negative consequences are more detrimental than others.

7. Make a Decision

Deliberation cannot go on forever. At some point a decision must be made. One common element to ethical dilemmas is that there are no easy and painless solutions to them. Frequently the decision that is made is one that involves the least number of problems or negative consequences, not one that is devoid of them.

At this point it will be helpful to return to the case that began this chapter in order to illustrate how the model can be used. This illustration will also help clarify what is meant by each of the elements in the model. Two additional cases will be presented and analyzed in the framework of this model to suggest how it can be used profitably.

Case Analysis

1. Gather the Facts

a. The patient had apparently attempted suicide, resulting in considerable facial damage but minimal brain damage. There were some questions about whether or not this was an attempted suicide, based on the following, unclarified matters: (1) How could the husband, who was in the home at the time and presumably heard the gunshot, and who was aware that the patient was sufficiently depressed to commit suicide, and then found her in her injured condition, not have immediately assumed that she had tried to take her life? (2) Was a simple misinterpretation of what had occurred plausible, and if so, was it the only reason the paramedics were called? (3) Where was the gun after the shot was fired and why had he not seen it? (4) If she was nonambulatory, how did she get access to a loaded gun? These are factual items that should be cleared up if possible, though at the end of the analysis there may still be some unanswered questions about the facts.

b. The patient was intubated temporarily with the expectation that she could be weaned off the respirator.

c. The patient is in poor health, and the family says she has a recent history of severe depression.

d. The patient's husband brought in her DPAHC, in which he was designated as the agent. His request was for emergency treatment to be stopped. He was insistent that he was reflecting the patient's wishes.

e. Terms of the DPAHC state that if the patient is recovering, she wants life-sustaining treatment. The DPAHC requires that the agent act after sufficient time for observation and diagnosis.

f. The initial consultation with family did not resolve conflict but rather intensified it.

g. The husband insisted that the written directive was a generic form that the patient was not really informed about.

h. The hospital staff had concerns about removing life-sustaining treatment being the equivalent of assisting in suicide. Staff also had concerns about removing life support from a clearly recovering patient.

i. The nursing staff was concerned that members of the patient's family might disconnect the respirator themselves. They were not allowed to see the patient without some supervision by hospital personnel. This served to further alienate family members and make them even more angry at how the case was progressing.

2. Determine the Ethical Issues

The issue here revolves around the conflict between the wishes of the agent, who insists he is reflecting the desires of the patient, and what seems to be in the best interests of the patient. It is a conflict between the autonomy of the agent to make decisions for the patient and the best interests of the patient. There is another conflict between the wishes of the agent and the stated wishes of the patient as expressed in her DPAHC. There is also a conflict between the institution (a Catholic hospital), which is bound by a set of ethical and religious directives for health care that do not allow physicians or nurses affiliated with the hospital to assist in suicide, and the family's *prima facie* request to "complete" the failed suicide attempt. The directives also discourage removal of life-sustaining treatment from patients who are clearly recovering, as was the case with this patient.

3. What Norms Have a Bearing on the Case?

The norms that have a bearing on the case include:

a. Patient autonomy, expressed both in the written terms of the advance directive and by the agent for the patient. Patient autonomy is rooted in the right to bodily integrity and the right to avoid unwanted medical interventions. The principles of autonomy and beneficence conflict, however, and are limited here by broader theological considerations such as the dignity of human beings created in God's image.

b. Beneficence toward the patient — to do what is in her best interest. This is ultimately grounded in the biblical norms mandating compassion, particularly for the most vulnerable, of whom this patient is clearly one.

c. Respect for human dignity, grounded ultimately in the biblical teaching of human persons made in God's image. This norm yields the moral guideline prohibiting assistance in suicide, a presumption toward the preservation of life, and thus the obligation not to remove life-sustaining treatment from a clearly recovering patient. These ethical commitments are expressed in the Catholic Church's Ethical and Religious Directives for Health Care, which are binding on the institution.

d. The long-standing ethical commitment of the medical profession to sustaining life (if possible) *and* relieving suffering — not relieving suffering at the expense of life itself. At stake here are the integrity of the profession and the moral character of its professionals.

4. List the Alternatives

- Alternative 1: Follow the agent's wishes and terminate life support.
- Alternative 2: Follow the written terms of the advance directive and continue life support.
- Alternative 3: Transfer the patient to a unit that would accommodate the agent's wishes.
- Alternative 4: Continue life support until the patient regains competence and can clarify her wishes.

302

5. Compare the Alternatives with the Norms

Until it is clear that the patient desires what the agent insists she does, it would seem that alternatives 2-4 would be consistent with our norms. Alternative 1 could be violating patient autonomy (i.e., the explicit terms of her advance directive) and the ethical and religious directives against assisted suicide and removal of life support from a clearly recovering patient.

6. Assess the Consequences

- Alternative 2: Patient lives and recovers. This alienates the family, perhaps violates the patient's wishes if the agent is accurately representing them, and perhaps violates ethical and religious directives.
- Alternative 3: Accommodate the family, follow the directives, and perhaps fail to protect the patient, who will presumably have life support turned off at another hospital; patient likely dies.
- Alternative 4: Temporarily (at the least) alienate the family; the patient lives and recovers, and gets a chance to clearly articulate her wishes; hospital follows ethical and religious directives.

7. Make a Decision

What recommendation should the hospital ethics committee make on this case? Which alternative is best? This case is a difficult one, since it pits the written wishes of a patient who can no longer speak for herself against the verbal and very emotional interpretation of someone who claims to know her wishes very well (her husband).[3]

3. Here is how the case was resolved. The patient was transferred from the hospital to a unit that specializes in ventilator-dependent patients on a Friday afternoon. She was ventilated during ambulance transfer. The plan was to review the matter with the husband and family, review all documents, and to terminate respiratory support on Monday. By Sunday morning the patient had awakened and was able to communicate, and by Sunday evening she was weaned off the respirator. In addition, her general medical condition was improving. The physicians spoke with her on Sunday, and she remembered the gunshot but denied pulling the trigger, though she was not absolutely sure. She also was vague whether she really wanted to commit suicide. She was seen by a psychiatrist, who stated that her memory generally was good, and she recalled another suicide attempt with pills in the mid-1970s. He felt she was currently mentally competent to make her own decisions. She stated that she wanted to live, and for the physicians to do everything necessary for her to recover. With regard to the

Case 2 — "Please Don't Tell!"[4]

A twenty-year-old Hispanic male was brought to a hospital emergency room, having suffered abdominal injuries due to gunshot wounds obtained in gang violence. He had no medical insurance, and his stay in the hospital was somewhat shorter than expected due to his good recovery. Physicians attending to him felt that he could complete his recovery at home just as easily as in the hospital, and he was released after only a few days.

During his stay in the hospital, the patient admitted to his primary physician that he was HIV positive, having contracted the virus that causes AIDS. This was confirmed by a blood test administered while he was hospitalized.

When he was discharged from the hospital, the physician recommended that a professional nurse visit him regularly at home in order to change the bandages on his still substantial wounds and to insure that an infection did not develop. Since he had no health insurance, he was dependent on Medicaid, a government program that pays for necessary medical care for those who cannot afford it. However, Medicaid refused to pay for home nursing care, since there was someone already in the home who was capable of providing the necessary care. That person was the patient's twenty-two-year-old sister, who was willing to take care of her brother until he was fully recovered. Their mother had died years ago, and the sister was accustomed to providing care for her younger siblings.

The patient had no objection to his sister providing this care, but he insisted that she not be told that he had tested HIV positive. Though he had always had a good relationship with his sister, she did not know that he was an active homosexual. His even greater fear was that his father would hear of his homosexual orientation and lifestyle.

The patient's physician is bound by a code of ethics that places a very high priority on keeping confidentiality. That is, information about someone's medical condition that he or she does not want known cannot be divulged by the physician. Some would argue that the responsibility of confidentiality is even greater with HIV/AIDS, since disclosure of someone's homosexuality normally carries devastating personal consequences for the individual who is forced "out of the closet."

---

husband, he has not appeared at the hospital since she was transferred. A daughter was extremely upset that the current hospital did not terminate the support promptly. There was supposed to be a conference with the family to decide on discharge planning Monday, but the family did not appear; neither did they appear at the postponement date on Tuesday. According to the administration, the police have been notified about all these new events.

4. Taken from the *Hastings Center Report* 22 (November-December 1992): 39-40.

On the other hand, the patient's sister is putting herself at risk by providing nursing care for him. Doesn't she have a right to know the risks to which she is subjecting herself, especially since she willingly volunteered to take care of her brother?

What should the physician do in this case? Should the physician breach the norm of confidentiality to protect the patient's sister, or keep confidentiality in order to protect the patient from harm that would come to him from his other family members, especially his father?

1. Gather the Facts

a. The patient is a young man, infected with HIV, and an active homosexual.

b. He suffered fairly severe abdominal wounds but is recovering well.

c. Homosexuality is looked down upon in Hispanic communities.

d. The patient has insisted that his physician maintain confidentiality about his HIV status.

e. The patient is afraid of rejection by his father if his homosexuality is discovered, an understandable fear given the way homosexuality is viewed in the Hispanic community.

f. He was wounded by gunfire in gang violence. It is not clear but is a reasonable assumption that he is a gang member. As a result, he likely fears rejection and perhaps retribution from his fellow gang members, especially if they discover that he is HIV positive.

g. He is uninsured and cannot afford home nursing care by a professional.

h. Medicaid refuses to pay for professional home nursing care.

i. The patient's sister is willing and able to provide the necessary nursing care for her brother. She is accustomed to providing maternal-like care for her brothers and sisters.

j. The patient has specifically requested that his sister not be told of his HIV status. She does not know that he is an active homosexual.

k. The patient's sister would be changing fairly sizable wound dressings for her brother, and the chances are high that she would come into contact with his HIV-infected blood. The probability of her becoming infected with the virus from this contact is difficult to predict.

2. Determine the Ethical Issues

The competing interests in this case are those of the sister who will provide the care and the patient who will receive it. Both have interests in being protected from harm. The patient fears being harmed in a psychosocial way if his homosexuality and HIV status are discovered. Thus he has put the physician in a difficult situation by demanding that his right to confidentiality be kept. Though she does not know it, his sister faces medical harm due to the risk of contracting the HIV virus from contact with her brother's blood. This could be stated as a conflict between confidentiality for the patient and his sister's right to know the patient's condition due to the risk she would be taking in giving him nursing care. The conflict could be summarized by the need for patient confidentiality versus the duty to warn the sister of risk of harm.

3. What Norms Have a Bearing on the Case?

Two moral norms that speak to this case come out of the way in which the ethical issue is stated. This case revolves around a conflict of rights, or, from a different moral angle, a conflict of duties that the physician has toward the patient and toward the sister. In other words, this is as much a matter of the physician's moral character as it is a question of ethical principles. The physician is called to exercise compassion toward both people, but what compassion (or the duty to "do no harm") demands depends on which individual in the case is in view. Thus two norms are paramount. First is the widely recognized norm that patients have a right to have their medical information kept confidential, particularly the information that could be used to harm them if it were disclosed. But a second norm that comes into play is the duty of the physician to warn interested parties other than the patient if they are at risk of imminent and substantial harm. This obligation is rooted in the biblical norms that command compassion (Luke 10:25-37) and looking out for the interests of others (Phil. 2:4).

A further norm in this case has to do with the virtue of the patient, who knowingly puts his sister at risk, particularly given her willingness to serve her brother at no compensation and seemingly without regard to her own interests. One might argue that the patient is acting in a way that is not consistent with the character traits of loyalty and love for his sister.

One of the difficult aspects of any ethical decision is knowing what weight to give the norms that are relevant to the case. The norm of confidentiality is considered virtually sacred in the medical profession, and most physicians will argue that it is necessary to keep confidentiality if patients are to trust their physicians and continue coming for treatment. But confidentiality is often considered subordinate to the duty to warn someone who will likely be harmed if that information is not disclosed. For example, if a psychologist believes that a patient will kill his wife, or beat her severely, the psychologist has a moral obligation to inform the wife that she is in danger from her husband. The duty to warn someone from imminent and severe harm is usually considered a more heavily weighted norm than confidentiality in cases like these.

The key question here in weighting the norm of confidentiality and the duty to warn (both fulfilling the biblical notion of compassion toward those in need of it) is the degree of risk that the patient's sister is taking by providing nursing care for her brother. If the risk is not substantial, then that weights confidentiality a bit more heavily. But if the risk is significant, then the duty to warn is the more heavily weighted norm. This is particularly so given the fact that the sister has volunteered to perform a very self-sacrificing service for her brother. Some would argue that her altruism is an additional factor that weights the duty-to-warn norm more heavily. Others would suggest that his contracting HIV is an example of "reaping what one sows," and that minimizes consideration of the patient's desire for confidentiality. An additional factor that should be figured into the deliberation is that the risk to the patient, though it may have a higher probability of happening, is not as severe as the risk to the sister. After all, if the worst-case scenario happened to the patient, his father would disown him and the gang would throw him out (though their action could be more severe than that). He would recover from all of that. But if his sister contracted HIV, she would not recover from that. Though the probability of the worst-case scenario is higher for the patient, the results of the worst case are clearly higher for the sister.

4. List the Alternatives

In this case, there are a number of viable alternatives that involve compromise on either the patient's part or his sister's. However, two alternatives do not involve compromise, and each reflects a weighting of the norms.

- Alternative 1: Tell the sister that her brother is HIV positive. This alternative comes out of taking the duty-to-warn norm as the higher priority. One way to do this is to request that the patient inform his sister of his condition. He could then request that she not tell any other family member or any of his friends. If he refused, then the next step might be for the physician to say to him, in effect, "If you don't tell her, I will."

- Alternative 2: On the other hand, a second alternative is to refuse to tell her that information, upholding the patient's request for confidentiality and taking the confidentiality norm as the one that carries more weight.
- Alternative 3: The physician could warn the patient's sister in general terms about taking appropriate precautions for caring for these types of wounds. She is to wear gloves and even a mask at all times when handling the bandages. Should she get any blood on her clothes or body, she is to wash immediately with a disinfectant soap. In other words, she is to take universal precautions that any medical professional routinely takes in caring for patients.

5. Compare the Alternatives with the Norms

In many cases the norms resolve the case. Depending on how one assesses the relative weight of the norms, that may be the case here. In fact, it may be that the alternative of encouraging universal precautions for the sister but not telling her why, comes very close to satisfying all the relevant norms. But certainly there are questions about the adequacy of those precautions. Will she follow them, or treat them casually? However, assume for the moment that appeal to norms does not resolve the dilemma.

6. Assess the Consequences

Here the task is to take the viable alternatives and attempt to predict what the likely consequences (both positive and negative) of each would be. In addition, one should try to estimate roughly how beneficial are the positive consequences and how severe the negative ones, since some consequences are clearly more substantial than others.

In many cases, when two opposing alternatives are presented, the consequences of one are the mirror image of the other. This is the case here with the alternatives of telling the sister or refusing to tell her of her brother's HIV status.

In alternative 1, that of *telling the sister (or insisting that the patient tell his sister),* the likely consequences include the following:

The sister would be properly warned about the risks of taking care of her brother, minimizing the risk of her contracting HIV and saving her from the risk of developing a fatal illness.

The brother's HIV status would be out in the open, leaving family and gang friends to draw their own conclusions about his homosexuality. Should they draw the right conclusion, which is likely, he suffers significant psychosocial harm from his gang members, and possibly (though not certainly) from his family. The patient's trust of the physician suffers, and he may refuse to see that physician, or any other one, again until a dire medical emergency arises. This would be unfortunate because, due to his HIV status, he will need ongoing medical care.

But with alternative 2, if the physician *refuses to disclose the information,* the following may be expected as the likely consequences:

The sister would not know about the risks she is taking, making her vulnerable to contracting an infection for which there is no cure. The degree of risk that she is taking is open to debate, but some would argue that if the degree of risk is any more than minimal, that justifies warning her since the virus produces a fatal disease.

The patient's HIV status remains a well-kept secret, as does his homosexuality. But it is not likely that either his HIV status or his homosexuality can be kept a secret forever, since, as HIV develops into full-blown AIDS, both are likely to come out at some point in the future.

Trust between the physician and patient is maintained.

If alternative 3 is taken, telling the sister to *take general precautions,* the following are the likely consequences:

She may exercise appropriate caution in taking care of her brother, but she may not. She may treat the precautions casually and unknowingly put herself at risk. If the physician tells her about the precautions in very strong terms to insure her compliance with them, that may start her asking questions about why the doctor was so insistent on her following these precautions. In fact, one of the motives of the physician might be to nudge her toward asking some of those questions of her brother, to further minimize the risk of contracting HIV.

In general, the patient's HIV status and homosexual orientation are kept secret and confidentiality is honored, but the question of how long it will remain a secret is unknown, and it will likely become known eventually.

Trust with the physician and patient is maintained. However, if the sister is nudged to ask her brother some pressing questions about why these precautions are so important, he may conclude that the physician has prompted his sister to ask these questions, leaving him feeling betrayed.

7. Make a Decision

What should the physician do in this case? Which norms are the most weighty? Are there others to include? Which alternatives are the most viable? Are there others to consider? Which consequences seem to be the most severe? Are there others that must be kept in view? It is important to realize that at some point deliberation must stop and a decision must be made, as uncomfortable as that may be.

Case 3 — Jehovah's Witnesses and Blood Transfusions

A twenty-seven-year-old male had been hit by a car while on his bicycle and had hit his head. At the time of the accident he did not think he had sustained a serious injury, but two days later he began to experience headaches and dizziness, and his wife brought him to the ER. After examination, a diagnosis of head trauma with alternation of level of consciousness was made. A CT scan of the head was performed and revealed a subdural hematoma (SDH). Lab work done upon his admission to the hospital identified an elevated blood alcohol level and a very decreased platelet level. The attending physicians recommended surgery to evacuate the subdural hematoma.

Recognizing the severely impaired ability of coagulation and the risk of further bleeding, the neurosurgeon ordered a platelet transfusion and anticipated that a blood transfusion would be necessary during surgery. The family, consisting of the patient's wife and two-year-old child (the wife was pregnant with their second child), informed the physicians that the patient was a Jehovah's Witness and was opposed to transfusions of any sort. At this point the patient was unable to make his own decisions. The family was informed of the severity of the patient's condition. They were told that without surgery the subdural hematoma could increase, resulting in further brain injury and eventually in death. With the surgery the patient had a very high probability of recovery to full health. They were also told that no substitutes for platelets existed. Church officials were brought in to try and help resolve the situation, but they appeared to reinforce the family's determination to avoid blood products. The family did consent to the surgery, but not to the blood products. The neurosurgeon refused to operate without platelet and blood transfusions, since without them the patient had slightly less than a 50 percent chance of surviving the surgery. The hospital looked for another neurosurgeon who would be willing to operate under the family's conditions of no blood products, but could not locate one.

Over the next few days the family remained firm in their decision, as the patient's condition progressively deteriorated; he died roughly five days after entering the hospital.

Was accepting the family's decision the correct one, since the patient was a young man who would be leaving behind a pregnant wife and small child? Or should the surgeon override the wishes of the family, even though they are based on the family's religious beliefs? Does it make a difference if the neurosurgeon is a Christian and disagrees with the tenets of the Jehovah's Witnesses, especially the part of their doctrinal statement that deals with blood transfusions?

Case Analysis

1. Gather the Facts

a. The patient is a twenty-seven-year-old male with a young, pregnant wife and preschool-age child to support.

b. He was involved in an accident that produced a serious head injury that requires surgery.

c. Blood transfusions are medically indicated for this kind of surgery, and the neurosurgeon will not operate without transfusions being available.

d. The patient's family indicates that the patient is a Jehovah's Witness, and part of that sect's doctrine mandates that adherents refuse all blood products, especially transfusions.

e. The patient had an elevated blood alcohol level at the time of admission to the hospital. Jehovah's Witnesses also prohibit drinking of alcohol. This raises a question of the patient's commitment to his faith and whether his wife is accurately representing his wishes for no blood transfusions.

f. Church elders were brought in and only reinforced the family's decision.

g. No other neurosurgeon is available to perform the surgery.

2. Determine the Ethical Issues

This case involves the classic conflict between patient *autonomy* (the right of patients or their appointed representatives to choose or refuse their own course of treatment) and the obligation of *beneficence* (the duty to act in the patient's best interests). This case is complicated by the life-or-death urgency to perform the surgery, so that the consequences of following the patient's wishes and not acting in the patient's best interests will result in his death, leaving three dependents without their means of support. It is further complicated by the fact that the patient cannot speak for himself at the time a decision about blood transfusions is needed. His wife is claiming to represent his wishes, but due to the presence of alcohol in the patient's blood at the time of admission, there are questions about his commitment to his faith. Perhaps his wife is not accurately portraying his wishes. One additional complication comes from the roots of the patient/family's wishes — their religious beliefs. It is widely held in bioethics that a patient's religious views are to be accepted as a given and not questioned. Except when the patient is a minor, decisions made on religious grounds are considered virtually sacred and overridden only in extreme circumstances.[5]

3. What Norms Have a Bearing on the Case?

This case involves a conflict of core norms. On one side is the norm of personal autonomy, which here is grounded in the couple's religious beliefs and is ultimately grounded in the biblical responsibility of individuals to make their own decisions about their lives. Even though the physician may disagree with their religious beliefs, and may desire to persuade them that another outlook is better, the physician's obligation ultimately is to accept their view of the world and allow them to make decisions they consider most consistent with their values. Of course, the physician may ask questions about the relevance of their views to the course of treatment under consideration and may even inquire about their openness to considering alternative views, but this inquiry must be done with respect and be free from coercion.

On the other hand, the competing obligation here to offer the treatment that violates the religious views of the patient is rooted in the norm to act in his best interests. This is grounded biblically in the obligations to love

5. For example, courts routinely override the religious beliefs of Christian Science parents who are denying medical treatment to their children. The right of autonomy is less weighty when others are harmed by the exercise of an individual's freedom, as is the case when children are harmed by denial of medical care that is the decision of Christian Science parents. However, in July 1997 a California court of appeals ruled in favor of parents who resorted to prayer and a Christian Science practitioner in order to treat diabetes. The child died and the parents were not held responsible, based on their First Amendment rights of religious freedom. See *Quigley v First Church of Christ, Scientist,* 1998 Cal. App. LEXIS 677 (29 July 1998).

and serve others, particularly those who are the most vulnerable. The physicians and hospital are emphasizing the obligation to do what is in the interests of the patient medically. The family argues that if he accepts blood products, he will be condemned to hell in the afterlife, according to Jehovah's Witness doctrine, and that is certainly not in his best interests.

The physician is in a difficult position, and considerations of virtue are relevant here. Is it virtuous to allow one's patient to die, when the family has consented to surgery but not to the transfusion? In other words, the physician is risking that the patient will not recover from surgery without the blood transfusion. This raises a question about how morally defensible is the surgeon's refusal to perform the surgery without the blood available for transfusion. Clearly the surgeon does not desire to put the patient at additional risk, and does not welcome the scrutiny that will ensue if the patient does not survive surgery. But might considerations of virtue suggest that such a risk is worth taking, since the patient will certainly die without the surgery? To answer this question the surgeon would have to assess if the surgery had a reasonable chance of succeeding without the transfusion.

4. List the Alternatives

- Alternative 1: Act in accordance with the family's wishes, accepting their religious beliefs, and, as difficult as it may be, care for this patient while he deteriorates and eventually dies.
- Alternative 2: Go to court in order to obtain a court order that will force the patient to accept the transfusion (forcing surgery with transfusion on the patient could not be done without a court order, since in many states that would constitute battery).
- Alternative 3: Perform the surgery with the transfusion, but do not document it nor tell the family about it.
- Alternative 4: Try to persuade the neurosurgeon to perform the surgery without the transfusion.

5. Compare the Alternatives with the Norms

Since this case involves a conflict of core ethical norms in medicine, it is unlikely that a clear decision can be reached at this point without weighting one norm more heavily than others. Generally in bioethics, autonomy carries more weight than beneficence, especially when it is grounded in religious views. However, one could argue that beneficence should carry more weight since we are not sure about the patient's commitment to his faith, given the alcohol in his blood. In addition, it should carry more weight because the consequences of upholding the patient's autonomy are so severe. But given the eternal element, that receiving blood products condemns one forever, one could argue that the consequences of overriding his autonomy are more severe.

It would appear that alternative 3 (performing the surgery with the transfusion and not telling anyone) might create less conflict with the family. But it violates another key norm in bioethics, and in ethics in general, that of truth telling, particularly given the relationship of trust that is supposed to exist between a patient and his or her physician. If that alternative were chosen and something went wrong in the operating room, the family would have valid grounds for a major lawsuit against the physicians, nurses, and hospital. Alternative 4 is another possibility, but given the way in which surgeons are investigated when someone dies on their operating table, the neurosurgeon's refusal to operate without the transfusion being available is certainly understandable. However, it does raise the question of whether in this case the neurosurgeon's refusal to operate is morally defensible, given the zero-percent probability that the patient will live without the surgery (as opposed to the nearly 50 percent chance that the patient will survive the surgery without the transfusion).

6. Assess the Consequences

If the neurosurgeon can be persuaded to operate without the availability of blood to transfuse, that alternative is the one that may well come closest to satisfying all of the important values that have a bearing on the case. If the surgeon remains unwilling, alternatives 1 and 2 are left. If alternative 1 is chosen, the results are clearly catastrophic. The patient dies, leaving a widow and two small children (one still in utero) and a demoralized nursing staff that has had to take care of this unnecessarily dying patient. However, in his religious system, his soul is saved and eternal condemnation is avoided. He is given the respect due him by adhering to his wishes. If alternative 2 is chosen, the family is alienated and may take the patient out of the hospital against medical advice, though that would be difficult to do in this case. However, if the court order is granted, the patient will recover and live and still be there for his family, though in a spiritually compromised state according to his religious views.

7. Make a Decision

What should the neurosurgeon have done? Should the neurosurgeon have operated without one of the critical tools (blood transfusion) necessary to insure that the patient has the best chance of recovery? Should the hospital have accepted the patient's wife's decision regarding blood transfusions? Or should the hospital have gone to court to attempt to override the wife's decision, since she may not have been representing her husband's religious commitments?

Conclusion

This model is a helpful way of insuring that all the relevant questions are asked in attempting to resolve an ethical dilemma. It is not to be used as a formula or as a computer program that will automatically enable a person to reach an easy decision when confronting an ethical dilemma. But it will give some direction to the decision-making process when a person is faced with what is often a confusing maze of facts and feelings. It can be used not only in the clinical ethics area, from which all three cases come, but is also suitable for dealing with ethical conflicts that arise in the health care organization, or in the business and public policy aspects of health care.

Conclusion

This past year the *Los Angeles Times,* Orange County edition, had a picture on the front page of Derek Humphry visiting local retirement and nursing homes. Humphry is the co-founder of the Hemlock Society, which is dedicated to bringing about legislation which would allow physician-assisted suicide in the United States. He is also the author of *Final Exit,* a slim book filled with detailed instructions for how patients might hasten their death. What was most arresting about Humphry's visits to these homes was the eager reception he received from the clientele. Most certainly each of these locations either had a chaplain on staff or had regular visits by local pastors and priests. Yet it did not appear from the article that these professionals were meeting people's needs to address the important issue of death and its relation to euthanasia. This little scenario involving Derek Humphry highlights several concerns of the authors of this book.

We believe that the Christian community needs to be informed about the complex biomedical issues of the day from a Christian perspective. In general, the Christian community and its Christian health care professionals find it extremely difficult to integrate the Christian worldview with the medical and ethical complexity surrounding biomedical issues. Thus adherents to a Christian worldview are forced to separate their faith from the questions raised by contemporary culture. Such an approach to the Christian faith reduces it to a faith which only addresses so-called spiritual matters like forgiveness, but has nothing to say about the rest of life. Therefore Christianity becomes only a religion of redemption instead of a total worldview or a lens by which to view, interpret, and understand all of reality. Consequently, one of the goals of this book has been to model the integration of the Christian faith with a careful and intelligent analysis of current issues facing the biomedical community. For the Christian, God is not only the Redeemer, he is also the Creator who has something to say about all of life.

Furthermore, we believe that Christianity can have an informing effect upon all discussions in the public arena. We understand the difficulty involved in such a project. As Robin Lovin has observed:

> Ethics in the modern world is fundamentally a discipline of giving public reasons for action. The way we respect the autonomy of persons in our social decisions is by inviting their consent on essential choices, rather than forcing them to conform or deluding them with propaganda. To make a moral argument is to state one's case in terms that require others either to concur in the choice or to offer better reasons for rejecting it. . . . Christians cannot surrender their distinctive claims. Yet the more clearly and directly they guide their actions by this "minority report," the greater the risk of finding their actions at odds with neighbors who make their choices only with reference to commonly held beliefs that can be checked against the facts.[1]

According to Lovin, the non-Christian world is interested in the "facts" of the matter more than theological assumptions. This is why we have carefully laid out the "facts" concerning each biomedical issue discussed here (*facts* meaning knowledge that virtually all would acknowledge about an issue regardless of their presuppositions). By scrupulously stating the "facts" regarding each issue, our aim is to provide the Christian layperson and Christian health care professional with the knowledge to begin interaction with those who do not share their theological presuppositions, certainties, or givens.

In addition, however, we are not ashamed or embarrassed by our theological position as Christians. We believe that the Christian worldview offers an important perspective to a pluralistic society. At times a purely rational, idealistic, or political solution appears thin or weak when juxtaposed with a Christian analysis. The overall concern and depth of consideration embodied in a Christian perspective can be refreshing and enlightening to the human spirit. Many times Christian insights can illumine the dark places of ethical decisions and dilemmas so that even those who do not accept the theological assumptions of the Christian faith are guided to make wiser decisions. Accordingly, we have produced a book which scrutinizes the biomedical issues of our time, both medical and practical, and explores what light a Christian

---

1. Robin W. Lovin, *Christian Faith and Public Choices* (Philadelphia: Fortress, 1984), pp. 3, 4.

perspective can bring to them. Faith can illumine our human experience, and in turn, our faith can be validated by experience.

A pluralistic, secular world needs the moral sustenance that a transcendent God brings to it. It is this Creator God who makes human beings both valuable and responsible. Moreover, the pluralistic, secular world needs to be provoked and unsettled by a Christian perspective. Pure secularity can degenerate into "whatever is happening ought to happen" or "whatever we can do we should do." It has no built-in devices or outside perspective by which to judge itself. This is an increasingly serious concern with the onset of such technologies as human cloning and genetic engineering. A Christian approach to bioethics offers a needed transcendent perspective that protects us from the worst in our natures and our world, while explaining and encouraging the best.

Index

abortion: autonomy and, 212-13; Catholic opposition to, 13; fetal tissue transplants and, 176-82; financial inducements and, 179-80; genetic testing and, 121-24; hardship and, 122; image of, 181; neutral arguments against, 281, 287-89; personhood and, 72-73, 170-71. *See also* unborn

advance directives: autonomy and, 198; content of, 144-45; discussion of, 220; need for, 236-37; overriding, 146, 236; types of, 235

afterlife, 227-28

agape, 21, 22-23, 48-49

age, criterion of, 268-69

agreement, 64-66, 69

AIDS. *See* HIV/AIDS

alpha-fetal protein blood test, 122

alternatives, 299-300, 302-3, 307-8, 313-14

amniocentesis, 120, 120n.45, 122

anencephaly, 123n.47

Annas, George, 223

anthropocentrism, 47, 50

Arant, Billy, Jr., 177

Aristotle, 84n.66, 85, 159n.4

artificial insemination, 92, 100, 103, 107

Atkinson, David, 131-32

authority of consent, 64-65

autonomy: abortion and, 212-13; abuse of, 194-99, 208; basis of, 83; beneficence and, 68, 194-97, 208; biblical perspective on, 203-7; defined, 199; drugs and, 211; Engelhardt on, 73; HIV/AIDS and, 214; limitations on, 203-4, 207, 210-11, 238; in modern medicine, 207-14; order and, 202; paternalism and, 16-17; peaceable community and, 67; physician-assisted suicide and, 213-14, 246, 302; priority of, 207-8, 210; reflective equilibrium and, 77; western tradition of, 199-202

Baby K, 218n.3

Baby M surrogacy case, 291n.18

baby selling, 109-10, 291, 292

balancing, 58, 59-60

Barth, Karl, 33

Basic Christian Ethics (Ramsey), 20

Beauchamp, Tom L., 56-61, 66-67, 68, 70, 74-78, 86-87, 96n, 299

behavior and illness, 43

beneficence: autonomy and, 67-68, 194-97, 208, 302; justice and, 70-71; nonmaleficence and, 70; ownership and, 71; restoration of, 215-16

bill of rights for patients, 198

Printed in the United States
84246LV00003B/65/A

9 780802 845955